D0146293

The Decline of Mortality in Europe

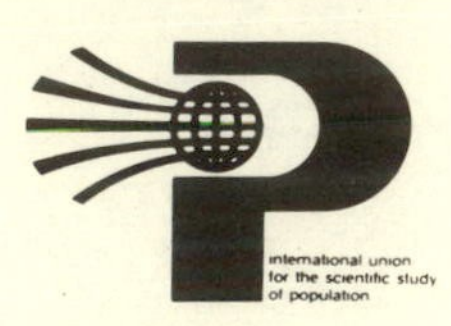

The International Union for the Scientific Study of Population Problems was set up in 1928, with Dr Raymond Pearl as President. At that time the Union's main purpose was to promote international scientific co-operation to study the various aspects of population problems, through national committees and through the work of individual members. In 1947 the International Union for the Scientific Study of Population (IUSSP) was reconstituted in its present form. It expanded its activities to:

- stimulate research on population
- develop interest in demographic matters among governments, national and international organizations, scientific bodies, and the general public
- foster relations between people involved in population studies
- disseminate scientific knowledge on population.

The principal ways in which the IUSSP currently achieves its aims are:

- organization of worldwide or regional conferences and operations of scientific committees under the responsibility of the Council
- organization of training courses
- publication of conference proceedings and committee reports.

Demography can be defined by its field of study and its analytical methods. Accordingly, it can be regarded as the scientific study of human populations with respect to their size, their structure, and their development. For reasons which are related to the history of the discipline, the demographic method is essentially inductive: progress results from the improvement of observations, more sophisticated methods of measurement, and the search for regularities and stable factors which lead to the formulation of explanatory models. In summary, the three objectives of demographic analysis are to describe, measure, and analyse.

International Studies in Demography is the outcome of an agreement concluded by the IUSSP and the Oxford University Press. This joint series is expected to reflect the broad range of the Union's activities and, in the first instance, will be based on the seminars organized by the Union. The Editorial Board of the series consists of:

THE DECLINE OF MORTALITY IN EUROPE

---

edited by

R. SCHOFIELD

D. REHER

A. BIDEAU

CLARENDON PRESS · OXFORD
1991

Oxford University Press, Walton Street, Oxford OX2 6DP
Oxford New York Toronto
Delhi Bombay Calcutta Madras Karachi
Petaling Jaya Singapore Hong Kong Tokyo
Nairobi Dar es Salaam Cape Town
Melbourne Auckland
and associated companies in
Berlin Ibadan

Oxford is a trade mark of Oxford University Press

Published in the United States
by Oxford University Press, New York

British Library Cataloguing in Publication Data
The Decline of mortality in Europe.
1. Europe. Man. Mortality rate. Social environmental factors, history—(International studies in demography).
I. Schofield, Roger S. II. Reher, David Sven
III. Bideau, A. (Alain) IV. Series
304.64094
ISBN 0-19-828328-8

Library of Congress Cataloging in Publication Data
The Decline of mortality in Europe/edited by R. Schofield, D. Reher, A. Bideau.
p. cm.—(International studies in demography)
Includes bibliographical references and index.
1. Mortality—Europe—History. I. Schofield, Roger, II. Reher, David Sven. III. Bideau, Alain, IV. Series.
HB1411.D43 1991 304.6'4'094—dc20 90-19692
ISBN 0-19-828328-8

Typeset by Colset Pte. Ltd., Singapore
Printed and bound in
Great Britain by Bookcraft (Batn) Ltd,
Midsomer Norton, Avon

Acknowledgements

In 1987, when the International Union for the Scientific Study of Population set up its new Committee on Historical Demography, one of the items during its first meeting was a proposal for a seminar on 'Medicine and the Decline of Mortality' to be organized jointly by the Committee and the Fondation Marcel Mérieux. A planning committee was set up which included Roger Schofield, Alain Bideau, David Reher, Jean-Pierre Bardet, and John Knodel to organize the scholarly aspects of the seminar. On the 22nd to the 25th June 1988 the participants met in the splendid surroundings of the Fondation Mérieux's Centre des Pensières on Lake Annecy in France. We would like to thank the Fondation Mérieux for the kind and generous way in which they supplemented the resources of the IUSSP and so enabled this seminar to take place.

The present volume contains a selection of papers which were given at the seminar, organized around the title *Decline of Mortality in Europe*. The three editors of this volume would also like to express their thanks to Professor E. Grebenik for his help in putting the manuscript in its final form. As a result of his work, a number of faults and inconsistencies in the original papers have been removed. The individual authors and the editors, of course, accept responsibility for any remaining errors or omissions.

Contents

Contributors

Jean Noël Biraben	Institut National d'Études Démographiques, Paris
Patrice Bourdelais	Centre de Recherches Historiques, Paris
John Burnett	Brunel University
Graziella Caselli	University of Rome
Roderick Floud	City of London Polytechnic
Michael R. Haines	Wayne State University, Detroit
Stephen J. Kunitz	University of Rochester Medical Center
Peter G. Lunn	MRC Dunn Nutritional Laboratory, Cambridge
Marie-France Morel	École Normale Supérieure de Fontenay-Saint-Cloud
Alfred Perrenoud	University of Geneva
Bi Puranen	Institutet för Framtidsstudier, Stockholm
David Reher	Universidad Complutense de Madrid
Roger Schofield	Cambridge Group for the History of Population and Social Structure
Jacques Vallin	Institut National d'Études Démographiques, Paris
Robert Woods	University of Liverpool

List of Figures

List of Tables

1 The Decline of Mortality in Europe

ROGER SCHOFIELD *Cambridge Group for the History of Population and Social Structure*

and DAVID REHER *School of Political Science and Sociology, University of Madrid*

1. Introduction

At first glance, the historical development of mortality in Europe can be easily and quickly summarized. Pre-decline patterns typical of most Ancien Régime societies were characterized by high overall levels, punctuated by periodic bouts with epidemics caused by infectious disease (plague, small-pox, typhus, etc.). During the eighteenth century, and chiefly thanks to ever more efficient government intervention, the incidence of crisis mortality diminished drastically in most of Europe. It was the 'stabilisation of mortality' as Michael Flinn called it, and was essential to the subsequent spurt in European growth rates.[1] With the reduction of epidemics, endemic infectious diseases became relatively more important and gains in life expectancy slowed considerably. It was not until the latter part of the nineteenth century that mortality once again declined sharply in most areas of Europe. Child mortality and, somewhat later, infant mortality were responsible for much of this decline, though gains in life expectancy affected all age groups. Mortality improvement was due mostly to the decline in diseases such as diarrhoea and tuberculosis. The third period of mortality decline began after World War II, spread throughout the world, and seems inextricably, though not exclusively, linked to the discovery and use of sulpha drugs and antibiotics.[2]

The classic interpretation for this evolution was given some years ago by the British physician, historian, and demographer, Thomas McKeown.[3] Briefly, he endeavoured to explain the long-term change in population

The authors of this chapter would like to thank Stephen Kunitz, Richard Smith, Sølvi Sogner, Josep Bernabeu-Mestre, Vicente Perez-Moreda, Dudley Baines, and George Alter for their helpful suggestions and ideas.

[1] Michael W. Flinn, 'The Stabilisation of Mortality in Preindustrial Western Europe', *Journal of European Economic History*, 3(2), (1974), pp. 285–318.

[2] For a brief review of this trend, see Stephen J. Kunitz, 'Mortality since Malthus' in David Coleman and Roger Schofield (eds.), *The State of Population Theory* (Oxford, 1986), pp. 279–302.

[3] Thomas McKeown, *The Modern Rise of Population* (London, 1976).

growth rates which started during the eighteenth century.[4] Using mainly data from England and Wales, McKeown came to the conclusion that population growth could not have come from any increase in fertility and was mainly the consequence of the secular decline in mortality.[5] This change, caused by the reduction in infectious diseases, can be attributed mainly to the improvement of nutrition which took place in Europe during the eighteenth and nineteenth centuries.

His interpretation is clear and strikingly simple. Much the same can be said of the basic pattern of decline we described earlier. Yet, historical reality has often proven intractable to facile interpretations, and there are indications that something similar might be happening to the historical decline of mortality in Europe. In recent years, theories which explain secular mortality change have become the hotbed of controversy, and, moreover, even the demographic parameters of mortality decline are still far from clear. The range of the debate and the, as yet, tenuous understanding of just what happened, will become clear in several of the chapters contained in this volume.

It would be only a small exaggeration to say that our understanding of historical mortality patterns, and of their causes and implications, is still in its infancy. Despite its importance, we probably know less of mortality than of fertility; there has been a European Fertility Project, but nothing similar exists for mortality. The complexities inherent in the methodological and substantive issues affecting its study have often daunted researchers and, together with data problems, have tended to limit progress in this field.[6]

2. Demographic Perspectives of Mortality Decline

A basic outline of the demographic characteristics of secular mortality decline in Europe can still only be sketched with very rudimentary lines. The

[4] For a recent thorough but somewhat critical summary of McKeown's theories, see Simon Szreter, 'The Importance of Social Intervention in Britain's Mortality Decline *c.*1850–1914: A Reinterpretation of the Role of Public Health', *Social History of Medicine*, 1(1) (1988), pp. 1-38, esp. pp. 7–17. Penetrating evaluations of McKeown's ideas within the context of intellectual tradition of medical science can be found in Stephen J. Kunitz, 'Explanations and Ideologies of Mortality Patterns', *Population and Development Review*, 13(3) (1987), pp. 379–408.

[5] More recent research into the population history of England has shown that the role McKeown attributed to mortality for the population growth of the 18th cent. is inaccurate. During that period, long-term total fertility trends were the key to population growth rates. It is doubtful whether this was the case in other European countries, especially those in the southern part of the continent. See E. A. Wrigley and R. S. Schofield, *The Population History of England 1541–1871* (2nd ed., Cambridge, 1989), pp. 228–48. Also R. S. Schofield, 'Population Growth in the Century after 1750: The Role of Mortality Decline', in Tommy Bengtsson, Gunnar Fridlizius, and Rolf Ohlsson (eds.), *Pre-Industrial Population Change: The Mortality Decline and Short-Term Population Movements* (Stockholm, 1984), pp. 17–39.

[6] There are signs that this situation is beginning to change. A very useful collection of articles on the subject of secular mortality decline can be found in Bengtsson *et al.*, op. cit. in n. 5. See also, R. I. Woods and J. H. Woodward (eds.), *Urban Disease and Mortality in Nineteenth-Century England* (London, 1984).

bulk of what we know is based on French, English, Scandinavian, German, and, to a lesser extent, Italian data. Elsewhere, the dearth of mortality studies is a serious obstacle to our understanding of the parameters of mortality decline.

The early phase of mortality transition, which stretches from the latter part of the seventeenth century to the beginning of the nineteenth, seems to have been characterized by the decline, or even disappearance, of crisis mortality caused by epidemic infectious diseases. The most noticeable of these were the epidemics of plague which had all but disappeared from the continent by the early part of the eighteenth century. A hundred years later, other epidemic diseases like smallpox and typhus had also declined substantially. The result was the gradual elimination of the characteristic 'peaks' on all mortality curves; a change which had important effects on population growth rates.[7] There are several as yet unresolved issues concerning this early decline in mortality. Whether or not it affected the entire continent is not at all clear. While the disappearance of the plague is unquestionable, crisis mortality continued to be common in certain areas until well into the nineteenth century.[8]

Moreover, any decline in prevailing levels of non-crisis mortality is still a matter of debate. During the first half of the eighteenth century, improvements, if any, in general mortality levels were only modest.[9] After 1750, there were striking gains in England, Sweden, and especially in France, though inadequate data from other countries make it unclear just how widespread or how new these were.

In England the changes during the eighteenth century may not have been 'secular' at all, and it was not until the first third of the nineteenth century that late sixteenth-century levels of mortality were equalled. Over the entire period, there were very large swings in prevailing mortality levels. Between 1580 and 1680 mortality worsened, with expectation of life at birth declining from nearly 40 years to just above 30. From 1680 to 1740 it is difficult to find any long-term trend. Between 1740 and 1820 mortality improved

[7] In the most comprehensive statement of this point, Michael Flinn, op. cit. in n. 1, devised a composite index of the importance of mortality crises, the 'crisis mortality aggregate', which measured both the intensity and prevalence of crisis. Using the more direct measure of percentage deviation from a 25-year moving average of deaths for a large sample of English parishes, Wrigley and Schofield (op. cit. in n. 5, pp. 314–16) have shown that, with the exception of the second quarter of the 18th cent., the major reduction in the intensity of mortality fluctuations in England and Wales took place between 1675 and 1800.

[8] An excellent example of this is central and southern Spain which was struck by a series of major yellow fever, typhus, and malaria epidemics between 1800 and 1804, easily the worst bout with crisis mortality since the end of the 16th and beginning of the 17th cent. See Vicente Pérez Moreda, *Las crisis de mortalidad en la España interior: Siglos XVI-XIX*, (Madrid, 1980). The case of Italy lies somewhere between the Spanish experience and that of northern Europe. See Lorenzo Del Panta, *Le epidemie nella storia demografica italiana: Secoli XIV-XIX*, (Turin, 1980).

[9] In England, mortality levels actually worsened during that period (Wrigley and Schofield, op. cit. in n. 5, pp. 235, 414).

sharply (e_0 rose from 31.7 years to 39.2), and levelled off during the mid-century.[10] Truly 'secular' improvements only took place after 1870.

The extent to which mortality in other countries showed similar fluctuations is largely a matter of speculation. In the few areas for which data are available, trends often differ. In France there was a marked though uneven decline in mortality during the eighteenth century, whereas in Norway and Sweden this did not take place until the first part of the nineteenth century, a positive period of decline almost everywhere.[11] The halt to mortality decline during the mid-nineteenth century, and the subsequent secular fall, seem to have been experienced in a number of countries. Elsewhere, insufficient data make any estimation of mortality trends largely a matter of guesswork. Yet in the southern and eastern parts of the continent life expectancy at birth was only very modest by the middle part of the nineteenth century (near or below 30 years), and any improvement over the conditions which applied a century earlier must have been marginal at best. The uniformity of secular changes in mortality in Europe may well be more apparent than real.

Another characteristic of mortality patterns in traditional Europe was the wide regional differences that existed at any given moment of time. Life expectancy, and especially infant and child mortality, varied substantially within countries. In 1860 in Spain, for example, life expectancy ranged from near 25 years to over 40; and there is reason to believe that these regional differences had been present for at least two or three centuries.[12] In other countries the situation was similar. In Sweden in 1861, infant mortality was above 290 per 1,000 in the city of Stockholm and below 100 per 1,000 in certain rural areas, and it varied between 97.9 per 1,000 and 160.3 in the adjacent rural provinces of Västernorrland and Jämtland.[13] In England and Wales, parish examples of infant mortality from 1650 to 1699 went from 45 per cent below the average in Hartland to 75 per cent above in Gainsborough.[14] One of the common characteristics of secular mortality change was the reduction of these cross-sectional regional differences, as well as of those between rural and urban areas. It is unclear, however, just when this reduction took place. In Spain it was really not before

[10] Ibid., pp. 230–31.

[11] Alfred Perrenoud, 'The Mortality Decline in a Long-Term Perspective', in Bengtsson *et al.* (eds.), op. cit. in n. 5, pp. 41–69, esp. pp. 44–50.

[12] Fausto Dopico, 'Regional Mortality Tables for Spain in the 1860s', *Historical Methods*, 20(4) (1987), pp. 173–79, esp. pp. 176–77.

[13] Erland Hofsten and Hans Lundström, *Swedish Population History: Main Trends from 1750 to 1970* (Stockholm, 1976), p. 119.

[14] Differences in mortality between Hartland and Gainsborough by a factor between two and three persisted throughout the 17th and 18th cents., and suggest that during that period life expectancy at birth in Hartland may have been 50 years or more, as opposed to Gainsborough where it was only about 30 years. See E.A. Wrigley and R.S. Schofield, 'English Population History from Family Reconstitution: Summary Results 1600–1799', *Population Studies*, 37(2) (1983), pp. 157–84, esp. pp. 178–79.

the beginning of the twentieth century, while in England the trend to convergence may have been taking place as much as a century earlier.

The causes of mortality decline are a source of ongoing controversy. McKeown insisted that improving nutritional status was at the core of the trend, but the improvement of nutrition during that period is far from clear. The creation of national grain markets precisely during the eighteenth and early nineteenth centuries contributed to evening out the ups and downs in grain consumption, though its effect on long-term mortality levels is still a matter for speculation. Other factors were also at work. Perrenoud in this volume feels that a colder climate helped mute the effect of disease, though this point is very difficult to substantiate, and runs counter to the conclusions of other studies in which colder winter temperatures have been shown to worsen mortality. The ability of national administrations successfully to isolate entire regions from epidemics like typhus, and especially the plague during the seventeenth century, was an important factor, as was their ability to contain the effects of subsistence crises.[15] But was it that 'critical variable' as Post called it?[16] On the other hand, there is little evidence that in most areas sanitation and public-health measures improved during the period.[17] Jenner's smallpox vaccination made a contribution to the reduction of childhood mortality, though the extent of its use and its exact demographic impact is still a matter for speculation.[18] As may have been the case with measles or scarlet fever, the evolution of certain diseases into less lethal maladies may also have had some impact on general mortality levels. In sum, mortality reduction seems to have been the result of several, often disconnected, factors.

In many European countries, this early and rather uneven decline in mortality was followed by a period of stable or even slightly rising mortality rates. This was the case in England, Scandinavia, France, Germany, and

[15] Post has argued that government intervention was decisive in limiting the consequences for mortality of the great dearth of the early 1740s in many areas of Europe. See John D. Post, *Food Shortage, Climatic Variability, and Epidemic Disease in Preindustrial Europe: The Mortality Peak of the Early 1740s* (Ithaca and London, 1985), pp. 28–29.

[16] See id., 'Famine, Mortality and Epidemic Disease in the Process of Modernization', *Economic History Review*, 39(1) (1976), pp. 14–37, esp. pp. 26–37. Also id., *The Last Great Subsistence Crisis in the Western World* (Baltimore and London, 1977), pp. 159–75.

[17] There are important exceptions to this. In cities like London during the 18th cent. there were important campaigns to improve the urban environment by paving and washing streets and by removing excrement. See James C. Riley, *The Eighteenth-Century Campaign to Avoid Disease* (London, 1987). Also R. Porter, 'Cleaning up the Great Wen', in W.F. Bynum and R. Porter (ed.), *Living and Dying in London* (London, 1991). In certain countries in the southern part of the continent there were also attempts to remove cemeteries outside town limits. The demographic implications of these measures are, of course, a matter of speculation.

[18] Where its use was widespread, it certainly played an important role. This seems to have been the case in Finland where, in a recent article, Pitkänen *et al.* have argued that vaccination was very important during the initial stages of decline. See K.J. Pitkänen, J.H. Mielke, and L.B. Jorde, 'Smallpox and its Eradication in Finland: Implications for Disease Control', *Population Studies*, 43(1) (1989), pp. 95–111, esp. pp. 98–101, 110.

possibly in Italy as well, during the middle part of the nineteenth century. Data from other areas show that even where decline can be perceived, it was halting and weak. With few exceptions we lack data on age at death by cause for this period, and so it is very difficult to pinpoint the exact reason for this reversal in the downward trend. The presence of cholera in Europe during the period was a contributing factor, though it is doubtful that it was the only, or even the major, reason. The social and economic changes at work in European society were also crucial. Increased concentration of population in towns during the nineteenth century tended to facilitate the spread of infections in an environment in which public health and sanitation were notoriously deficient and mortality rates traditionally higher than in rural areas.

During the latter part of the nineteenth century mortality once again began to decline, this time with far-reaching consequences. Save for the momentary interruptions of the influenza epidemic of 1918 and both world wars, the secular trend has not been reversed. This transition in mortality, which raised life expectancy in many countries by more than ten years over a period of only three decades, parallels the almost simultaneous transition in fertility.[19] Even though mortality in wealthier countries was lower and declined at somewhat faster rates, the entire process took place nearly everywhere on the continent during a very short period of time, much as had occurred with fertility.

As Vallin points out in his contribution to this volume, in most areas the mortality of children aged between 1 and 14 years declined first and most, and was followed by that of infant mortality which proved to be somewhat more resistant to change.[20] Despite moderate increases in adult survival, between 1870 and 1930 most gains in life expectancy were due to decreased death rates among children. In this volume, Caselli has argued that infectious diseases, especially respiratory tuberculosis, declined most and, at least in England and Italy, accounted for over half the gains in life expectancy between 1871 and 1911, and for nearly 40 per cent of the mortality improvement between 1871 and 1951.[21] Decreases in respiratory ailments (pneumonia, bronchitis, and influenza) and in the prevalence of diarrhoea and enteritis also made significant contributions to the length of life, though

[19] This has prompted many scholars to consider declining fertility as a cause of improving survivorship, particularly during the younger years of life. Here, however, it is most difficult to define the direction of causation, because declining infant and child mortality is also a clear fertility depressant. For a discussion of this issue, see Robert I. Woods, P. A. Watterson, and J. H. Woodward, 'The Causes of Rapid Infant Mortality Decline in England and Wales', pt. 1, *Population Studies*, 42(3) (1988), pp. 343–66, and pt. 2, *Population Studies*, 43(1) (1989), pp. 113–32, esp. pp. 121–26.

[20] Ibid., pt. 1, pp. 350–52.

[21] Preston has argued that the English experience analysed by McKeown was highly untypical. See Samuel H. Preston, *Mortality Patterns in National Populations with Special Reference to Recorded Causes of Death*, (New York, 1976), p. 20.

in the initial stages of transition their impact was minimal. The differing age and cause structures of mortality among, say, the Italian and the French or English populations, as noted by both Caselli and Vallin in this volume, suggest that there may well have been multiple paths to mortality transition which have yet to be unearthed by scholars.[22] As research progresses, the patterns sketched here are likely to undergo important modifications.[23]

3. Explanations of Mortality Change

The causes of the secular decline in mortality are the source of ongoing debate among historical demographers, historians of medicine, economic historians, and others who have attempted to understand the dynamics involved. Many of the papers in this volume participate either directly or indirectly in a controversy which, rather simply stated, pits nutrition against public health, living standards against social organization, and levels of income against scientific advance. Proponents of these positions often seem to give persuasive but mutually exclusive accounts of the mortality transition anchored in their respective viewpoints.[24] One of the reasons for this is our, as yet, incomplete knowledge of the processes involved. For example, where deaths by age and cause are known for only a very few countries, little is understood of the relationship of morbidity to mortality during the transition, and next to nothing of the biological and genetic determinants of exposure and resistance to disease. Even so, these contrasting positions may not be so exclusive as many of their proponents seem to suggest.

It is only reasonable to start with the ideas of McKeown, as expressed in *The Modern Rise of Population* (1976). His forceful argumentation was based on the unique data of the returns of deaths classified by age and certified cause of death available for the entire population of Britain from July 1837 onwards. He observed that the category of cause of death which contributed most to mortality decline between 1848 and 1971 had been that of air-borne micro-organisms (especially tuberculosis), followed by water- and food-borne micro-organisms (ch. 3).[25] Making use of these results, he

[22] A major contribution to our understanding of the structure of cause of death, albeit during a more recent period, is to be found in the recent study of French mortality by Vallin and Meslé. See Jacques Vallin and France Meslé, *Les Causes de décès en France de 1925 à 1978* (Paris, 1988).

[23] A number of alternate patterns have been sketched by Preston, op. cit. in n. 21.

[24] See S. Ryan Johansson and Carl Mosk, 'Exposure, Resistance and Life Expectancy: Disease and Death during the Economic Development of Japan 1900–60', *Population Studies*, 41(2) (1987), pp. 207–36, esp. pp. 209–11. See also Carl Mosk and S. Ryan Johansson, 'Income and Mortality: Evidence from Modern Japan', *Population and Development Review*, 12(3) (1986), pp. 415–40.

[25] Szreter has recently attempted to reassess McKeown's emphasis on airborne micro-organisms, and especially respiratory tuberculosis, as the key group of diseases that declined during the period. Apart from problems with defining tuberculosis, he points to important

proceeded to minimize the contribution of different factors to this trend by means of a rather liberal use of reductive logic. On the one hand, medical advances could not be credited with the decline in mortality since, with the exception of smallpox and diphtheria, most other diseases (whooping cough, measles, scarlet fever) were declining long before effective chemotherapy or other scientific techniques had become available (ch. 5). Sanitary and public-health measures were certainly effective after the middle of the nineteenth century, but he surmised that mortality had been declining earlier and, furthermore, they were only effective against water- and food-borne micro-organisms which ultimately accounted for only a minority of the decline in mortality (ch. 6).

Air-borne micro-organisms (especially tuberculosis) had accounted for the majority of the decline of mortality during the nineteenth and the twentieth centuries, and these were largely unaffected by advances in public health. McKeown put forward the hypothesis that exposure to these diseases could not possibly have been limited during the mortality transition, and therefore resistance to them must have grown on account of the improved nutritional status of the population (ch. 7). In this *tour de force* of reasoning by exclusion, he placed economic and nutritional factors at the centre stage of mortality improvement. He also reasoned, with little empirical basis, that a reduction in the prevalence of infectious diseases had also characterized the mortality decline of the eighteenth and early part of the nineteenth centuries, long before any improvements in public health had taken place. Therefore, nutrition became the single most important causal explanation of mortality change over the past three centuries.

His insistence on the unchallenged importance of nutrition runs against a long-standing tradition of social and medical historians, as well as the views of most contemporaries, who felt improvements in public health and sanitation had been at the source of declining mortality. According to this idea, the State fulfilled a key role in effectively organizing public defence against disease, providing basic health facilities and educating the population in accord with scientific advances in health care. Perhaps the clearest demonstration of the validity of this widely held theory was given by Preston when he estimated that income, nutrition, and other indicators of the standard of living cannot have been responsible for more than 25 per cent of the rise in life expectancy at birth in a number of national populations during much of the twentieth century.[26] Therefore, according to Preston,

---

inconsistencies in his argument. E.g. among the declining airborne diseases some, like scarlet fever and smallpox, were unrelated to nutritional levels, and others, such as bronchitis and pneumonia, actually showed an increase between 1848 and 1901. See Szreter, op. cit. in n. 4, pp. 10–17.

[26] See Preston, op. cit. in n. 21. Also Samuel H. Preston, 'Causes and Consequences of Mortality Decline in Less Developed Countries during the Twentieth Century', in R. E. Easterlin (ed.), *Population and Economic Change in Developing Countries* (Chicago, Ill., 1980), pp. 289–360.

the efficiency of public-health technology becomes the most important, albeit residual, explanation for declining mortality. This idea has received considerable support in much of the developing world in recent years, where mortality has been reduced drastically despite few improvements in the standard of living.[27]

Both positions are convincing, both have readily apparent defects, both have very long-range implications for our view of the historical process of change, and neither is able to explain mortality transition fully on its own. Rather than clearly drawn landscapes, they are more like signposts indicating the areas of potentially fruitful enquiry for researchers delving into the subject of mortality decline. Both approaches have clear weaknesses. For example, McKeown's insistence on nutrition as the sole factor of mortality decline before the second half of the nineteenth century is based on non-existent data on cause of death during the earlier period and ignores the important medically induced decline of smallpox during the early part of the century. More importantly, however, it is based on the supposition that nutrition and living standards were improving between 1700 and 1850, when there is no evidence of improved nutritional levels, and indirect proof that living standards were in fact worsening during that period.[28] On the other hand, convincing statistical evidence of the pre-eminence of public health for mortality is only available for twentieth-century societies at a time when the development of medical science and the existence of information systems makes present-day societies quantitatively and qualitatively different from those of a century ago. Furthermore, it is very difficult to argue in favour of the importance of public-health measures in Europe before the second half of the nineteenth century. This would leave the earlier part of the decline of mortality largely unexplained, except as a fall back to an earlier level of mortality such as occurred in England and in Geneva before 1820.

Our purpose here is certainly not to pass judgement on the relative merits of each position. It seems fairly clear that the positions involved are not mutually exclusive and that a viable understanding of mortality decline must necessarily make use of both. By concentrating on nutrition and public

[27] In areas like Kerala (India), Costa Rica, or China, Caldwell has identified provincial health services, women's education, and the political will to make health care the most efficient possible as important for rapid decline in mortality in the absence of improved standards of living. See John C. Caldwell, 'Routes to Low Mortality in Poor Countries', *Population and Development Review*, 12(2) (1986), pp. 171–220, esp. 200–03.

[28] Massimo Livi Bacci has argued that there is very little evidence to suggest an improvement in levels of nutrition over the, 18th cent., and that mortality improvement probably took place in its absence. See Massimo Livi Bacci, *Population and Nutrition. An Essay in European Demographic History* (Cambridge, 1991), esp. pp. 79–111. In the standard-of-living debate for England, the 1820s are generally considered to be have been a pivotal moment, after which rising real wages superseded the stagnating ones of the long period since 1750. See P. H. Lindert and J. G. Williamson, 'English Workers' Living Standards during the Industrial Revolution: A New Look', *Economic History Review*, 36(1) (1983), pp. 1–25.

health, they synthesize an array of factors which influenced mortality patterns and transitions in past societies. Nutrition, living standards, public health, and sanitation are included among these, but so are others directly or indirectly associated with them, such as living conditions, the workplace, urbanization, education, the aetiology of old and new diseases, physicians and medical science, mothers, infant-feeding practices and hygiene, politicians, planners and reformers, and even climate. If we cannot understand these aspects of mortality, our view of the field will be skewed and it will be very difficult to participate judiciously in the debate on the causes of decline.

One of the major difficulties with McKeown's theory of the importance of nutrition was the fact that it can only be proved inferentially. Finding more convincing proof has become a major task for many historians. One of the most conventional ways of doing this has been to generate information on real incomes or living standards, though this has also shown itself to be an imperfect measure, since it is based on the supposition of the existence of a pattern which does not hold invariably; that is, that increases in income are immediately and uniformly used to improve the nutritional levels of the population. Research on heights has proven to be a far more rewarding line of enquiry, because heights seem to be a good indicator of nutritional status during childhood.[29] In this volume Floud is careful to distinguish between nutrition (food intake) and nutritional status (which also included the disease environment and thus is partially the consequence of public health). Traditionally heights have been strongly correlated with child mortality levels though, as Floud points out, this does not necessarily give any support for McKeown's thesis expressed in terms of food intake rather than nutritional status.[30]

The relation between nutrition and the disease environment is taken further by Lunn in this volume in his paper based on data from developing countries. He affirms that while low body-weight increases a child's susceptibility to diarrhoea, progressive and lasting bouts of diarrhoea tend to stunt growth and decrease resistance to infection.[31] In this way, nutrition is both

[29] For examples of recent work on this topic see Roderick C. Floud, Kenneth W. Wachter, and A.S. Gregory, *Height, Health and History: Nutritional Status in Britain 1750–1980* (Cambridge, 1990); Roderick C. Floud, 'Anthropometric Measures of Nutritional Status in Industrialised Societies: Europe and North America since 1750', in A. Sen and S. Osmani (eds.), *Poverty, Undernutrition and Living Standards* (Oxford, 1989).

[30] In a recent paper, Robert Fogel has convincingly emphasized the remarkable parallels in long-term evolution of heights and mortality. He has also suggested that the differences between French and British mortality levels toward the later part of the 18th cent. can be predicted from height differentials. See Robert W. Fogel, 'Second Thoughts on the European Escape from Hunger: Famines, Price Elasticities, Entitlements, Chronic Malnutrition, and Mortality Rates' (National Bureau of Economic Research, Working Paper Series on Historical Factors in Long Run Growth, 1989), esp. pp. 49–53.

[31] See N.S. Scrimshaw, C.E. Taylor, and J.E. Gordon, *Interaction of Nutrition and Infection* (WHO, Monograph Series, 57, Geneva, 1968).

the cause and the consequence of a generalized diseases environment, and thus is intricately bound up with public health and sanitation. The work of Lunn and others seems to indicate that, at least during the first years of life, there is no simple way of separating nutritional from public-health factors. Here the gap between McKeown and his opponents may be more apparent than real.[32]

In a number of recent studies nutritional levels have also been indirectly linked to mortality in adult populations. The most traditional way of doing this has been by showing class-specific differences in life expectancy in pre-industrial and industrializing societies, where mortality levels in the wealthier sectors are consistently lower than in other social groups.[33] Analyses of short-term fluctuations in grain prices and adult mortality have shown, for the most part, positive and significant links between both, during the year when a rise in prices takes place, and during the subsequent year.[34] What is more, when social group or income have been controlled within the same general disease environment, it has been apparent that the poorer groups in society suffered more from price fluctuations than did the richer ones.[35] In both these types of analysis there seems to exist a significant negative correlation between nutrition and mortality. Unfortunately, however, as so often happens in this field, it is exceedingly difficult to specify the links between the two adequately. Thus, we are left with a doubt about

[32] Despite the fact that McKeown insisted on the pre-eminent position of nutrition, he also recognized the importance of a multi-causal approach to mortality decline. This was especially evident in some of his later writings. See e.g. Thomas McKeown, 'Food, Infection and Population', *Journal of Interdisciplinary History*, 14(2) (1983), pp. 227–47, esp. pp. 244–46.

[33] An example of these differences can be found in a recent study on mortality in the city of Paris during the 19th cent. where life expectancy at 20 years of age (e_{20}) was between four and eight years higher among the propertied classes than among day labourers. See Alain Blum, Jacques Houdaille, and Marc Lamouche, 'Éléments sur la mortalité différentielle à la fin du XVIIIe et au début du XIXe siècles', *Population*, 44(1) (1989), pp. 29–54, esp. pp. 38–39. Similar results can be found in other studies of differential mortality. See e.g. Jean-Pierre Bardet, *Rouen aux XVIIe et XVIIIe siècles: Les Mutations d'un espace social*, (2 vols., Paris, 1983); Alfred Perrenoud, 'L'Inegalité sociale devant la mort à Genève au XVIIème siècle', *Démographie historique* (*Population*, 30, special issue (1975)), pp. 221–39.

[34] For examples of this type of work, see Ronald Demos Lee, 'Short-Term Variation: Vital Rates, Prices and Weather', in Wrigley and Schofield, op. cit. in n. 5, pp. 356–401; Patrick R. Galloway, 'Basic Patterns in Annual Variations in Fertility, Nuptiality, Mortality, and Prices in Preindustrial Europe', *Population Studies*, 42(2) (1988), pp. 275–302; David R. Weir, 'Markets and Mortality in France 1600–1789', in J. Walter and R. Schofield (eds.), *Famine, Disease and the Social Order in Early Modern Society* (Cambridge, 1989), pp. 201–34. Other authors have rejected any direct causal link between subsistence crises and mortality. See Jacques Dupâquier, *La Population rurale du Bassin parisien à l'époque de Louis XIV* (Paris, 1979), p. 265.

[35] See e.g. Patrick R. Galloway, 'Differentials in Demographic Responses to Annual Price Variations in Pre-Revolutionary France: A Comparison of Rich and Poor Areas in Rouen 1681 to 1787', *European Journal of Population*, 2 (1986), pp. 269–305; David S. Reher, 'Population and Economy in Eighteenth-Century Mexico: An Analysis of Short Term Fluctuations', Paper given at the Conference on the Population History of Latin America organized by the IUSSP Committee on Historical Demography in Ouro Preto, Brazil; David S. Reher, *Town and Country in Preindustrial Spain* (Cambridge, 1990) esp. ch. 4.

the possibility that higher mortality among the poor might have been tied more, say, to population densities or migratory in-flows, than to nutritional levels themselves.[36] Disentangling the weights of different factors is a recurrent problem when attempting to understand mortality and its transition in Europe.

A traditional and fruitful area of research into past mortality patterns has been the study of specific diseases, their aetiology, incidence, lethality, and development over time. As the importance of some declined, the proportional weight of others increased, with changing shares in total mortality or morbidity rates as a consequence. Plague, yellow fever, malaria, typhus, and smallpox were among those which declined or disappeared from Europe before the middle of the nineteenth century. All of them were normally the cause of crisis mortality and most of them, with the exception of typhus, are relatively insensitive to nutritional levels.[37] Their decline has been ascribed to many factors which range from changing climates to government intervention; and nutrition probably played little or no role in this process.

When analysing diseases, it is essential to distinguish between exposure to contagion and resistance to infection. This is quite clear when we look at diseases which led the mortality decline during the nineteenth and early twentieth centuries, when the situation was quite different from that during the eighteenth century. Those which declined most over the period were diphtheria, whooping cough, scarlet fever, cholera, tuberculosis and, somewhat later during the first part of the twentieth century, diarrhoea, pneumonia, influenza, and others. All of these can be more or less directly related to nutritional status, mainly because resistance to them is lower among the malnourished. On the other hand, exposure to these diseases was often strongly influenced by public-health and sanitation measures. The case of cholera and other water-borne diseases is unquestionably evidence for a combination of both factors as Bourdelais argues in this volume. Something similar, however, can also be said of others like tuberculosis where, as Puranen shows in her contribution to this volume, exposure was a consequence of living conditions, hygienic standards, as well as place of residence and the isolation of patients in sanatoria. While it seems an impossible task

[36] Walter and Schofield, and Dupâquier have given strong arguments for the importance of migration for mortality fluctuations. See John Walter and Roger Schofield, 'Famine, Disease and Crisis Mortality in Early Modern Society', in Walter and Schofield (eds.), op. cit. in n. 34, pp. 1–73, esp. pp. 52–57; Jacques Dupâquier, 'Demographic Crisis and Subsistence Crises in France 1650–1725', in Walter and Schofield (eds.), op. cit. in n. 34, pp. 189–99, esp. pp. 198–99. Walter and Schofield (on p. 72) stated that 'it may be reasonable to conclude that the large differences between societies in the case of mortality owed little to biological or behavioural mechanisms linking availability of food directly with death, but were largely created by the different operation of social, economic, and political factors that were systematically related to the level of economic development'.

[37] See R.I. Rotberg and T.K. Rabb, *Hunger and History* (Cambridge, Mass., 1985), p. 308.

to ferret out the exact weight of each one, a disease-by-disease analysis tends to suggest that declines in mortality were often achieved by both public-health measures and nutritional improvement.[38]

When discussing the decline in importance of certain diseases it is useful to distinguish between the incidence of a particular disease and its lethality. The fact that the case-fatality rate may have decreased does not necessarily mean that there was also a decline in its prevalence. In the case of tuberculosis, once called 'the captain of the men of death', exposure to the tubercle bacillus continued to be widespread until well into this century, and probably the case-fatality rate declined well before the incidence of the infection. With typhoid fever it seems that just the opposite occurred, with prevalence declining more rapidly and earlier than the case-fatality rate. Where morbidity and mortality have been compared systematically within the same population, they have often proved to have been negatively related; moments of low and declining mortality have been characterized by relatively high morbidity rates, and conversely.[39]

The overall disease environment may also have had far-reaching effects. Many researchers have argued that exposure to disease during early life is related to mortality patterns later on. For some, mortality in certain 'stressed' generations, tends to have been higher than normal later in life;[40] and for Alter and Riley: 'past health status is a good predictor of future health status'.[41] This could be the case with tuberculosis, where sanitary reforms which affected the young have been linked to declining rates of deaths from tuberculosis, thus suggesting that an improved health environment and nutritional status during the first years of life enables people to be more resistant to tuberculosis later on. On the other hand, it is also true that a certain amount of infection is necessary in order to allow the immune system to develop; measles, smallpox, and poliomyelitis are examples of this. The question is: just how much is enough?[42] Preston and van de Walle have argued that the cohort-specific mortality gains after the mid-nineteenth century in France may well have been due to a more benign disease environment during the early stages of life resulting from improvements in public hygiene and possibly nutrition, which ended up by having a positive effect

[38] There were also a number of diseases the importance of which increased dramatically in industrializing Europe towards the latter part of the nineteenth century. Many of them, like pellagra, rickets, or infantile scurvy, were the consequence of living conditions or nutritional deficiencies and imbalances; and infantile scurvy even tended to affect the wealthy more than other groups in society. See e.g. Massimo Livi Bacci, 'Fertility, Nutrition, and Pellagra: Italy during the Vital Revolution', *Journal of Interdisciplinary History*, 16 (1986); K. I. Carpenter, *The History of Scurvy and Vitamin C* (Cambridge, 1988).

[39] George Alter and James C. Riley, 'Frailty, Sickness, and Death: Models of Morbidity in Historical Populations', *Population Studies*, 43(1) (1989), pp. 25–46.

[40] Graziella Caselli and Ricardo Capocaccia, 'Age, Period, Cohort and Early Mortality: An Analysis of Adult Mortality in Italy', *Population Studies*, 43(1) (1989), pp. 133–54, esp. 152–53.

[41] Alter and Riley, op. cit. in n. 39 above, p. 32.

[42] We would like to thank Stephen Kunitz for sharing some of these ideas with us.

on mortality later in life.[43] The issue is a new one, and further research on the subject is needed before these cohort effects of morbidity on mortality can be estimated more accurately.

For both the emerging diseases, and for many of those which declined late, the rapid process of industrialization and urbanization in nineteenth-century European society created new obstacles to improved health. Towns had always been characterized by higher mortality rates due mainly to greater population densities which facilitated infection and filth; and during the nineteenth century increasing proportions of the population were living in those urban centres. The poor living conditions of the age were probably one of the principal reasons why mortality ceased to improve during most of the central decades of the century. This was certainly apparent to contemporary observers like Chadwick, Dickens, Zola, and many others.[44] Overcrowded housing conditions were ideal sources of disease transmission. New types of job in industry, and especially the massive use of child labour, were also detrimental for the general health of the population. For many, the new liberal bourgeois society had yet to yield many concrete benefits. There is an entire field of social history centred on the study of living conditions of early industrializing nineteenth-century society. For the purposes of the analysis of mortality transition, however, the implications of, say, working conditions cannot be readily separated from those of social group, income, and perhaps living conditions, as Haines and Burnett show in their contributions to this volume. This has made any estimation of the precise demographic implications of these different aspects of society and life very difficult.

The role of medicine and medical science in the decline of mortality has been belittled by McKeown and many other scholars. But was their contribution as insignificant as it is often made out to be? Before the discovery of antibiotics and sulpha drugs during the middle part of the present century, physicians had almost no effective weapons with which to combat disease and infection directly; and by then much of the battle against infectious disease had already been won. For the most part, hospitals were more agents for the spread of contagion than centres of cure, and medical practitioners were the frequent butt of jokes. Yet the situation is not nearly as simple as it might seem. Jenner's smallpox vaccine, the use of the diphtheria antitoxin, the establishment of tuberculosis sanatoria to isolate patients, and the discoveries of Pasteur, all led either directly or indirectly to significant declines in mortality, as is shown by Biraben in this volume. Medical men were also important in so far as they were behind most public-health and sanitation policies, and were leaders in the movement for reform and

[43] Samuel H. Preston and Etienne van de Walle, 'Urban French Mortality in the Nineteenth Century', *Population Studies*, 32(2) (1978), pp. 275–97, esp. pp. 290–91.

[44] E. Chadwick, *Report on the Sanitary Condition of the Labouring Population of Great Britain*, ed. M.W. Flinn (1842; Edinburgh, 1965).

education in these areas. Even though the direct role of medical science may have been limited, the importance of its indirect contribution to mortality decline and to the quality of life in industrializing society should not be underestimated.

Spurred on the one hand by the appalling squalor of urban industrial life and on the other by a vocal and influential reform movement, European governments played an increasingly active role in regulating public health and sanitation. Medical and scientific discoveries in the field of health were used by the reformers to call for action from political leaders. Concrete public-health measures were often opposed by local business interests who felt that they were an unnecessary hindrance to economic growth. As Bourdelais and Woods argue below, the case of the cholera epidemic in Hamburg in 1892 is unquestionably the most eloquent example of this entire process. There, despite the discovery some years earlier of the cholera bacillus, the public authorities, under pressure from local economic interests, had neglected to establish a system of filtered water for the city and, when the epidemic first appeared, vacillated as long as possible before declaring a state of epidemic. The result was that 1.4 per cent of the population died of cholera that year, whereas in the nearby port of Bremen where many precautionary measures had been taken only 6 persons died.[45] Until local economic interests and political powers were convinced of the usefulness of preventive measures counselled by medical science, progress could only be uneven and slow.

Efforts in the field of public health ranged from the installation of sanitation and sewage systems to the education of mothers on the importance of breast-feeding, food purity, and household sanitation. As Morel argues in her contribution to this volume, the implementation of ideas and practices based on medical research at a household level was a major factor for the decline of many diseases, especially those which affected infancy and childhood. Yet acceptance of new ideas at a local level often took a considerable amount of time and education. The smallpox vaccine, or the importance of extreme care in the preparation of food given to infants, only became effective practices many years after Jenner's and Pasteur's discoveries. The process of health education was probably subject to cultural and educational constraints which differed by region and by social group. These are variations that comprise a subject which warrants further research.

Infant feeding practices could enhance or diminish the chances for survival of the very young. As is now generally accepted, breast-feeding affords the child added protection not only because of the nutrients in the mother's milk, but also because it results in decreased dependence on

[45] See Richard J. Evans, *Death in Hamburg: Society and Politics in the Cholera Years 1830–1919* (Oxford, 1987), p. 275.

potentially impure sources of food.[46] The extent and duration of breast-feeding played a key role in infant mortality, and some authors have attributed the relatively low levels of infant mortality in England to the widespread practice of breast-feeding.[47] Also, more hand- or bottle-fed children tended to die during warm summers than those who were breast-fed, and in some European countries seasonality and age at weaning could enhance or diminsh the probability of survival.[48] Unfortunately, our knowledge of infant feeding practices is still too sketchy in most areas to allow us to evaluate its impact on mortality patterns adequately.

A number of studies have pointed to the importance of climate in determining both long- and short-term fluctuations of mortality in Europe. Periods of global warming have been associated with lower mortality and faster population growth;[49] while warmer summers or colder winters have been linked to higher-than-average mortality especially among the very young children.[50] As Caselli points out, infant and especially child mortality patterns in Europe show considerable similarities with summer climates: areas of hot, dry summers seem to be plagued by high levels of child mortality, where diarrhoea and other intestinal diseases are relatively more important than in other parts of the continent. The peculiar structure of pre-transitional childhood mortality patterns, which can be seen in Coale and Demeny's 'South' tables where child mortality ($_4q_1$) is as high or higher than infant mortality (q_0), may well be related to summer climate and its consequences for food and water purity.[51]

Yet the potentially negative effects of climate were eventually overcome; parents began to take care not to give rotten food or contaminated water to their children. In the long run, cultural factors were essential for the breakthrough in the fight against high mortality. Once people, and local and national authorities, became aware of the importance of health and sanitation, numerous obstacles to the decline of mortality were removed. Education and culture may not have been the only elements in the mortality transition, but their importance was far from negligible. One of the major

[46] For more on infant feeding practices, see Valerie A. Fildes, *Breasts, Bottles and Babies: A History of Infant Feeding* (Edinburgh, 1986).

[47] Woods *et al.*, op. cit. in n. 19, pp. 115–19.

[48] See e.g. John Knodel and Hallie Kintner, 'The Impact of Breast-Feeding on the Biometric Analysis of Infant Mortality', *Demography*, 14(4) (1977), pp. 399–419; Hallie J. Kintner, 'Trends and Regional Differences in Breast-feeding in Germany from 1871 to 1937', *Journal of Family History*, 10(2) (1985), pp. 163–82; and David S. Reher, *Familia, población y sociedad en la provincia de Cuenca 1700–1970* (Madrid, 1988), pp. 102–13.

[49] Patrick R. Galloway, 'Long-Term Fluctuations in Climate and Population in the Preindustrial Era', *Population and Development Review*, 12(1) (1986), pp. 1–24.

[50] See e.g. Patrick R. Galloway, 'Annual Variations in Deaths by Age, Deaths by Cause, Prices, and Weather in London 1670–1830', *Population Studies*, 39(3) (1985), pp. 487–505; Woods *et al.*, op. cit., in n. 19, pp. 361–62; Lee, op. cit. in n. 34, pp. 386–98.

[51] Ansley J. Coale and Paul Demeny, *Regional Model Life Tables and Stable Populations*, (Princeton, NJ, 1966).

conclusions which can be derived from reading the papers included in this volume is that there was no simple or unilateral road to low mortality, but rather a combination of many different elements ranging from improved nutrition to improved education. Simplistic and simplifying explanations of the mortality transition ultimately yield biased viewpoints and limited results.

Another major conclusion stemming from this volume and from much of the existing literature in the field, is that any thoroughgoing understanding of the mortality transition will necessarily be an interdisciplinary one. Demographic knowledge, which is still far from complete, will help define the dependent variable in a complex equation including social, economic, cultural, geographical, and even climatological variables. The present volume is a fitting testimony of this need. As an interdisciplinary approach is refined, there is a good chance that we shall be able to achieve an adequate understanding of the mortality transition, because mortality, unlike fertility, depends on genes, biology, and the environment rather than on human choice. Demographers, historians of medicine, social and economic historians, biologists, nutritionists, and geneticists will all be essential to this process of discovery of the past.

2 The Attenuation of Mortality Crises and the Decline of Mortality

by ALFRED PERRENOUD *Department of Economic History, University of Geneva*

If this chapter had been written a few years ago, the questions with which I am concerned in this paper would have appeared simple; it seemed self-evident that the secular fall in mortality had been caused primarily by a reduction in the importance of mortality crises, which were a fixed feature of the old demographic regime. It was also thought that these crises played an important part in the determination of population growth, 'the regulator *par excellence*—perhaps better termed the destroyer of population growth'.[1]

When looked at from this point of view, the old demographic regime seems to have been subject to periodic fluctuations in mortality, which appeared as a dynamic variable in the interaction between the economy, population, and society. Equilibrium between population and resources seemed to be determined as much by ecological constraints as by food supplies, technology, and social organization. The forces which acted as a brake on population growth were inherent in the system and closely dependent on one another. They were:[2]

1. Epidemics, which were themselves the result of the 'microbial unification of the world' that had followed the expansion of trade[3] and improvements in communications;
2. the formation of nation states which resulted in widespread wars which, in their turn, caused periods of shortage and the spread of epidemics;
3. the agricultural system, where the substitution of commercial monoculture for a traditional polyculture of subsistence, itself a result of the increasing complexity of the social system, made man much more dependent on climate and commerce. Moreover, according to Bernard,

[1] M. Livi Bacci, *La Société italienne devant les crises de la mortalité* (Florence, 1978), p. 5.

[2] A. Perrenoud, 'Le Biologique et le humain dans le déclin séculaire de la mortalité', *Annales ESC*, 40(1) (1985), pp. 113–35.

[3] E.R. Ladurie, 'Un concept: L'Unification microbienne du monde (XVIe–XVIIe siècles)', *Revue suisse d'histoire*, 23(4) (1973), pp. 627–96.

monoculture resulted in anaemias, as poor nutrition implied absence or insufficiency of some essential constituents of the blood.[4]

Fundamentally, this ecological-demographic model is Malthusian, because even though it stresses biological factors, these are endogenous to the system as a whole which is subject 'to subsistence crises as well as to microbial short-circuits'.[5]

However, more recently we have acquired new knowledge. Data relating to the population of England have made it possible to re-evaluate the classical doctrines and have provided a more detailed account of the part played by crises in the development of mortality and of population growth. During recent years, there has been a wide-ranging discussion of the factors that determined the first stages of the mortality decline between the seventeenth and nineteenth centuries.

1. The Determinants of Mortality Decline

The question is complex. All kinds of speculations and different explanations have been put forward. A logical presentation, in which McKeown's arguments are used, provides four possible reasons. First, there were improvements in standards of living, nutrition, and housing. Secondly, there were advances in sanitation and health (particularly in public health) adopted as a result of both governmental and private initiatives. In the third place, increases in medical knowledge and better treatment could have contributed to a reduction of both morbidity and mortality. Lastly, biological factors, independently of any human intervention, could have modified the relationship that existed between man and the parasites that cause disease, and reduced the virulence of some diseases. Clearly, however, these four explanations are interdependent.

The first explanation is the one most commonly accepted today. It was McKeown who first put forward the view that the reduction of mortality could only have been caused by an improvement in the general level of living of the population.[6] Progress in agriculture and transport led to improvements in nutrition, and the decline in mortality was caused by increased resistance of the organism to infectious disease.[7] Modern epidemiological research has shown that in contemporary populations there is a clear relationship between malnutrition, particularly protein–energy malnutrition,

[4] J. Bernard, *Le Sang et l'histoire* (Paris, 1983).

[5] E. R. Ladurie, 'L'Histoire immobile', *Annales ESC*, 29(3) (1974), pp. 673–92.

[6] T. McKeown, *The Modern Rise of Population* (London, 1976).

[7] Id., 'Food, Infection and Population', in R. I. Rotberg and K. T. Rabb (eds.), *Hunger and History* (Cambridge, 1985), pp. 29–49.

and susceptibility to infectious diseases and to mortality.[8] It is possible, however, to question the relevance of these comparisons. The severe malnutrition suffered by the populations studied cannot easily be compared with that of modern European populations.

More recently, Galloway has studied some ten European countries and has related demographic variables to cereal prices and climate. His studies confirm the existence – at least in the short term – of both Malthus's preventive and positive checks. In particular, he has shown 'that the structure and magnitude of the preventive check is similar across all countries and time periods', but that 'the strength of the positive check varies widely and in accord with measures of socio-economic development'.[9] Contrariwise, at the level of a city like Rouen, there is little difference between the responses to changes in prices of the mortality of the rich and the poor, but the strength of the preventive check depends on the social position of individuals'.[10] Extending his researches, Galloway has suggested that variations in climate could, through their effect on food supplies, explain long-term variations in the world's population.[11]

The study by R. W. Fogel and others on the impact of long-term changes in nutrition on health and demographic, economic, and social behaviour was undertaken to support McKeown's thesis. It was designed to establish a relationship between the standard of living, the level of nutrition, and the heights of individuals, and to show that changes over time in average stature were correlated with mortality. This would have been a weighty argument in favour of the proposition that nutritional status is a primary determinant of mortality.[12]

However, the problem of synergy between nutrition, mortality, and

[8] N.S. Scrimshaw, C.E. Taylor, and J.E. Gordon, *Interactions of Nutrition and Infection* (WHO Geneva, 1968); R.K. Chandra, 'Nutritional Deficiency and Susceptibility to Infection', *Bulletin of the WHO*, 57(2) (1979), pp. 167–77.

[9] P.R. Galloway, 'Population, Prices and Weather in Preindustrial Europe', Ph.D diss., (Univ. of California, Berkeley, Calif., 1987).

[10] Id., 'Differentials in Demographic Responses to Annual Price Variations in Pre-Revolutionary France: A Comparison of Rich and Poor Areas in Rouen 1681 to 1787', *European Journal of Population*, 2(3–4) (1986), pp. 269–305.

[11] Id., 'Long-Term Fluctuations in Climate and Population in the Preindustrial Era', *Population and Development Review*, 12(1) (1986), pp. 1–24.

[12] R.W. Fogel, 'Nutrition and the Decline of Mortality since 1700: Some Additional Preliminary Findings', National Bureau of Economic Research, Working Paper 1802 (1986); id. *et al.*, 'Secular Changes in American and British Stature and Nutrition', in Rotberg and Rabb (eds.), op. cit. in n. 7, pp. 285–304; A.G. Carmichael, 'Infection, Hidden Hunger, and History', in Rotberg and Rabb, op. cit. in n. 7; J. Komlos, 'Stature and Nutrition in the Habsburg Monarchy: The Standard of Living and Economic Development in the Eighteenth Century', *American Historical Review*, 90 (1985), pp. 149–61; L. Sandberg, and R. Steckel, 'Heights and Economic History: The Swedish Case', *Annals of Human Biology*, 14(2) (1987), pp. 101–10; R.C. Floud, 'The Heights of Europeans since 1750: A New Source for European Economic History', National Bureau of Economic Research, Working Paper 1318, (1984); see also R.C. Floud, Ch. 8 in this vol.

morbidity in past populations has become a controversial subject.[13] A major conclusion of the conference held in Bellagio which was attended by historians, demographers, and nutritionists was a recognition that almost all present interpretations of the evidence are not sufficient to explain the facts. In summarizing the many problems raised by the study of the relationship between nutritional status and mortality Livi Bacci concluded that the supposed relation between these two variables could not have been the only, nor even the most important, in its effect on the survival of human beings in the past.[14]

Public-health measures and the part played by medicine have rarely been mentioned as important factors in mortality decline before the introduction of pasteurization and the provision of a clean water supply towards the end of the nineteenth century. However, there are some exceptions. There were local measures taken during the seventeenth and eighteenth centuries to control plague, which were later extended to a national level. Quarantine, isolation, *cordons sanitaires*, in particular that imposed by the Habsburg monarchy on the 1500 km. border with Turkey are not sufficient to explain the disappearance of plague by themselves, but it cannot be denied that they played an important part in this process. As regards treatment, it is clear that vaccination against smallpox in the country, and even inoculation during the eighteenth century, contributed not only to the fall in mortality, but that these measures also reduced the severity of mortality fluctuations.[15]

Although, except for vaccination, medicine was not very successful in the struggle against disease before the twentieth century, the miasmatic and atmospheric theories of disease which formed part of medical thinking during the eighteenth century served to modify the conditions which determined the pathological state of any given population. Measures which have been recognized by environmental medicine since the end of the seventeenth century and which were supported by public authority, such as improvements in the atmosphere and dealing with stagnant water, and particularly efforts at drainage, must have led to changes in the environment which reduced the impact of the zoonoses, and, in particular, of diseases spread by insects, and will have altered the equilibrium. Riley has suggested that although these measures were not primarily directed against insect populations, whose part in the transmission of disease was as yet unrecognized, they

[13] C.E. Taylor, 'Synergy among Mass Infections, Famines and Poverty', in Rotberg and Rabb (eds.), op. cit. in n. 7, pp. 285–304; Carmichael, op. cit. in n. 12.

[14] M. Livi Bacci, 'The Nutrition–Mortality Link in Past Times: A Comment', in Rotberg and Rabb (eds.), op. cit. in n. 7, pp. 95–100.

[15] A. J. Mercer, 'Smallpox and Epidemiological Demographic Change in Europe: The Role of Vaccination', *Population Studies* 39(2) (1985) pp. 287–307; P. Razzell, *The Conquest of Smallpox: The Impact of Inoculation on Smallpox Mortality in Eighteenth-Century Britain* (Firle, 1977).

did serve to reduce the density of arthropod populations, a significant factor in contamination, and may thus have exercised a significant influence on mortality in Europe.[16]

There remains the last factor. Helleiner and Chambers have suggested that epidemics followed a law of their own, independent of human intervention.[17] McNeill has demonstrated how complex pathogens appear and either remain or disappear, depending on whether circumstances are favourable or unfavourable. Every ecological niche is characterized by its own equilibrium, which is, however, unstable and changes all the time. However, the incidence of a disease will depend on the presence or absence of antibodies in the human bloodstream, and simultaneously natural selection can result in a change in the behaviour of a disease. Exogenous factors, such as climate, nutritional status, population density and movements constantly upset these fragile equilibria.[18]

This view is not shared by Kunitz who does not accept that 'increasing inherited resistance to infection was *the* or even a major factor' in the decline of mortality. He attributes the biological changes to increased State intervention on one hand, and to the decline in military activity on the other. The 'increasing integration of national economies led to a change in human crowd diseases, notably measles and smallpox, transforming them into more benign childhood diseases', which affected mortality in childhood in the first instance.[19]

Wrigley and Schofield have shown, however, that long-term variations in mortality tend to be exogenous and were influenced by natural or biological factors, rather than by social and economic ones.[20] Other authors, particularly in Scandinavia, have reached the same conclusion, namely that the beginning of mortality decline can be explained only in terms of immunological changes and the establishment of a new equilibrium between pathogenic agents and their human hosts.[21]

It would be extremely difficult to measure the true effect of these factors, but it seems clear that long-term variations in mortality can only be understood if biological factors are taken into account. The analysis requires 'a

[16] J.C. Riley, 'Insects and the European Mortality Decline', *American Historical Review*, 91 (1986), pp. 833–58.

[17] K.F. Helleiner, 'The Vital Revolution Reconsidered', in D.V. Glass and D.E.C. Eversley (eds.), *Population in History* (London, 1965), pp. 79–86; J.D. Chambers, *Population, Economy and Society in Pre-Industrial England* (Oxford, 1972).

[18] W. McNeill, *Plagues and Peoples* (New York, 1976).

[19] S.J. Kunitz, 'Speculations on the European Mortality Decline' *Economic History Review*, 36 (1983), pp. 349–64.

[20] E.A. Wrigley and R.S. Schofield, *The Population History of England 1541–1871* (Cambridge, 1981).

[21] G. Fridlizius, 'The Mortality Decline in the First Phases of the Demographic Transition: Swedish Experiences', in T. Bengtsson, G. Fridlizius, and R.H. Ohlsson, *Pre-Industrial Population Change* (Stockholm, 1984), pp. 74–114.

more explicitly biological analytic framework',[22] which would result in an integration of genetic and immunological factors within the specific aetiology of each disease, its mode of transmission, and its fatality rate, and which would take account of both individual and environmental factors and nutritional status, but also of the synergistic effects which can exist between different diseases[23] and of the physiological damage that they inflicted on survivors and which lessened their resistance.[24]

2. Normal Mortality and Crisis Mortality

As we are interested in the nature of mortality decline and the part played in this by the attenuation of crisis mortality, we must in the first place attempt to measure the extent of the latter phenomenon in a long-term context. But, whereas at the national level (which is what we are interested in), information on crisis mortality goes back a long way, data relating to the long-term trend in mortality are, with one exception, available only from the eighteenth century onwards.

By drawing on these data, I shall in the first place dispose of the conventional view that the decline in mortality which has been recorded since the eighteenth century was due mainly to the attenuation, or even the disappearance of mortality crises, whereas mortality in 'normal' years remained unchanged until the nineteenth century. This stability of 'normal' mortality is far from evident, and we could well ask whether in France, as well as in Europe as a whole, 'the expectation of life at birth during the preceding century was in mild years similar to that observed between 1750 and 1789'.[25]

The example of England also leads us to revise this point of view. There are two major conclusions. The first relates to the relatively low level of mortality in England, compared with that in France; above all the very low levels at the end of the sixteenth and the beginning of the seventeenth centuries when there were no crises. We must wait until 1870 before again finding as high a value for life expectancy as the 41 years observed during the 1580s. These surprising results have naturally aroused some scepticism.[26] Is it really possible that during these somewhat remote periods, before the health transition was under way, life expectancy had reached the

[22] S. R. Johansson and C. Mosk, 'Exposure, Resistance, and Life Expectancy: Diseases and Death during the Economic Development of Japan 1900–1960', *Population Studies*, 41(2) (1987), pp. 207–35.

[23] Carmichael, op. cit. in n. 12.

[24] G. Alter and J. C. Riley, 'Frailty, Sickness and Death: Models of Morbidity and Mortality in Historical Populations', *Population Studies*, 43(1) (1989), pp. 25–46.

[25] M. Dupâquier, (ed.), *Histoire de la population française* (Paris, 1988), vol. ii, p. 155.

[26] L. Henry and J. D. Blanchet, 'La Population de l'Angleterre de 1541 à 1871', *Population*, 38(4–5) (1983), pp. 781–826.

levels of the late nineteenth century? If this were really the case, would it not be necessary to revise completely our views of the factors which have generally been associated with the first phase of mortality decline?

Unfortunately, data for these remote periods are scarce. Longitudinal information about élite groups (religious, nobles, or patricians) are not comparable, and are in any case not very useful as a representation of the general mortality of the period. There remain only local sources. I have already drawn attention to the astonishing similarity between the mortality trends of England and Geneva, where long-term trends were identical. Beginning at a low level, in both cases mortality increased during the seventeenth century. Between 1591 and 1690, the slopes of the trend lines were virtually the same (In England: $y = 23.8 + 0.069x$, in Geneva: $y = 36.9 + 0.077x$). This period is followed by a discontinuity during the 1690s, and, after a recrudescence during the 1720s, by a turn which was slow at first and accelerated towards the end of the century. The most surprising finding is that in Geneva, too, we must wait until 1810 before we find a death rate lower than 25 per 1,000 in non-crisis years. Such rates were recorded on a number of occasions towards the end of the sixteenth and the beginning of the seventeenth centuries.[27] I would add that in the Genevan countryside, even on the most pessimistic assumptions,[28] life expectancy at birth had already reached 45 years in the middle of the eighteenth century and had risen to 51 years for children of couples who were married between 1790 and 1819. This example shows that a relatively high level of life expectancy could be achieved even under the 'old' demographic regime.

Moreover, at times when there were violent surges in mortality caused by epidemics or hunger, the selection effect of mortality crises in which the least resistant died resulted in a reduction of mortality during periods of recuperation. The very important crises that occurred between the fourteenth and sixteenth centuries must necessarily have been accompanied by very low levels of 'normal' mortality, if the population was not to have been reduced considerably.

Consider the example of Italy. Livi Bacci has identified nine crisis years between 1340 and 1399 for every 100 years of observation, i.e. a crisis occurred on average every eleven years. The median intensity of mortality during these years was nine times the level recorded in 'normal' years. Assuming a birth rate of 40 per 1,000 and a 'normal' mortality of 30 per 1,000, the loss of population during this period would have amounted to 53 per cent and—other things being equal—this figure may be regarded as a maximum. Therefore, during the periods of recuperation, life expectancy at birth must have been of the order of 35 years. A similar rough calculation

[27] Perrenoud, op. cit. in n. 2.

[28] On the assumption that all children whose fate was unknown died before reaching their fifth birthday.

for the period 1400–50 (when crises were equally frequent, but excess mortality was smaller—five times the normal level) would result in a stationary population, with a 'normal' crude death rate of 30 per 1,000, or in a growth of 40 per cent if the death rate were 25 per 1,000. The true situation lies somewhere in between, and it is perfectly possible for life expectancy at birth to have exceeded 35 years. Clearly, with these mortality levels, populations had a large capacity for recuperation, and the rate of natural increase probably exceeded 1 per cent per year. These calculations make it possible to understand the strong recovery that occurred after 1450, when the frequency of crisis years was reduced to 3 in 100 years, and the median excess over 'normal' mortality was reduced to four times.[29]

The second conclusion that follows from the English data is the absence of an unequivocal relationship between the frequency and intensity of mortality crises and the general level of mortality on one hand, and the stabilization and decline of mortality on the other. Weaker crises during the seventeenth century were, in fact, accompanied by an increase in the general level of mortality which lasted until 1680.

In Table 2.1 we show variations in annual death rates for different quarter-centuries. The figures demonstrate that there is no correlation between the mean level of mortality and its variability, certainly not before 1750. The coefficient of variation for 1625–49 at 17 per cent was three times higher than for 1775–99, when it was 5.7 per cent, whereas the average level

Table 2.1 Variation of crude death rates in England for 25-year periods

Period	Mean	Standard Deviation
1541–74[a]	28.55	7.20
1575–99	24.24	3.58
1600–24	24.81	3.38
1625–49	26.23	4.45
1650–74	28.14	4.69
1675–99	30.28	3.44
1700–24	27.87	2.46
1725–49	30.49	4.99
1750–74	27.24	1.91
1775–99	27.86	1.54
1800–24	25.36	1.48
1825–49	22.66	1.14
1851–71[b]	22.31	0.85

[a] 35 years
[b] 20 years

[29] Livi Bacci, op. cit. in n. 1.

of mortality was nearly the same, or even a little lower, during the earlier period.

Wrigley and Schofield have calculated the frequency of crisis years per month of observation at the parish level. Between 1550 and 1674 this index declined from 14.6 to 10.8 per 1,000 months of observation. Thereafter, it fell only a little further and somewhat irregularly until the 1770s when its value stood at 9.8, continued to decline until 1820 (5.0) before rising again to 10.7 for 1830–38. If the decades are ranked by frequency of crisis years at the parish level and by the expectation of life for the country as a whole, there is no correlation between these two variables. (Spearman's ρ comes to 0.2266, $t = 1.2278$, d.f. = 28.)

Wrigley and Schofield attributed this difference in trend between crises (which were diminishing) and mortality (which was rising) to 'long-term changes in the relationship between micro-organisms and their human hosts'. Widespread but sporadic epidemics which resulted in large numbers of deaths but allowed for periods of recuperation 'gave way to a less hectic endemic phase, in which the relationship was more continuous and the general level of mortality consequently higher'. This pattern is well illustrated by the example of smallpox during the second half of the eighteenth century. The different phases of the disease may be followed in Sweden. In certain countries regular epidemics occurred every five or six years and resulted in very high death rates, whereas in others fluctuations were moderate, but at the cost of an endemicity which was just as lethal. From 1780—i.e. well before the introduction of vaccination—smallpox was in retreat in all the areas studied. Its cyclic character had not disappeared, but the disease had become much less virulent.[30]

At present, England is the only country for which there exist reconstituted data that make it possible to follow the general trend in mortality before the eighteenth century. It would be premature to generalize from this single example. However, a number of hypotheses can be put forward.

3. The Frequency and Chronology of Mortality Crises

It is probable that mortality increased after 1550. This becomes apparent from the return of the major epidemic diseases, at first sporadically, later with greater frequency. They arrived at a time when 'normal' mortality rates were favourable and this made it possible for the population to grow during the sixteenth century, before general conditions began to deteriorate. In the half-century from 1620 there were great and continuing disturbances with increasing numbers of crises and higher morbidity. In the Italian cities the

[30] G. Fridlizius and R. Ohlsson, 'Mortality Patterns in Sweden 1751–1802: A Regional Analysis', in Bengtsson, Fridlizius, and Ohlsson (eds.), op. cit. in n. 21, pp. 299–328.

Table 2.2 Smallpox mortality rates in Geneva

Period	q_0	$_4q_1$	$_5q_5$
1580–99	26.1	69.3	18.8
1600–49	21.2	79.0	20.0
1650–99	11.7	52.4	16.5
1700–49	7.4	41.9	16.7
1750–99	13.9	34.9	11.3

Source: A. Perrenoud, 'Contribution à l'histoire cyclique des malidies: Deux cent ans de variole à Genève 1580–1810', in A. E. Imhof (ed.), *Mensch und Gesundheit in der Geschichte* (Husum, 1980), pp. 175–98.

number of years in which deaths were more than 50 per cent above the 'normal' level came to 34 per 1,000 between 1580 and 1619, rose to 84 per 1,000 between 1620 and 1659, and fell back to 27 per 1,000 between 1660 and 1699.[31] Seven of the 20 most important mortality crises in England and which affected the whole country occurred between 1540 and 1620, seven between 1620 and 1670, and only five during the whole of the eighteenth century.

This resurgence of mortality was caused mainly, but not entirely, by the plague and by diseases transmitted during wartime (particularly typhus), associated with periods of shortage, and occurred at a time when morbidity from non-epidemic diseases, too, was increasing. Smallpox, a disease which is not strongly affected by the socio-economic environment, is generally believed to have become more prevalent during the seventeenth, and to have raged particularly during the eighteenth century. However, it seems, on the contrary, to have been especially virulent since the sixteenth century. In Geneva, the eight most serious epidemics, in which age-specific mortality rates from smallpox for children exceeded 300 per 1,000, all occurred before 1690. However, towards the end of the seventeenth century, and particularly after the 1690s, epidemics became less lethal at a time when mortality was tending to fall. In the long run, there was a considerable decline. Roughly 107 children out of every 1,000 died of smallpox at the end of the sixteenth century, 96 during the seventeenth, and 64 during the eighteenth century, but epidemics were most lethal during the first half of the seventeenth century.

This period of disturbance ended during the 1670s with the disappearance of the plague. It was followed by a prolonged period of transition which lasted until 1780 and which was characterized by an attenuation of mortality

[31] L. Del Panta and M. Livi Bacci, 'Chronologie, intensité et diffusion des crises de mortalité en Italie 1600–1850', *Population*, 32, special issue (1977), pp. 401–40.

crises, though the magnitude and timing of this differed in different countries. In Italy mortality stabilized after 1660, in England after 1690 (with a final recrudescence during the 1720s), in France, according to Lebrun, the excess mortality during the years 1709 and 1710 marked the end of the old mortality crises,[32] but mortality only stabilized slowly. Although the frequency of crises did not diminish, their lethality did. If we apply the crisis index established by J. Dupâquier[33] to the annual numbers of deaths estimated by D. Rebaudo for the French rural population between 1670 and 1740[34] (he dealt with burials of individuals who died at ages exceeding five years), the distribution of 480 region-years (eight regions between 1680 and 1739) was as follows:

386 non crisis years;
24 crises of size 1, spread over 28 years;
16 crises of size 2, spread over 26 years;
13 crises of size 3, spread over 22 years;
6 crises of size 4, spread over 16 years;
1 crisis of size 5, spread over 2 years.

There were thus 94 years with crises, or 19.6 per cent of the total. These figures may be compared with Dupâquier's sample in the INED survey for the years 1750–92:[35]

337 non-crisis years;
28 crises of size 1, spread over 34 years;
16 crises of size 2, spread over 31 years;
9 crises of size 3, spread over 24 years;
1 crisis of size 4, spread over 4 years.

There were altogether 93 crisis years out of 430, or 21.6 per cent. Major crises of size 4 or larger effectively disappeared after 1710, with the sole exception of the crisis which occurred between 1789 and 1792 in Aquitaine–Pyrénées. However, even though the crises tended to be less severe, those of moderate severity (sizes 3 and 4) lasted for longer; their average duration increased from 2 to 2.8 years.

[32] F. Lebrun, 'Les Crises démographiques en France au XVIIe et XVIIIe siècles', *Annales ESC*, 35(2) (1980), pp. 205–34.

[33] Dupâquier's Index is $i = (D - M)/s$, where D is the number of deaths in the year concerned, M is the mean number of deaths during the ten preceding years, and s the standard deviation of deaths during the same ten years. A scale is used, which goes in geometric progression from a value of 1 for a minor crisis to one of 6 for a catastrophe, when the value of the index exceeds 32.

[34] D. Rebaudo, 'Le Mouvement annuel de la population française rurale de 1670 à 1740', *Population*, 34(3) (1979), pp. 589–606.

[35] J. Dupâquier, 'L'Analyse statistique des causes de mortalité', in H. Charbonneau, and A. Larose, (eds.), *The Great Mortalities: Methodological Studies of Demographic Crises in the Past* (Liège, 1979), pp. 83–112.

The decline in cyclical fluctuations came much later in the Scandinavian countries, except in Finland where an 'archaic' mortality regime persisted until the end of the nineteenth century. But even in Norway and Sweden mortality did not begin to become more stable until the beginning of the nineteenth century. In both these countries the epidemic of 1773 increased mortality by 90 per cent over its trend value. Similarly, in 1809 mortality again rose to 60 per cent above normal. In Denmark, the malaria epidemic of 1829–31 was similar in severity to the crises of 1762–63 and 1772–73.

In Italy, too, the series of numbers of deaths collected by Del Panta and Livi Bacci shows that the attenuation of crises varied greatly in different regions.

In Fig. 2.1 we show the inequality in the size of fluctuations until the middle of the nineteenth century for a number of countries for which data are available. They are given as percentages of the trend value. The figure for England never exceeded 20 per cent after 1750. In France, this value was exceeded three times, with a peak of 35 per cent in 1794; in Denmark four times, with two recurrences during the nineteenth century when the excess was greater than 30 per cent; and in Sweden and Norway the value of 20 per cent was exceeded nine times, with peaks of 89 per cent in 1773, and 59 per cent in 1809.

Whereas in England, France, and also in Norway, a new mortality regime appears to have begun after 1815, this was not the case in Sweden or Denmark, where the variability of mortality remained high until 1860, even though there were no more major crises. In Fig. 2.2 the coefficients of variation of mortality rates in different quinquenniums are shown, and it will be seen that an attenuation of fluctuations can be found only in France between 1780 and 1830. This was, however, followed by an increase which culminated in the crisis of 1871.

The fluctuations of mortality in different countries did not run in parallel. The size of fluctuations differed, their attenuation varied in time, and it was exceptional for crises to occur simultaneously in different countries. None

Table 2.3 Frequency of crisis years in which mortality exceeded the 'normal' level by 50 per cent or more, per 1,000 years of observation

Period	Northern Italy	Tuscany	Central and Southern Italy	Total
1669–99	35.0	73.7	77.6	62.1
1700–39	69.0	47.2	69.7	62.0
1740–79	16.7	51.4	63.6	43.9
1780–1819	45.9	34.4	51.0	43.8

Source: L. Del Panta and M. Livi Bacci, 'Le componenti naturali dell'evoluzione demografica nell'Italia del Settecento' in ids. (eds.), *La popolazione italiana nel Settecento* (Bologna, 1980), pp. 71–139.

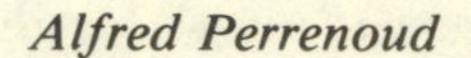

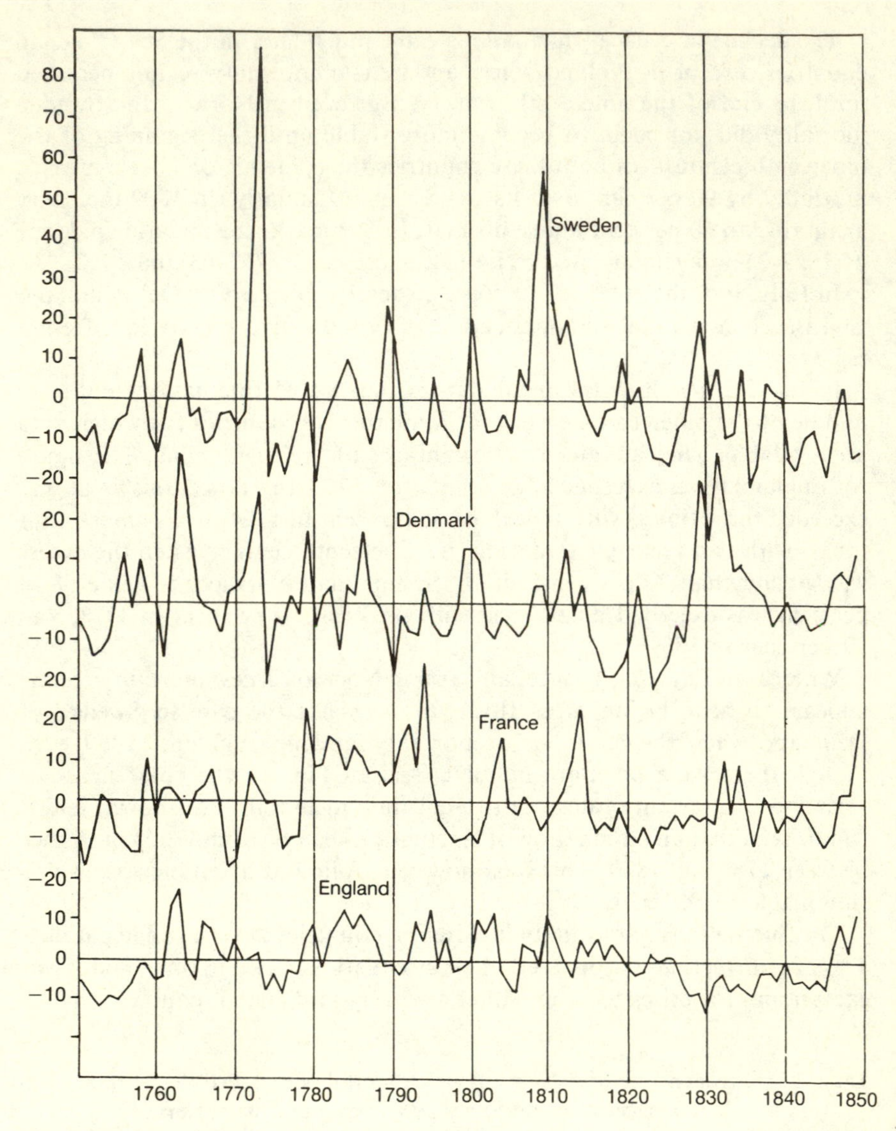

Fig. 2.1 Annual fluctuations in crude death rates, as a percentage of the trend values: Sweden, Denmark, France, England

the less, as the slopes of the trend lines show, mortality decreased everywhere, but the extent of the decline was not related to the degree of variation. Between 1750–59 and 1840–49, mortality in France declined by 34 per cent (on the basis of data collected by INED in which an allowance is made for under-registration of deaths), the analogous figure for Denmark was 29 per cent, for Sweden and Norway approximately 25 per cent, and for England 12 per cent.

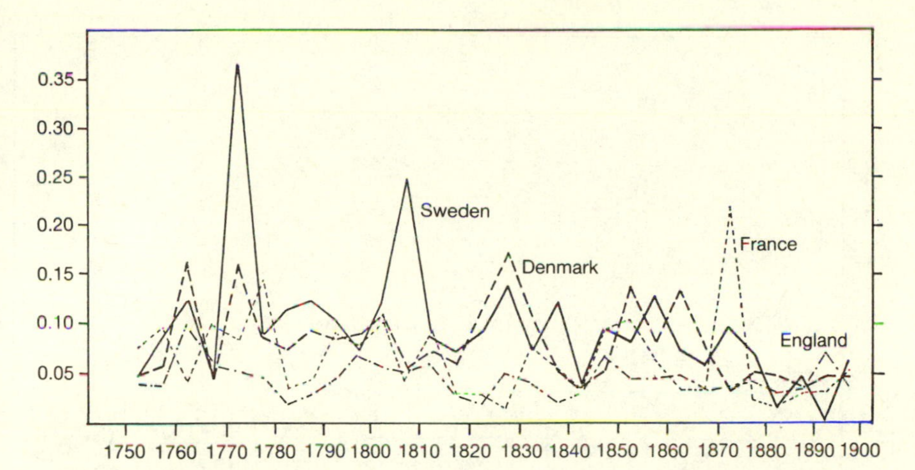

Fig. 2.2 Coefficient of variation of crude death rates for five-year periods: Sweden, Denmark, France, England

We appear to have reached two main conclusions. The secular decline in mortality was due not so much to the attenuation or disappearance of fluctuations in mortality, but rather to a decline in 'normal' mortality. This was evident even between 1780 and 1820 when the underlying decline of mortality was more pronounced than between 1820 and 1850, although there were fluctuations that were caused mainly by political disturbances. Whereas mortality fell considerably everywhere, the decline was neither continuous nor regular, but occurred in successive bounds which were grafted on to a curve of slow decline.[36] Observation of these discontinuities should illuminate the action of explanatory variables.

4. The Stages of Mortality Decline

If we consider periods longer than the short term, is it possible to find the points of inflexion of discontinuity on the curve which shows the trend of mortality? It is not easy to establish a chronology of phases of progress or stagnation. Short-term fluctuations obscure the general picture and make it difficult to establish the underlying trends. We can obtain trend values that will yield 'normal' mortality, purged of fluctuations, by using the method of moving averages, omitting extreme values. This was the method used by Del Panta and Livi Bacci,[37] who calculated a moving average of eleven values, omitting the two largest values n_{10} and n_{11} and the two smallest values n_1 and n_2 and, therefore, effectively used a seven-term

[36] J.C. Chesnais, *La Transition démographique: Étapes, formes, implications économiques* (Paris, 1986), p. 79.

[37] Del Panta and Livi Bacci, op. cit., in n. 31.

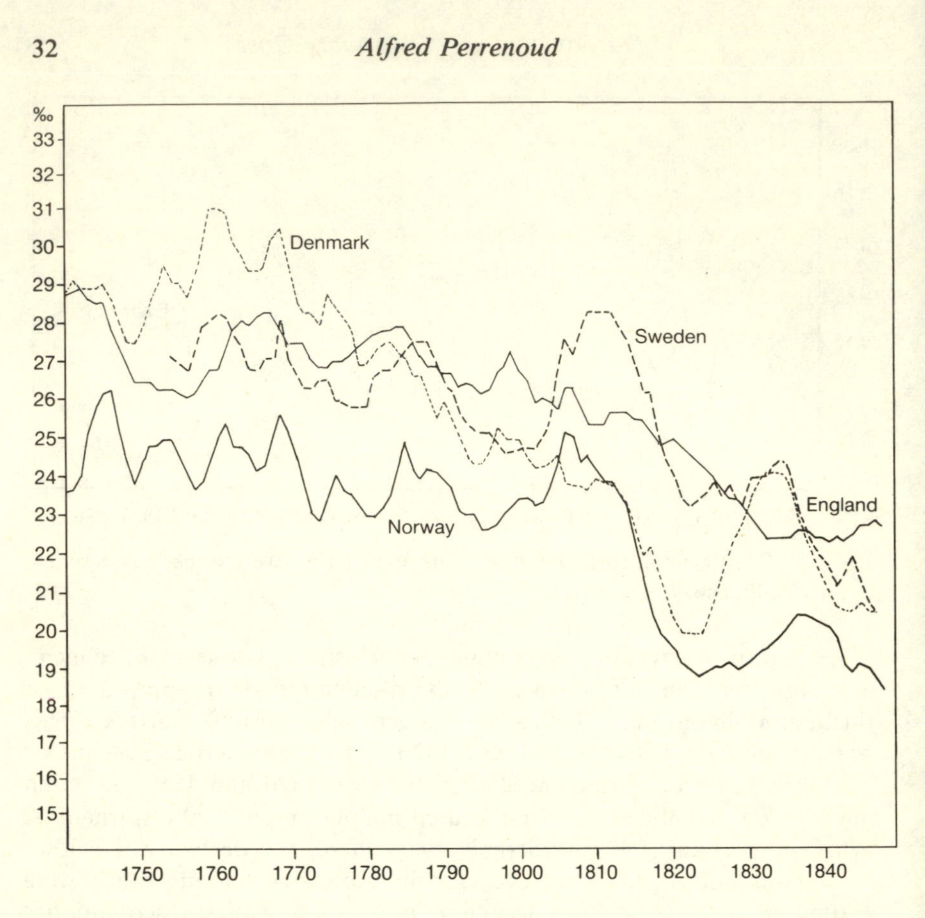

Fig. 2.3 Truncated moving averages (11 terms) of crude death rates: Sweden, Norway, Denmark, England

moving average. The advantage of this method consists in the elimination of the two largest values which often relate to abnormal situations, and of the two lowest values which were generally recorded during years that immediately followed a crisis. However, this method only eliminates short-term disturbances, and when a crisis lasts for more than two years, the moving average will reflect the high mortality of crisis years.

A chronology of these trends shows changes between years of rising and falling mortality that occurred, often simultaneously, in different countries. The years 1750, 1795–1805, and 1815–25 were years of low mortality almost everywhere, whereas the decades of the 1780s, 1805–1815, and 1825–40 were all marked by a remarkable recrudescence of mortality. However, the most important feature is the underlying general and strong decline in mortality rates since the end of the eighteenth century. Even though these declines were not completely synchronized throughout Europe, their general movement is clear, the slopes are comparable in size, and the occasional disturbances, amplified by the moving average which extends their duration, not mask the trend. The decline began between 1780 and 1800; perhaps a little earlier in Scandinavia (where the recovery following the catastrophic mortality of 1772–73 affected the trend), and was complete by 1830. After that year, the trends diverged: in France, England, and a number of other European countries, mortality stagnated until 1870–80, though in Scandinavia it continued to fall.

Until 1790 the fall was only slight. When crude death rates are considered, the slope of the regression lines is very low. Between 1735 and 1789, the values were: England: $y = 28.6 - 0.03x$; Denmark: $y = 29.5 - 0.03x$; Norway: $y = 26.0 - 0.015x$; Sweden (1750–89): $y = 27.7 + 0.006x$. It is known that the crude death rate in France was very high during the 1740s and remained high until 1795, but then fell uninterruptedly until 1825.[38] When smoothed means are used, the values of the slopes are a little more pronounced, except for England. Between 1740 and 1785 the values were: England: $y = 27.4 - 0.004x$; Denmark: $y = 29.4 - 0.034x$; Norway: $y = 25.0 - 0.03x$; Sweden (1754–1785): $y = 27.5 - 0.04x$. These figures go to show that the impact of crises on the underlying trend was weak and that the fall in mortality recorded during the period had little to do with the attenuation of crises.

However, if it were true that nothing had radically changed during the eighteenth century, what is the explanation for the growth of population after a long period of stagnation? Population dynamics during the pre-industrial demographic regime cannot be explained entirely in terms of changes in mortality. It would be wrong to suggest that the full potential of fertility was achieved in agricultural societies and that fertility could not, therefore, vary. But, if it is true that in England population growth owed more to an increase in fertility than to a decrease in mortality, it has not yet been shown that the same is true of other European countries. There must have been significant changes before 1740.

I believe that it was towards the end of the seventeenth century, and more particularly around the 1690s, that a new mortality pattern emerged. This happened after the plague had disappeared and during a period when climatic conditions, from an agricultural point of view, were on balance unfavourable. The change can be clearly seen in England which was spared the crisis of the 1690s; it can also be seen in Geneva where it mainly affected infant mortality, and, in Italy, in the suburbs of Bologna, where again infant mortality was affected.[39] In France, as far as can be judged from figures on burials, there was a relative trough between 1690 and 1720, which does not

[38] A. Blayo, 'La Mortalité en France de 1740 à 1829', *Démographie historique* (*Population*, 30, special issue (1975)), pp. 123–42.

[39] A. Bellettini and A. Samogia, 'Évolution différentielle du mouvement saisonnier de la mortalité infantile et enfantine dans la banlieue de Bologne XVIIe–XIXe siècles', *Annales de démographie historique*, (1983), pp. 195–207.

appear in figures for baptisms during that period. Even in Japan, in a village studied by Hayami, life expectancy on the second birthday increased by nearly eight years between the cohorts of 1671–1700 and those of 1726–50.[40]

It is clear that this first instance of a decline in mortality, which occurred at the turn of the seventeenth century (and which shows the same features as the decline that occurred a century later in completely different economic, social, and medical circumstances)[41] reinforces the view that mortality was autonomous, and that biological factors played an important part in its determination.

A search for the causes of mortality decline cannot ignore these coincidences. We regard the concept of uniformity as essential, and as a preliminary to any analysis we must determine the similarities that extended beyond national or regional particular cases, not only as regards changes in crude death rates, but also changes in their socio-demographic components, and particularly in the age structure.

5. The Age Pattern of Deaths

If the medium- and long-term consequences of mortality crises are to be measured, it is necessary to take account of the age distribution of crisis deaths. Depending on whether it was the young or the old who were mainly affected, long-run population growth will have been influenced by the effect of losses in different generations, or stimulated by a replacement of elderly couples, who had reached the end of their reproductive lives, by the younger generation.[42]

The attenuation of mortality crises will, therefore, have to be studied in terms of age structure. But data are hard to come by. Some information is available for Geneva (Fig. 2.4) and suggests some interesting results. The decline in mortality fluctuations, measured by a coefficient of variation which is the ratio of the standard deviation to a moving average, antedated the eighteenth century, and can be discerned as early as the sixteenth. The fluctuations were particularly pronounced among children less than 15 years old. This age group was strongly affected by crises until 1690, whereas the curve of adult deaths in Geneva stabilized considerably earlier with the disappearance of the plague in 1640. However, the decline occurred earliest in the oldest age groups, in which members were little affected by the major

[40] A. Hayami, 'Aspects démographiques d'un village japonais 1671–1871', *Annales ESC*, 24(3) (1969), pp. 617–39.

[41] Perrenoud, op. cit. in n. 2.

[42] Livi Bacci, op. cit. in n. 1; J. Dupâquier, 'De l'animal à l'homme; Le Mécanisme autorégulateur des populations traditionnelles', *Revue de l'Institut de sociologie*, 2 (1972) pp. 197–207.

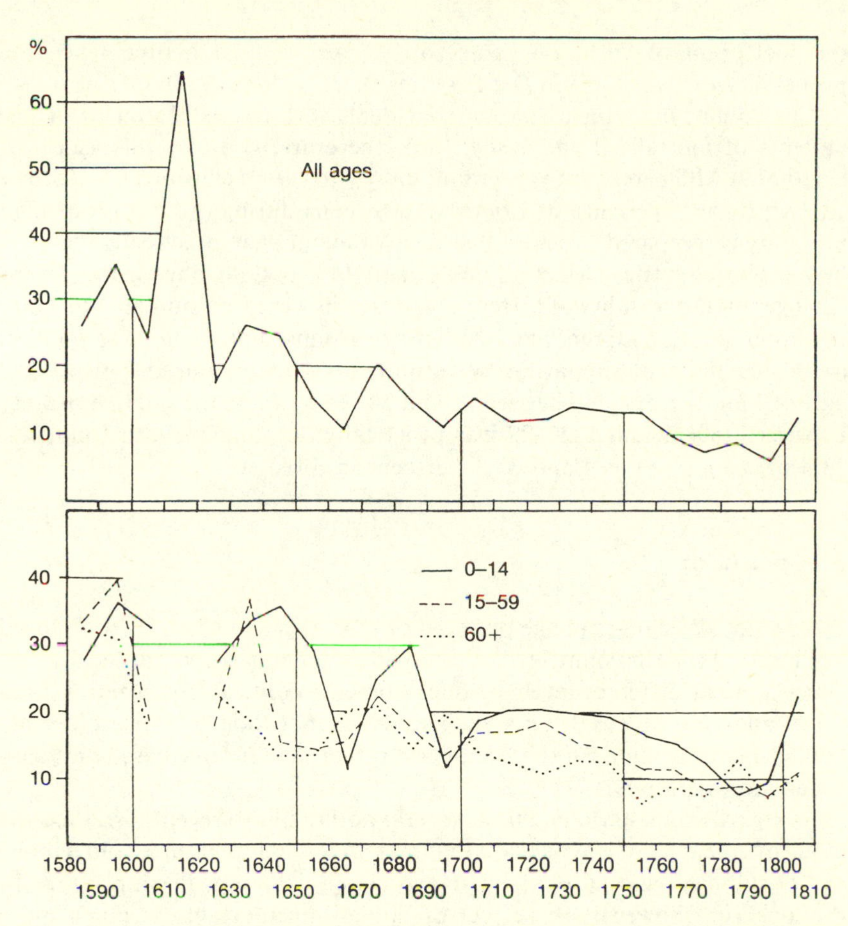

Fig. 2.4 Reductions in the amplitude of mortality cycles as measured by coefficient of variation

Source: A. Perrenoud, *La Population de Genève au début du dix-neuvième siècle: Étude démographique*, i (Geneva, 1979).

epidemics. Beginning with the eighteenth century, the contrasts become less pronounced, but the lags remain: variations in mortality disappear after 1750 among those aged 60 and over, after 1770 for those aged 15–59, and between 1780 and 1789 for those aged 14 or younger. And at all ages there was a recrudescence of cyclical mortality between 1800 and 1809.

However, once again a decline in variability does not necessarily imply a decline in the level of mortality. The value of ${}_{10}q_0$ was nearly the same between 1760 and 1769, as between 1780 and 1789, (0.378 compared with 0.373), but the variations were twice as large in the former period as in the latter (15 per cent and 7.8 per cent respectively), and between 1730 and 1739, the coefficient of variation came to 19.8 per cent at a time when the probability of dying within the first ten years of life was 0.361.

This volume contains a chapter that deals with the development of age patterns of mortality[43] and I shall not, therefore, consider this aspect at length, but will merely draw attention briefly to the conclusions of a former study.[44] If the experience of France and Sweden during this period of high mortality is compared, we note that developments were practically identical in the two countries. Mortality began to fall in both during the 1790s. Changes in the mortality of different age groups were very similar. Mortality fell faster among children than in other age groups, and the fall was smaller, the higher the age. Similarities were particularly pronounced between the ages of 1 and 4 years, and between 5 and 14 years, where the fall in mortality between 1760–69 and 1820–29 was practically the same in both countries: 33.4 per cent in France and 33.1 per cent in Sweden.

6. Conclusion

If the study of changes in age patterns of mortality shows such pronounced similarities between countries that are widely separated geographically and which were at different levels of development, political organization, and social and cultural characteristics, should we not look for an ecological-biological explanation for these changes, rather than for one based on socio-economic conditions?

As regards short-term changes, several authors have recently studied the effect of climate, and have shown that extremes of temperature, cold winters or hot summers and autumns were associated with rises in mortality.[45] In the long run, however, the effect of climate on mortality is much more difficult to measure. The relationship between climate and harvests is clear, but the demographic effects of famines, scarcities, or of nutritional deficiencies are much more difficult to assess. As Galloway has written: 'Climatic change can affect vital rates in two ways: through its influence on food supply *per capita*, and through direct biometeorological effects of deteriorating climate'.[46]

The arguments invariably relate to the negative effects of a cooler climate, but would it not be preferable to reverse the causal chain? By relating demographic changes too exclusively to changes in agriculture and short-term climate it has been overlooked that periods of mortality decline correspond to periods during which the climate became cooler (curiously these periods

[43] J. Vallin, Ch. 3, in this vol.

[44] Perrenoud, op. cit. in n. 2.

[45] For a synthesis of recent work and a comparison on the European scale, see Galloway, op. cit. in n. 9.

[46] Galloway, op. cit. in n. 11, p. 20.

were concentrated at the turns of centuries) and historians have shown that 'every hundred years, there were hard winters during the nineties of each century' (the decades 1490–99, 1590–99, 1690–99, 1790–99, and 1890–99).[47] The trend of mortality in England clearly illustrates this change of view. Between 1560 and 1609 all the climatic indicators point to a period of cooler weather, and life expectancies increased to a level which was not achieved again until the nineteenth century. Conversely, the progressive warming after 1650 which became more pronounced between 1676 and 1686, when there was much heat and drought,[48] coincided with a continuous rise in mortality which reduced life expectancy below 30 years, the secular minimum. Moreover, during the very bad years at the end of the seventeenth and the beginning of the eighteenth centuries, which through their effects on harvests might have been expected to lead to rising mortality, mortality levels in fact declined, and not only in England. The comparison can be continued until the eighteenth century, which, though cooler as a whole, contained two periods when the climate became warmer: 1718–37 and 1773–83. These years were renowned throughout Europe for their summer temperatures, and during both these periods mortality increased. There followed a new cooling, comparable to the little ice age of the end of the seventeenth century, which affected the first third of the nineteenth century and which again led to an increase in life expectancy.

Scholars who were blinded by the crises in agriculture have not given sufficient attention to 'normal' mortality and to the independent alternation of good and bad periods, to the waxing and waning of epidemics, and to fluctuations which cannot always be explained in agricultural or political terms. Nor has sufficient weight been given to the equilibrium between parasite and host during periods when the climate became cooler or warmer, nor to variations in the amount of rainfall or in droughts. For, though cooler periods may have a deleterious effect on harvests, they were also unfavourable to the development of microbes and their vectors, insect and others, which flourish during warmer periods.

It is possible that climate may after all have been an important factor in infant mortality which could explain differences in development between north-eastern and southern Europe,[49] or between plains and mountainous regions. However, for the time being at least, we lack data at the national level and comparisons are only possible in the nineteenth century, but a history of mortality can only be written from a long-term perspective.

[47] E. R. Ladurie, *Histoire du climat depuis l'an mil* (Paris, 1983), vol. ii, p. 129.

[48] Ibid. vol. i, p. 72.

[49] M. Breschi and M. Livi Bacci, 'Saison et climat comme contrainte de la survie des enfants: L'Expérience italienne au XIVᵉ siècle', *Population*, 41 (1986), pp. 9–35; J. Landers, and A. Mouzas, 'Burial Seasonality and Causes of Death in London 1670–1819', *Population Studies*, 42(1) (1988), pp. 59–83; V. Perez-Moreda and D. S. Reher, 'Demographic Mechanisms and Long Term Swings in Population in Europe 1200–1850', in IUSSP, *International Population Conference, Florence, 1985*, iv (Liège, 1985), pp. 313–37.

3 Mortality in Europe from 1720 to 1914
Long-Term Trends and Changes in Patterns by Age and Sex

JACQUES VALLIN *Institut National d'Études Démographiques, Paris*

On the eve of the First World War the demographic transition in Europe was far from complete and, in particular, the decline in mortality had a long way to go: indeed, it had hardly begun. However, though we are well aware of what has happened since that time, our knowledge of earlier developments is often vague, sometimes confused, and always incomplete. Regular reliable statistics on mortality only became available in Europe towards the end of the nineteenth century. Social scientists know that there is often a time-lag between the appearance of a particular phenomenon and the construction of instruments designed to measure it. In spite of the long history of burial registers this is also true of mortality, whose course altered radically between the eighteenth and nineteenth centuries. It is easily understandable that the historical demographers responsible for the organization of this volume are interested in an analysis of mortality over this extended period, when the conditions for demographic transition first appeared. But I would ask for sympathy for the difficulties faced by a demographer (who is not a historian) and who has been asked to provide a synthetic view based on very diverse material within a relatively short space, and for his frustration at having to omit the most recent period in which the decline of mortality was most pronounced, and for which there exists an abundance of statistical information to document the transition.

At the national level, annual statistics based on registrations go back furthest in Finland, where they extend as far back as 1722.[1] Those for Denmark, Iceland, and Norway go back to 1735,[2] and for Sweden to 1736.[3] Except in these five Nordic countries, statistics do not go back

[1] H. Gille, 'The Demographic History of the Northern Countries in the Eighteenth Century', *Population Studies*, 3(1) (1949), pp. 3–65.

[2] Ibid. B. R. Mitchell, *European Historical Statistics 1750–1970* (London and New York, 1978); Statistisk Sentralbyra, *Historisk Statistikk 1968* (Oslo, 1969).

[3] Gille, op. cit. in n. 1; Statistika Centralbyrån, *Historisk Statistik för Sverige*, pt. i. *Befolkning: Andra upplagan 1720–1967* (Stockholm, 1969).

beyond the nineteenth century (France, 1801; Austria, 1820; Belgium 1830; England and Wales, 1839; Netherlands, 1840) and most of these series relate only to the situation during the second half, or even the end, of that century. Moreover, in many instances only the total number of deaths is available. Information relating to age and sex patterns for that period is even scarcer.

It is only through the reconstitution studies undertaken by historical demographers with such remarkable success in recent decades that it is possible to complete the picture given by administrative sources. Unfortunately, most of these studies relate to very limited geographical areas.[4] There are only two countries for which reconstitution at a national level has proved possible—France as a result of work by Henry,[5] based on a nationally representative sample of parish registers for the period 1740–1829, and England, where Wrigley and Schofield have used techniques of retrospective projection to trace the demographic history of their country between 1541 and 1871.[6]

These two reconstitutions, together with the available official national statistics form the basis for this outline of the development of European mortality during the eighteenth and nineteenth centuries.

1. The First Stages of Mortality Decline in Europe

In Fig. 3.1 we trace the development of crude death rates in the five countries for which the longest series are available, and which provide information for an appreciable part of the eighteenth century: France and England on one hand, and Finland, Norway, and Sweden on the other.

The figures for France for the period 1740–1829 are taken from the study by Louis Henry[7] as adjusted by Jean-Noël Biraben.[8] For the years 1830–1920, the rates have been calculated directly from civil registration statistics.[9] The period 1801–29 is covered by both these series and no significant differences have been found between them. For England, the

[4] Several studies for Italy during the 18th and 19th cents. have been reviewed by Del Panta and Livi Bacci. L. Del Panta and M. Livi Bacci, 'Le componenti naturali dell'evoluzione demografica nell'Italia del Settecento', in *La popolazione Italiana nel Settecento* (Bologna, 1979); L. Del Panta, *Evoluzione demografica e popolamento nell'Italia dell'Ottocento 1794–1914* (Bologna, 1984). But even at the level of different states which constituted Italy before 1860, much work remains to be done before long annual series of mortality rates can be obtained.

[5] *Démographie historique* (*Population*, 30, special issue (1975)).

[6] E. A. Wrigley and R. S. Schofield, *The Population History of England 1541–1871* (London, 1981).

[7] See Y. Blayo, 'Mouvement naturel de la population française de 1740 à 1829', *Démographie historique* (*Population*, 30, special issue (1975)), pp. 15–64.

[8] Institut national d'études démographiques, *Sixième rapport sur la situation démographique de la France* (Paris, 1977), prepared by Jean-Noël Biraben.

[9] INSEE, *Annuaire démographique de la France: Résumé rétrospectif 1966* (Paris, 1966).

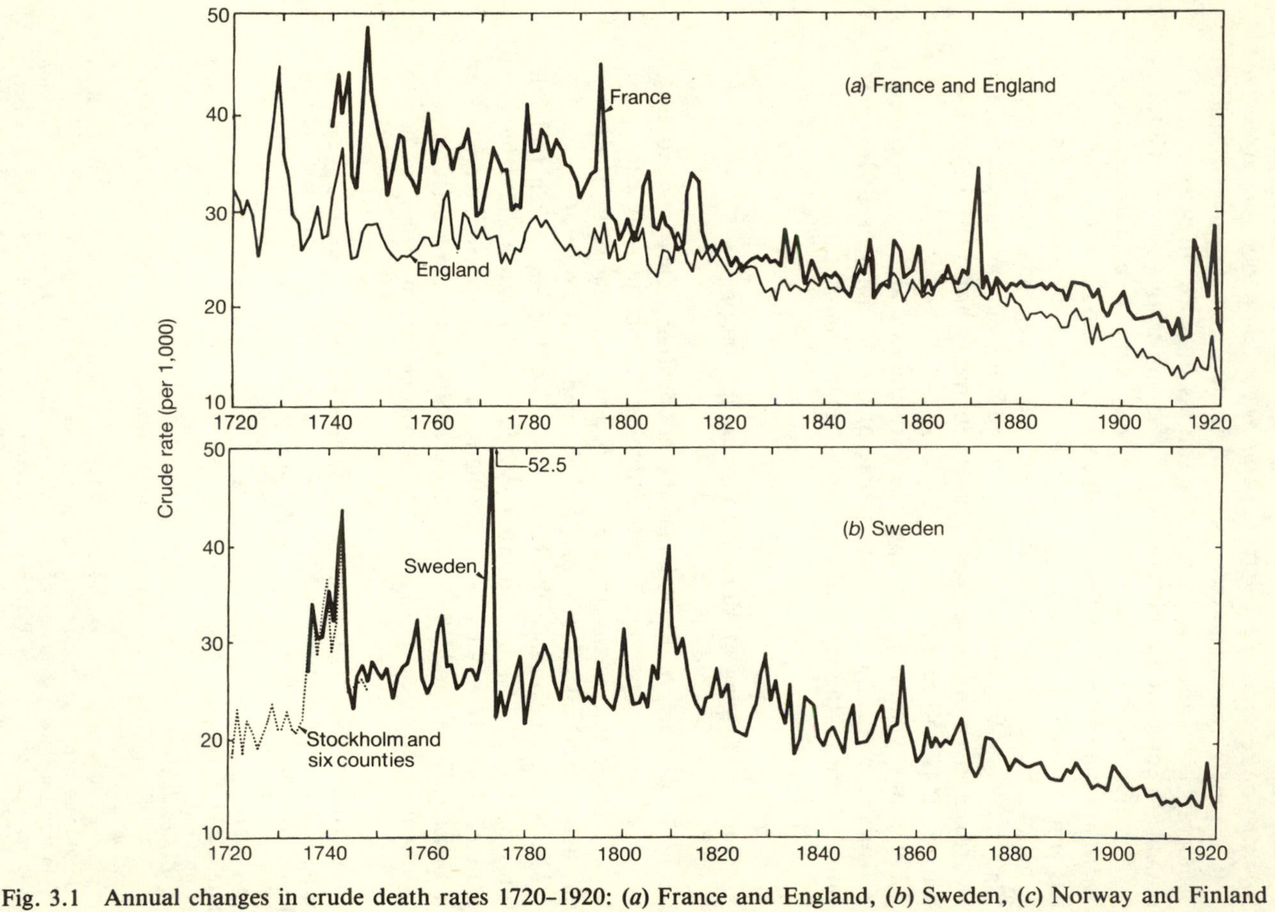

Fig. 3.1 Annual changes in crude death rates 1720–1920: (*a*) France and England, (*b*) Sweden, (*c*) Norway and Finland

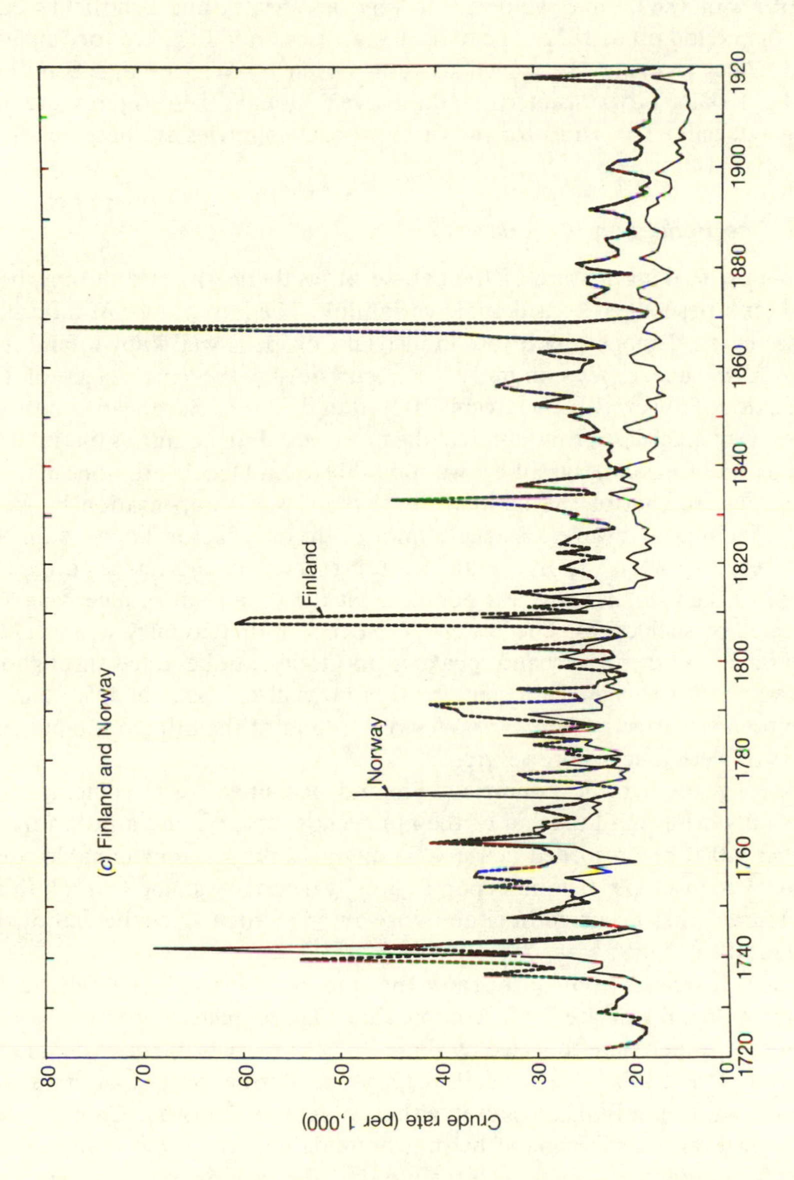
(c) Finland and Norway
Finland
Norway
Crude rate (per 1,000)
80
70
60
50
40
30
20
10
1720
1740
1760
1780
1800
1820
1840
1860
1880
1900
1920

data for 1720–1871 are those given by Wrigley and Schofield[10] and for 1872–1920 are official statistics.[11] Although these latter figures go back as far as 1839, it is known that death registration in England was incomplete until about 1860,[12] and we prefer to rely on Wrigley and Schofield's data for the period up to 1872. The official statistics after 1872 are for England and Wales, but may be joined to those given by Wrigley and Schofield without danger of misinterpretation, even though their figures are for England only. The series for the three Nordic countries are based entirely on official data.

1.1 The Reduction of Variability

The most striking feature of the course of crude death rates during these two centuries is their considerable variability. The importance of mortality crises in the demography of pre-industrial Europe is well known, and it is clear that such crises continued to occur during the first stages of the transition. However, their effects differed in different European countries. They were much less pronounced in the more populous countries (in this case France and England), because it was possible to find local variations in these countries, so that at the national level there was compensation between different areas. However, chance cannot be the only factor that explains the difference between the five countries represented in the figure. England, though much smaller and less populous at the time than France, was less affected by such crises. The last crisis to occur in that country was in 1729. In France, on the other hand, peaks in mortality can be noted throughout the whole of the eighteenth century; there was also a peak in 1871 and, in addition, the effects of the First World War and of the influenza pandemic of 1918 were much more severe.

Among the Nordic countries, Finland remained very vulnerable to mortality crises until the end of the nineteenth century, and a peak rate of 78 per 1,000 was recorded in 1868. Today it is almost unimaginable for a country to lose 8 per cent of its population by death in a single year. Nothing comparable has occurred in either Norway or Sweden since the end of the eighteenth century.

Such differences obviously raise the question whether the statistics in different countries are truly comparable. Those relating to the Nordic countries, which were collected by similar methods are probably comparable *inter se*. It is doubtful that death registration during periods of crisis was more complete in Finland than in either Sweden or Norway. Comparisons between France and England before the middle of the nineteenth century are more dubious. It is not impossible that the technique of retrospective

[10] Wrigley and Schofield, op. cit. in n. 6.

[11] *Statistical Abstract of the United Kingdom* (London).

[12] Mitchell, op. cit. in n. 2.

projection used by Wrigley and Schofield may have underestimated the true variability, whereas the methods used by Henry, based on a respresentative sample of parish registers may have exaggerated them. However, even allowing for these doubts, it would seem that the course of mortality has been very different in the five countries considered. Climatic differences may have played an important part; from this point of view a comparison between Norway and Finland is particularly revealing. However, it is also of interest to consider these differences within a social and economic context.

Whilst the size of fluctuations in annual death rates is impressive, the reduction of these fluctuations towards the end of our period – one might almost say their elimination – is hardly less so. But elimination is probably too strong a term to use. Even if the losses caused by the First World War were to be left out of account, it is impossible to ignore the effects of the pandemic of Spanish influenza in 1918. However, in each of the five countries considered, the mean size of fluctuations between 1880 and 1913 was lower than that found in any other consecutive 30-year period. When looked at in this way, the effect of the influenza pandemic of 1918 may be regarded as almost a belated epidemiological accident. With the benefit of hindsight we can say that it constituted the last major mortality crisis in peacetime Europe, and that it was almost an anachronism. The end of the nineteenth century, and more particularly the 1880s, appear to mark the beginning of a new mortality regime, in which chance factors no longer play as large a part as they did previously.

1.2 Phases of Progress and Phases of Stagnation

Clearly, one of the phases of the public-health transition (the elimination of major mortality crises) has occurred during our period. This is not, however, true of the second most important aspect of the transition – the secular decline of mortality. The reduction and later elimination of large annual fluctuations in mortality will in itself have led to a reduction in the level of mortality. Fluctuations in mortality may be regarded as 'crises' which interrupt the 'normal' regime of mortality; they do not indicate a swing between 'good' and 'bad' years. By removing crisis years from consideration, the mean level of mortality is automatically lowered and annual death rates are kept nearer to 'normal' levels.

The elimination of crisis years coincided with a change in 'normal' mortality levels. Although, in each of the five countries the secular trend of mortality was declining throughout the centuries studied, it emerged at different times in different countries, and the rate of decline varied. A comparison between the experience of England and France is particularly instructive (Fig. 3.1(*a*)). In France, there is evidence of a clear decline in the crude death rate between 1750 and 1845 (we have no data for earlier years), but during the following 40 years the death rate did not change appreciably and only resumed its decline towards the end of the 1880s. In England, on the other hand, to judge by the information in Fig. 3.1(*a*), 'normal' mortality appears to have been constant throughout the eighteenth century until the 1820s when there followed a brief period of decline which lasted for about ten years and which was succeeded by a renewed period of near-constancy that lasted until the 1870s. After that date, however, decline became rapid and continuous.

The most surprising feature of this comparison, however, is the lower mortality which England seems to have enjoyed, when compared with France, at the beginning of the period. Between 1740 and 1749 the French crude death rate was of the order of 32 to 35 per 1,000, and a peak value of 49 was reached in 1747. In England, the corresponding level was only about 25 to 28 per 1,000, and a peak value of 37 was reached in 1742. During the following half-century, health standards improved in France but not in England, so that by the end of the second decade of the nineteenth century, mortality levels in the two countries were similar. Thereafter, the two curves are very similar, save for one or two crisis years, until about 1875, when mortality in England fell both earlier and more rapidly than in France towards the end of the nineteenth century and gave the former a decisive advantage. Whilst it is indisputable that on the eve of the twentieth century mortality in England was lower than in France, the question remains whether the advantage supposedly enjoyed by England at the beginning of the period was real. If it was, either death rates of the order of 40 per 1,000 had never been experienced in England, or there must have been an earlier first stage in the health transition in that country. Wrigley and Schofield's results suggest that the first explanation is true, because, according to them, crude death rates in England have oscillated around a mean value that was lower than 30 per 1,000 ever since 1541. It is possible that climatic factors may have favoured England during that period. Temperate, cool countries are less exposed than those with a warmer climate to the spread of some infectious diseases, particularly diseases of the digestive system. This may have an important effect on infant mortality, but could also influence the mortality of adults.

However, we might also ask whether it is really likely that mortality in France was higher than in England during the middle of the eighteenth century. Louis Henry and Didier Blanchet have pointed to two important reasons that suggest why deaths in England may have been underestimated.[13] First, the under-registration of burials of very young children was taken into account in the French estimate, but seems to have been neglected in the retrospective projection for England. In the second place,

[13] L. Henry and L.D. Blanchet, 'La Population de l'Angleterre de 1541 à 1871', *Population*, 38(4–5) (1983), pp. 781–826.

the high level of emigration from England during the seventeenth and eighteenth centuries would automatically have led to an underestimation of adult deaths. It is, in fact, likely that an important part of the difference between mortality in England and in France was apparent rather than real, that mortality may have declined in both countries from the middle of the eighteenth century, and that mortality levels were nearly the same in both countries during the nineteenth century, when the registration of deaths had become more complete.

Under-registration of the deaths of very young children, which has been noted in England, may also have played a part in the mortality estimates for the three Nordic countries shown in Fig. 3.1 at the beginning of our period. It is possible that mortality in those countries may have been somewhat higher at the beginning of the eighteenth century, and the decline in mortality larger. It is, however, clear that throughout the nineteenth century the fall in mortality in both Norway and Sweden was more regular than in either England or France, where there was a period of stagnation. This period of stagnation which occurred later in France than in England (1845–90 compared with 1830–75) seems to have coincided with the years of greatest social hardship caused by industrialization under a capitalist system.

1.3 Some Very Different Histories

Limiting ourselves to five countries only might, of course, have resulted in very biased views about the course of mortality in Europe during the period studied. But, in spite of the differences which we have outlined above, the history of four of these five countries (leaving Finland out of account for the time being) is not dissimilar. The common feature is a relatively early start of the decline in mortality. Although we have no comparable long series for other countries, it would seem that almost everywhere else, the decline began later. This appears to have been true, at least for the five additional countries, for which we have figures that relate to the second half of the nineteenth century (see Fig. 3.2).

Except in the Netherlands, where the course of mortality during this period was very similar to that in England, levels appear to have been higher in the four remaining countries. In Germany and Italy the decline seems hardly to have begun by the middle of the nineteenth century; in Russia it began only towards the end of the 1890s, and Spain was in an intermediate position. Partial data for Italy for the period before political unification indicate that crude death rates during the eighteenth and the beginning of the nineteenth century were of the order of 35 to 40 per 1,000.[14] However, by the end of the nineteenth century mortality had begun to decline

[14] Del Panta, op. cit. in n. 4.

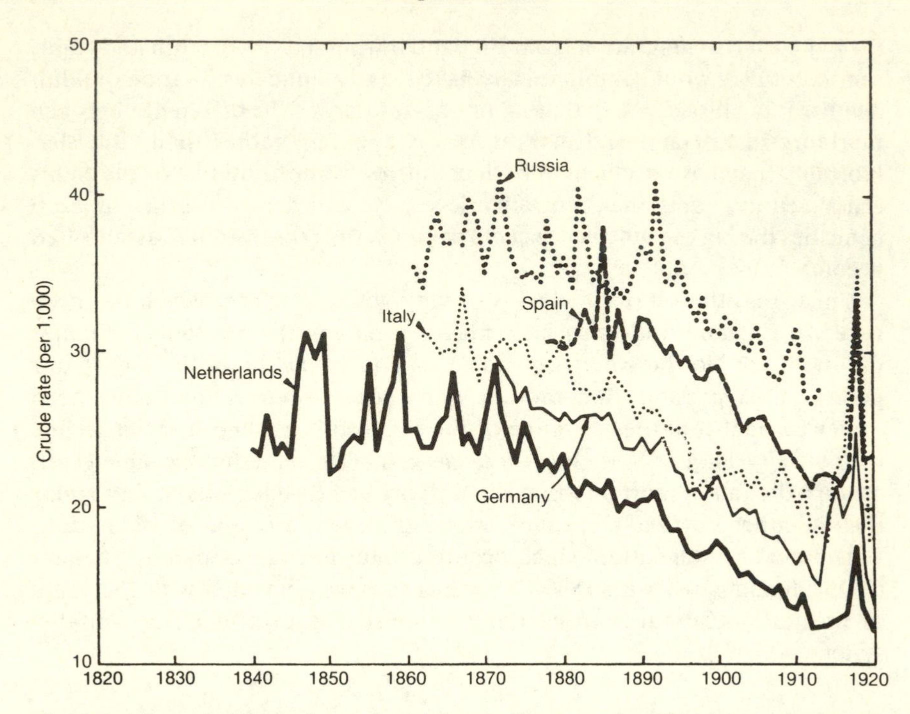

Fig. 3.2 Annual changes in crude death rates between the mid-nineteenth century and 1920 in five European countries

throughout Europe, though the rate of decline was no faster in countries in which the fall started later than in those in which it had begun earlier, and differences which had become apparent during the middle of the nineteenth century persisted and (in a relative sense) even increased on the eve of the First World War.

1.4 Striking a Balance over Two Centuries

We return to the early starters. If we consider the crude death rate (an index studied by historical demographers because, together with the crude birth rate, its level determines the rate of natural growth), the two centuries that we are looking at seem to have been decisive. For instance, in France average death rates for successive quinquenniums fell from 40.2 per 1,000 in 1740–44 to 15.4 in 1909–13. By 1980–84 the rate was 10.1 per 1,000. The bulk of the decline – more than 80 per cent – had thus been achieved by the end of the First World War.

However, it would not be right to judge changes in the public's health during these two centuries from these figures. During the twentieth century, the decline in the crude death rate was slowed down by the progressive ageing of the population. It would also be wrong to conclude that the health transition was complete, because crude death rates had remained stationary at a level of about 10 per 1,000. Life expectancies at birth continued to increase, and there is no reason to believe that this increase will not continue in the future.

Between 1740–45 and 1909–13 expectation of life at birth in France rose from 24.7 to 50.4 years (see Fig. 3.3), i.e. by 25.7 years. In 1983–85 the figure was 74.7 years, an additional gain of 24.3 years. In other words, only half the increase in life expectancy since 1740–45 occurred during the eighteenth and nineteenth centuries, the remainder occurred during the 70 years since the First World War. This takes no account of possible future gains. If life expectancy at birth were to approach more and more closely to the human life-span of, say, 100 years, this change would herald a third stage of the mortality transition which could be as important as the two previous stages have been.

Even in Sweden and Norway, where mortality was lower than in France on the eve of the First World War (Fig. 3.3), life expectancy at birth at that time was only about 58 years, compared with the present value of nearly 77 years. Moreover, we are dealing here with the early starters. Life expectancies for the bulk of the population of Europe at the end of the two centuries that we have considered were still considerably lower (Table 3.1).

Life expectancy at birth at the beginning of the 20th century was highest

Table 3.1 Life expectancy at birth on the eve of the First World War in European countries for which life tables are available

Country	Period	e_0
Denmark	1911–15	57.7
Norway	1911–21	57.2
Sweden	1911–20	57.0
Netherlands	1910–20	56.1
Ireland	1910–12	53.8
England and Wales	1910–11	53.5
Switzerland	1910–11	52.3
France	1908–13	50.4
German Empire	1910–11	49.0
Italy	1910–12	46.9
Finland	1911–20	46.3
Spain	1910	41.7
Bohemia, Moravia, Silesia	1889–1902	40.3
Bulgaria	1899–1902	40.2
Austria	1900–01	40.1
Hungary	1900–01	37.5

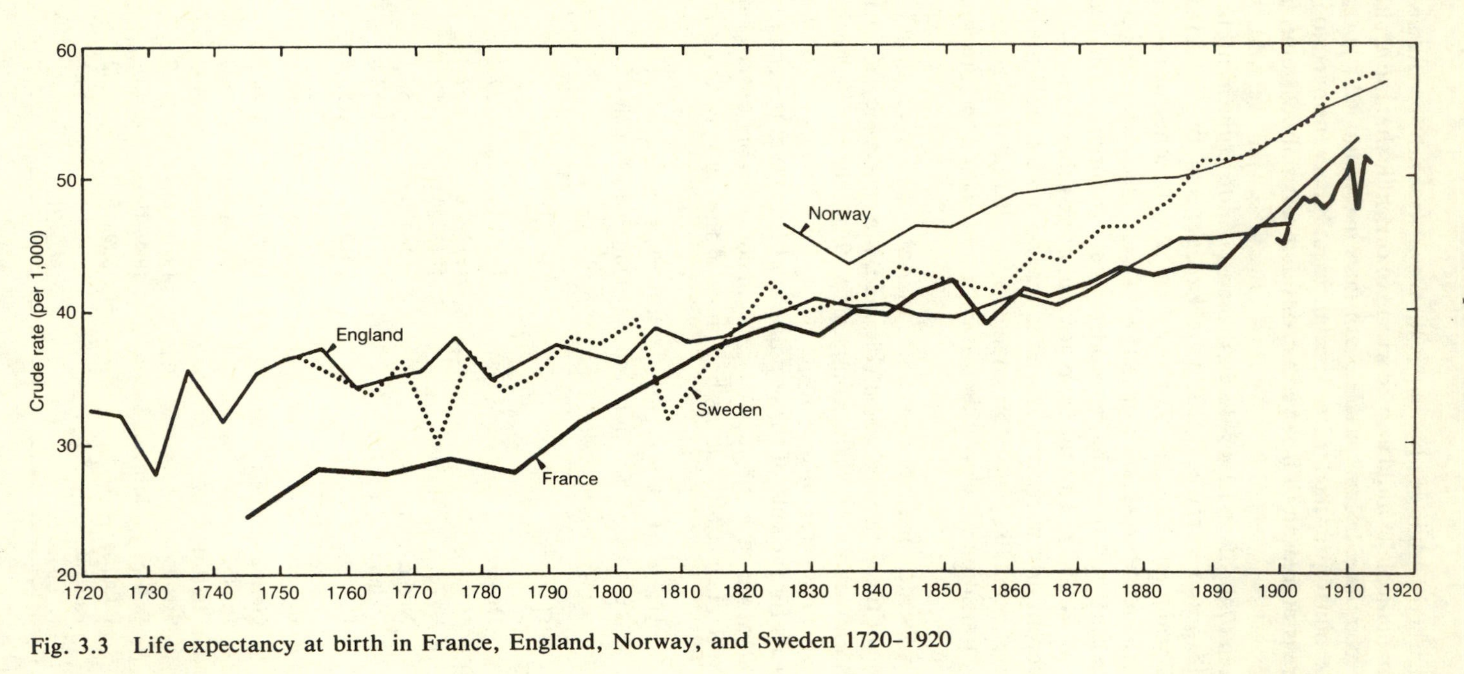

Fig. 3.3 Life expectancy at birth in France, England, Norway, and Sweden 1720–1920

in countries with the most advanced statistical systems. The list given in the first part of Table 3.1 which shows the countries in which life expectancy at birth exceeded 50 years on the eve of the First World War is reasonably complete. This is not true of the second part of the table which contains a list of countries in which life expectancies fell short of 50 years and for which the necessary information is available. In this group we find Italy, the German Empire, Spain, and some of the most important parts of the Austro-Hungarian monarchy. The difference between the country with the highest expectation of life (Denmark: 57.7 years) and that with the lowest (Hungary: 37.5 years) is of the order of 20 years, nearly as large as the total gain realized by the early starters over two centuries. We must also draw attention to the absence of Russia from the countries listed in Table 3.1. As the infant mortality rate in that country was of the order of 250 per 1,000 in about 1910, it is probable that life expectancy at birth was less than 30 years. These figures show the very large variability of the situation in Europe towards the end of the first stage of the health transition, as well as the importance of developments which occurred later.

It is, therefore, of some interest to investigate changes in the sex and age patterns of mortality during the first stage of the transition, and particularly among the early starters.

2. Changes in the Sex and Age Pattern of Mortality

2.1 The Course of Infant Mortality

In pre-industrial Europe mortality during the early stages of life was very high, and had a considerable effect on life expectancy at birth. Thus, in France in 1740–44, the chance of dying within the first five years of life was nearly one-half (0.474). If this mortality could have been eliminated by the touch of a magic wand, life expectancy at birth would immediately have increased by 21 years from 24.2 to 45.7 years. The principal feature of the first stage of the mortality transition, therefore, was the reduction in mortality at early stages of life.

In Fig. 3.4 we illustrate the information available on the course of infant mortality in different European countries between 1720 and 1920.

Only for Sweden do we possess a long annual time series, but the infant mortality rates for England and France can be completed with decennial or quinquennial figures taken from the works of the historical demographers that we have cited earlier. Changes are similar to those that we have traced in the crude death rates, though there are some slight differences. There is little value in stressing again the underestimation of infant mortality in England (and possibly also in Sweden) at the beginning of the eighteenth century. It is more interesting that between 1845 and 1890 when the crude

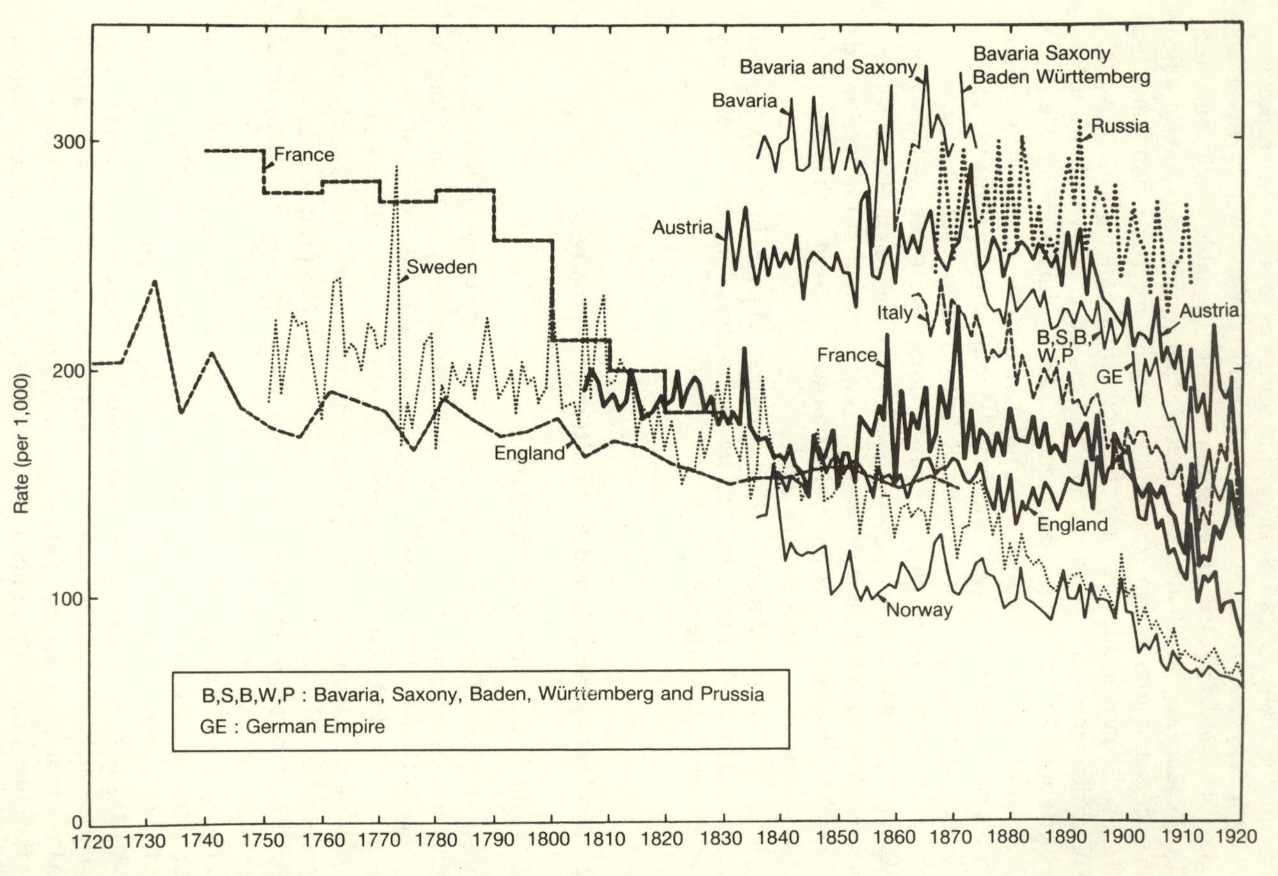

Fig. 3.4 Annual changes in infant mortality 1720–1920 in different European countries

death rate in France remained stationary, the curve that describes infant mortality was dome-shaped. Infant mortality increased considerably between 1850 and 1870 and did not resume its decline until 1895. It is true that the most severe period of industrialization in France occurred during the period of the Second Empire, and led to a deterioration in the health conditions of an increasing proportion of young children, namely those belonging to the industrial working class. Long hours of work and the need for young mothers to work outside their homes, forced them to give out their children to be nursed, often in very poor conditions.

In England, the movement of infant mortality until 1875 was almost exactly the same as that of the crude death rate, which had remained on a plateau since 1830. However, the gains that were made between 1875 and 1885 were cancelled by an equivalent increase between 1885 and 1900, and it was only after that date (five years later than in France) that a real new decline occurred. More clearly than the crude death rate, the course of infant mortality suggests that the first stage of the public-health transition was limited to the end of the eighteenth and the beginnings of the nineteenth centuries. From then, we would have to wait until the end of the nineteenth century to discern the great wave of mortality decline which was to continue throughout the twentieth. The First World War did not mark the limit of a period of transition, and the cut-off points that have been chosen are, to some extent, arbitrary.

It should also be noted that the division of the transition into two distinct stages, which was typical of England and France (and possibly also of Norway, though data for that country are lacking) did not apply to Sweden. In that country, infant mortality fell continuously, except for year-to-year fluctuations, from the middle of the eighteenth century onwards, and there was no change during the period of the First World War.

Fig. 3.4 complements the information shown in Figs. 3.1 and 3.2 which illustrate the variability of the situation in different countries. In about 1850, when the first stage of the decline was beginning in England and France, infant mortality in these two countries and in Sweden was only about 150 per 1,000, whilst it amounted to 300 per 1,000 in Bavaria, the only state in Germany for which information is available, and in which the transition did not appear even to have begun. It was a little lower in Austria, but remained at a level of about 250 per 1,000 from the beginning of the statistical era until about 1895. If there had, indeed, been an earlier first stage of transition in that country, the decline can only have been small, and must, in any case, have been followed by a long period of stability throughout the nineteenth century, just as in England and France. The situation in Russia seems to have been intermediate between that of Bavaria and Austria, but it is perfectly possible that the registration of infant deaths there was less complete during the first decades of the statistical era (1870s and 1880s).

The situation in Italy is of some interest. Although statistics only began to be collected in 1863, there is reason to believe that infant mortality rates were roughly the same as in Austria during the first half of the nineteenth century.[15] The rate declined continuously and rapidly from 1863 onwards and reached the same level as in England and France by about 1900. However, a gap opened again after that date, particularly between infant mortality rates in England and Italy, as progress in England was more rapid. Unlike the situation in other European countries, there was no check to the decline of the infant mortality rate in Italy during the second half of the nineteenth century.

Differences between infant mortality rates in different European countries were probably largest around 1850. By that time important progress had already been achieved in some countries (Norway, Sweden, England, and France), whereas in others there had been practically none (Bavaria, Russia), or very little (Austria, Italy). Recorded rates ranged between 100 per 1,000 in Denmark to 300 in Bavaria, and possibly in Russia. On the eve of the First World War, the decline had begun everywhere, except in Russia, and the range (if Russia is again excluded) was from 70 per 1,000 in Norway and Sweden to 140 in Germany and 180 in Austria.

2.2 Inequalities in the Decline of Mortality at Different Ages

Although in the countries in which it started early, infant mortality had fallen considerably during the 200 years studied, the largest falls in the risks of dying were not found during the first year of life. Data that make it possible to study the course of mortality in different age groups since the eighteenth century are hard to find and are of very different kinds. Only for Sweden and France is reliable information available at the national level for the whole of this period. The reconstitution studies in England rely overmuch on model tables and cannot be considered as giving a true picture. We shall, therefore, take France as an example.

In Fig. 3.5 we show five-year probabilities of dying for different age groups for five periods separated by approximately 40 years: 1740–49, 1780–89, 1820–29,[16] 1877–81,[17] and 1913.[18] For comparison we also show a recent life table, that for 1983–85.[19]

Between 1740–49 and 1913 mortality fell considerably at all ages. However, the achievements between 1913 and the present day are even more

[15] Del Panta put them between 0.245 and 0.319 in different regions during the Napoleonic period, and between 0.215 and 0.293 during the second quarter of the 19th cent.: Del Panta, op. cit. in n. 4.

[16] Blayo, op. cit. in n. 7.

[17] INSEE, op. cit. in n. 9.

[18] J. Vallin, *Tables de mortalité du moment et par génération 1899*–1981: Mise à jour provisoire des tables annexes du cahier 63. (3 vols., Paris, 1984).

[19] B. Faur and Y. Court, *La Situation démographique en 1985: Mouvement de population* (INSEE, Paris, 1987).

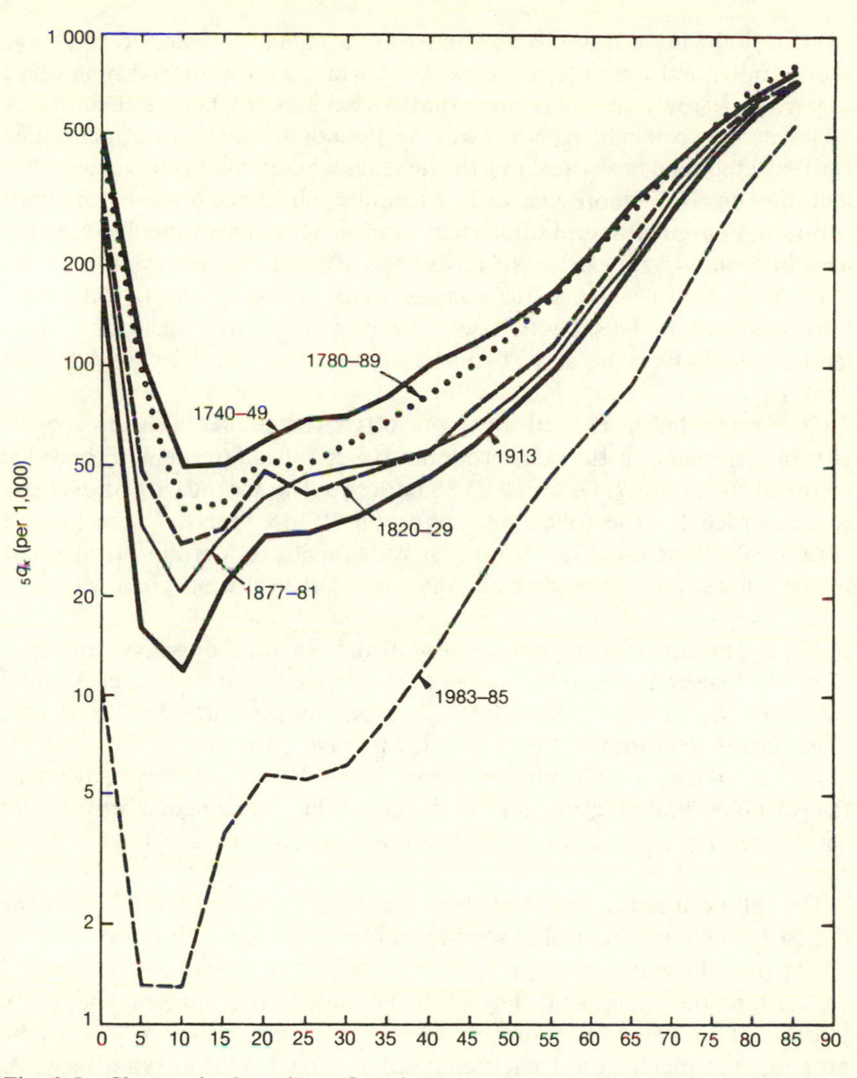

Fig. 3.5 Changes in the values of $_5q_x$ in France between 1740–1749 and 1913: both sexes

impressive, and this should be borne in mind when the relative importance of the period for the demographic transition as a whole is considered.

By looking at the tables for periods between 1740–49 and 1913, it is possible to trace the two main stages which have already been described earlier. Between 1740–49 and 1780–89 and further on to 1820–29, there are falls at all ages, even though they differ in size in different age groups. The same is true for the period 1877–81 to 1913. However, between 1820–29 and

1877–81, falls in mortality were comparatively small, applied to some age groups only, and were often neutralized by increases in mortality in other age groups. However, the periods that we have used when calculating the tables do not coincide exactly with the periods of stagnation mentioned earlier. If they had been the same, the declines would have been even smaller, and the increases more marked. Mortality appears to have remained constant, or even increased somewhat, at most ages. Only those between the ages of 5 and 15 appear not to have been affected by this trend.

For the period as a whole, the decrease in mortality was most pronounced in this age group. To show this, we have plotted the data in Fig. 3.6, with levels in 1740–49 taken as 100 and have shown these values for different periods.

The largest fall in the risk of dying was recorded between the ages of five and ten years. In 1913 this probability was only 15 per cent of the value recorded for 1740–49, i.e. a fall of 85 per cent. The second-largest decrease was recorded for the following age group (10–15 years), where the fall since 1740–49 exceeded 75 per cent. It was, therefore, during this phase of life, when risks of dying were already low, that health progress was most pronounced.

The age group 0–5 years only comes third, with a fall of 66 per cent since 1740–49. However, this lower rate of decline applies to a much higher initial value, and the effect of this fall on life expectancy at birth was, therefore, much larger than that in the two following age groups.

Between the ages of 20 and 55, mortality in 1913 was approximately half that of 1740–49. At higher ages, the reduction becomes smaller and smaller with increasing age, and amounted to less than 10 per cent at ages 80 and over.

The fall occurred in different stages. Between 1740–49 and 1780–89 the largest reductions in mortality were found among older children and young adults (i.e. those between the ages of 15 and 45). Between 1780–89 and 1820–29, on the other hand, they applied mainly to the youngest ages (0–10 years) and to those in mature middle age (35–65 years). As we know, progress was much slower between 1820–29 and 1877–81. What progress there was benefited the young (between the ages of 0 and 25), and those over the age of 45. During the decades that preceded the First World War, mortality fell at all ages below 45, and the fall tapered off at higher ages.

In Fig. 3.6 mortality levels in 1983–85 are also shown as a ratio of those experienced in 1740–49. Except at ages 5–10 and 10–15, mortality in 1913 was still considerably higher than at present. Progress after 1913 was particularly marked among young adults, but there was also progress during the first five years of life, and among the elderly. Thus, between the ages of 75 and 80, mortality only fell by 15 per cent over a period of two centuries, whereas in 1983–85 the probability of dying at that age was only 45 per cent of the value for 1740–49, i.e. a reduction of 55 per cent.

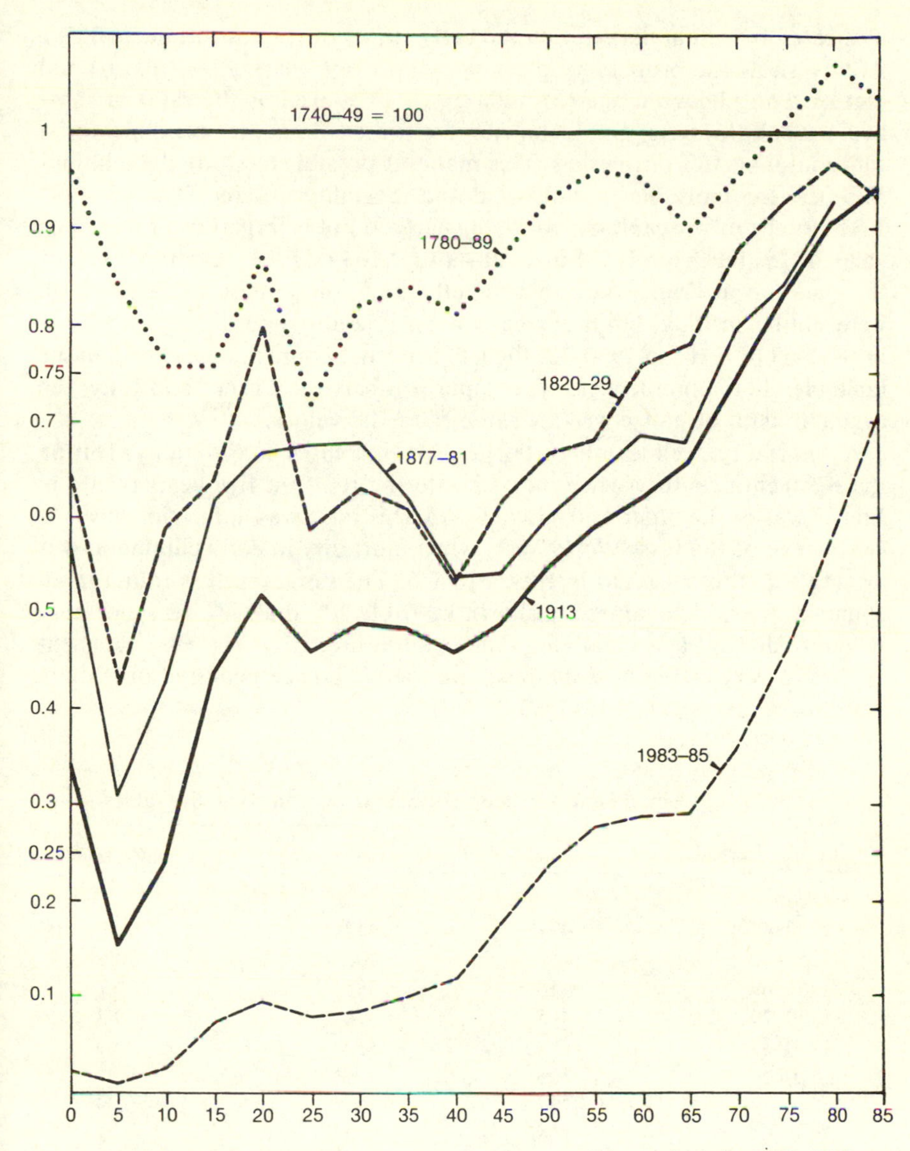

Fig. 3.6 Values of $_5q_x$ at different ages in France, taking values in 1740–1749 as 100: both sexes

2.3 Persistence of Differences in Patterns of Age-Specific Mortality

Following the publication of model life tables by Coale and Demeny, it has become customary to distinguish between different patterns of age-specific mortality (Models North, South, East, and West). The differences can be illustrated by actual data during the early stages of the transition. In Table 3.2, we show the probability of dying within five years of birth ($_5q_0$) and that of dying between ages 25 and 55 ($_{30}q_{25}$) as well as the ratio of these two probabilities for five countries for which data are available for a substantial part of our period. This makes it possible to study the relationship between mortality in childhood and mortality in later life.

The range of probabilities for dying early in life is largest in France. The value of $_5q_0$ fell from 0.474 in 1740–49 to 0.163 in 1913. A comparison of the situation in France with that in Italy is of some interest. Rates of fall were similar in Italy, but occurred at a considerably later date, from 0.467 in 1862–63 to 0.165 in 1930–32. Figures for other countries are shown in the table merely to complement the comparison between France and Italy; the available data do not cover the same range of values.

As mortality declines, the ratio $_{30}q_{25}/_5q_0$ increases considerably. During the eighteenth century when mortality during the first five years of life in France was of the order of 0.450 to 0.475, this ratio was approximately 0.9. On the eve of the First World War, when mortality in early childhood was around 0.2, the ratio had increased to 1.6. The same result is found in all countries for which values are shown in Table 3.2 in all of them mortality fell more during early childhood than in adult life. However, this statement applies to very different situations, and the difference persisted over time. An illustration is given in Fig. 3.7.

Table 3.2 Comparison of values of $_5q_0$ and $_{30}q_{25}$ in some life tables

Country Period	$_5q_0$ (1,000)	$_{30}q_{25}$ (1,000)	$_{30}q_{25}/_5q_0$
France:			
1740–49	474	457	0.96
1750–59	450	402	0.89
1760–69	458	398	0.87
1770–79	445	366	0.82
1780–89	451	402	0.89
1820–29	306	309	1.01
1840–59	277	301	1.09
1861–65	306	283	0.92
1877–81	270	298	1.10
1898–1903	209	277	1.32
1908–13	170	264	1.56
1913	163	255	1.55
England and Wales:			
1838–54	263	338	1.28
1871–80	252	338	1.34
1891–1900	234	290	1.24
1910–12	162	227	1.40

Country Period	$_5q_0$ (1,000)	$_{30}q_{25}$ (1,000)	$_{30}q_{25}/_5q_0$
Sweden:			
1757–63	344	377	1.10
1816–40	250	357	1.43
1841–55	232	324	1.40
1891–1900	161	224	1.39
1901–10	126	206	1.63
Norway:			
1846–50	200	282	1.41
1851–55	166	277	1.67
1856–60	168	259	1.54
1861–65	212	249	1.17
1866–70	181	266	1.47
1871–75	183	264	1.44
1876–80	169	251	1.43
1881–85	177	248	1.41
1886–90	171	245	1.44
1891–95	159	253	1.59
1896–1900	141	239	1.69
1901–05	118	231	1.97
1906–10	101	321	2.18
1911–15	94	214	2.27
Italy:			
1862–63	467	382	0.69
1881–82	365	302	0.83
1899–1902	286	247	0.86
1910–12	238	285	0.95
1930–32	165	177	1.07

[a] Calculations from data from Natale and Berbassola

Sources: *France* 1740–1829: Blayo, op. cit. in n 7; 1840–59: J. Bertillon, 'Des diverses manières de mesurer la durée de la vie humaine', *Journal de la société de statistique de Paris*, 3 (1866), pp. 45–64; 1861–65: Statistique de la France, *Mouvement de la population 1861–1865* (Strasbourg, 1870), pp. lxxxix–cxlvii; 1877–81: Statistique de la France, *Statistique annuelle 1881*; 1898–1903: Service de recensement, *Résultats statistiques du recensement général de la population effectué le 24 mars 1901*, iv (Paris); 1908–13: Statistique générale de la France, *Annuaire statistique 1921* (Paris); 1913: Vallin, op. cit. in n. 18. *England and Wales, and Sweden*: Statistique générale de la France, *Statistique internationale du mouvement de la population d'après les registres de l'état civil: Résumé rétrospectif depuis les origines jusqu'au 1905* (Paris, 1907).
Norway: J. K. Borgan, *Cohort Mortality in Norway 1846*–1980 (Oslo, 1983).
Italy 1862–63: Computed from data published by M. Natale, *La Mortalitá per causa nelle regione italiane: tavole per contemporanei 1965–66 e per generazioni 1790–1964*. (Rome, 1973); 1881–1932: Istituto centrale di statistica, *Annali di statistica* 6, viii (Rome, 1926), and ibid. 7, i (Rome, 1936).

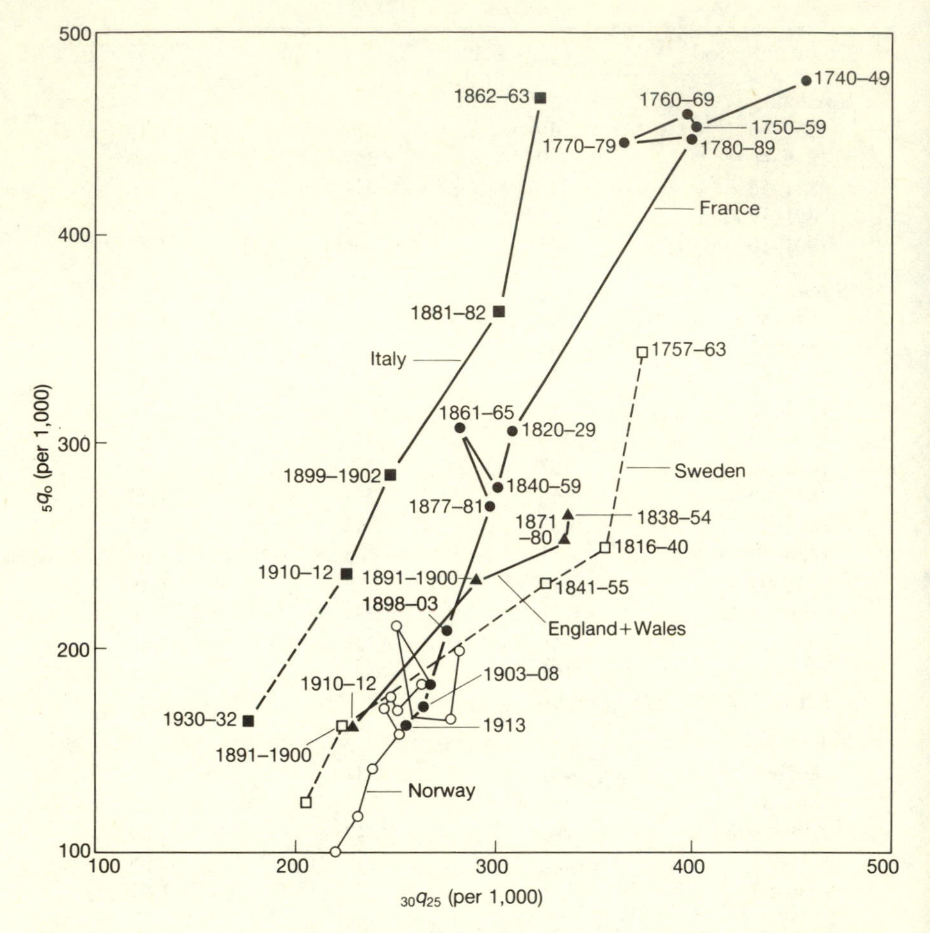

Fig. 3.7 Values of $_5q_0$ plotted against values of $_{30}q_{25}$ 1750–1914: England and Wales, France, Italy, Norway and Sweden

At comparable levels of child mortality, the mortality of adults was much higher in France than in Italy. To show the range of values, we have extended Fig. 3.7 and Table 3.2 to 1930–32, considerably later than the end of the period studied. The persistence of the difference between the two countries is noteworthy. The only exception found is the French table for 1861–65, which is closer to the pattern found for Italy. However, this period is exceptional in the development of French mortality as shown in Fig. 3.7. We have seen that infant mortality increased in France between 1850 and 1870, whereas mortality at other ages tended to remain constant. This has resulted in an approximation of the French pattern to that found in Italy, but this convergence was transitory; by 1877–81 the French life table had returned to the pattern of 1840–59, and mortality had resumed its previous trend.

In none of the other countries shown in Fig. 3.7 did mortality during the first five years of life reach a level as high as 0.450. If such levels have been experienced elsewhere, we are ignorant of the pattern of which they formed part. The highest values found for $_5q_0$ (0.340 in the Swedish tables for 1757–63, and between 0.250 and 0.260 for the earliest English tables, and that for Sweden for 1816–40) form part of a pattern of age-specific mortality which is even further removed from that of Italy than that of France. When mortality during the first five years of life was of the order of 0.250, the risk of dying between the ages of 25 and 55 was 0.230 in Italy, 0.290 in France, 0.340 in England and Wales, and as high as 0.360 in Sweden.

At lower levels of childhood mortality the patterns in England and Sweden are more like that in France. Together with the data for Norway, they form a reasonably consistent pattern, which is, however, very different from that found in Italy.

These three patterns (Italy, France, and England–Sweden–Norway) correspond to three different types of the health transition. In England, Norway, and Sweden the transition began fairly early, but except in crisis years, mortality in these countries—and childhood mortality in particular—had never been very high. In France, too, the transition began fairly early, but mortality at the onset of the transition—particularly infant mortality—was considerably higher than in the first group. Finally, in Italy, the transition only began in the middle of the nineteenth century, but the initial level of infant mortality had also been high in that country. Could this have been cause and effect? For example, could the Italian age pattern of mortality have been different because mortality began falling later in that country? It is also possible that progress in France and northern Europe applied to all age groups, but particularly to children, whereas in Italy it was at first confined to adults. However, it should be noted that the relative advantage enjoyed by Italian adults over children has persisted. Or is it the case that the health of adults was better preserved in Italy, because of differences in lifestyle? There may be specific cultural or climatic factors in Mediterranean countries which work to the disadvantage of children, and favour adults. Thus, the later start of industrialization may have been achieved at a lower cost to public health.

The difference between England and Sweden on one hand, and France on the other, may be due to similar reasons, but could also have been caused by differences in the quality of the data for earlier periods. If infant mortality had been underestimated in the former two countries until the middle of the previous century, the difference in Fig. 3.7 could have been a statistical artefact. Otherwise, it would be necessary to explain why the difference between mortality in France and Sweden tended to disappear when childhood mortality had fallen to 0.200, whereas this did not happen to the difference between the childhood mortality of France and of Italy.

In Fig. 3.8 we show a more complete comparison between quinquennial

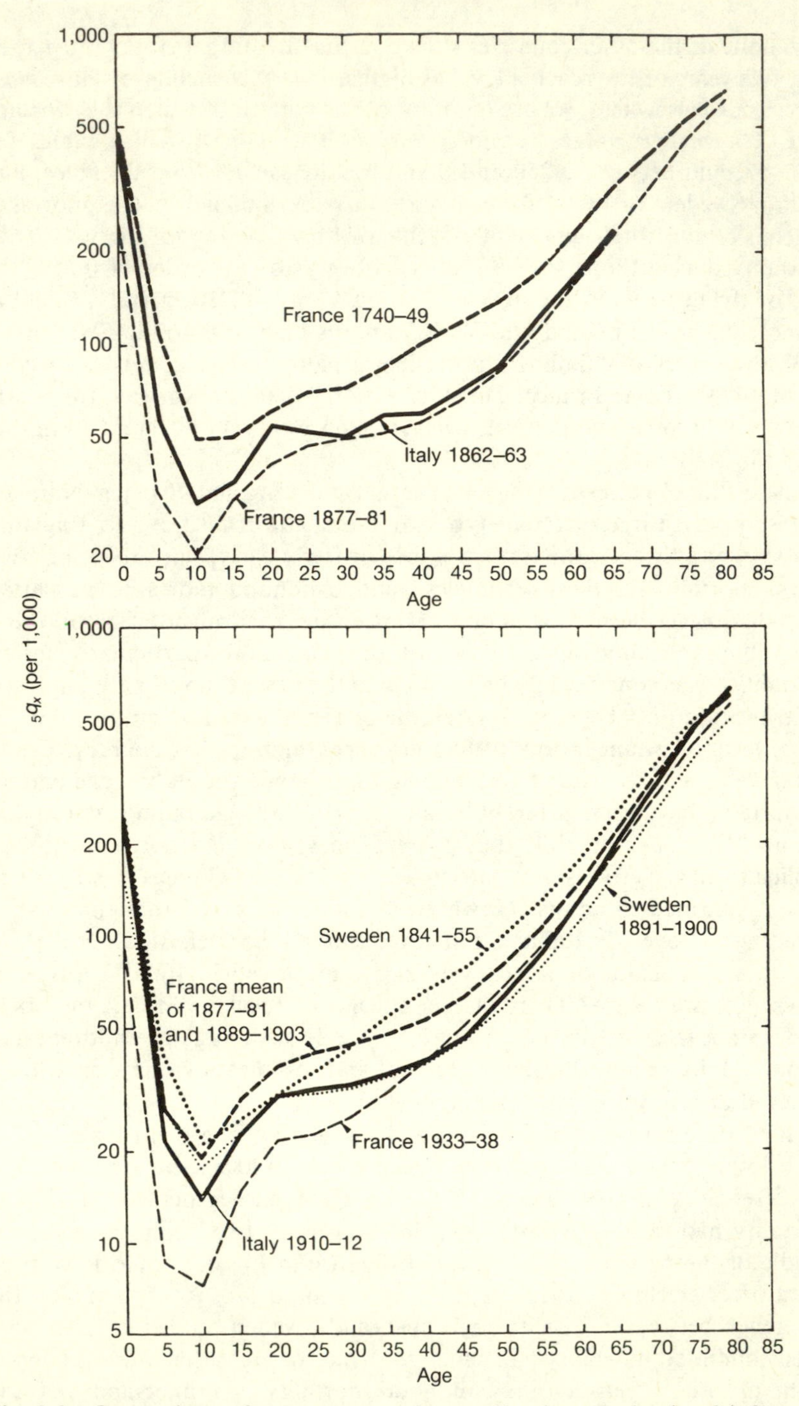

Fig. 3.8 Comparison of age patterns of mortality for two levels of infant and childhood mortality: France, Italy, and Sweden

probabilities of dying at different ages in Italy, and those in France and Sweden for two different levels of childhood mortality. (Tables 3.3 and 3.4.)

At the highest mortality levels it is only possible to compare France and Italy (French table for 1740–49 and Italian for 1862–63). The value of $_5q_0$ in these tables was practically the same in both countries (0.474 and 0.467 respectively). At all other ages, the probabilities in the French table were higher than in the Italian, except between the ages of 20 and 25 where there was a peak in the Italian table which is absent in the French. Thus in 1862–63 when the transition is supposed to have begun in Italy, mortality during the first five years of life stood at a level which had been experienced in France a century earlier, but at ages exceeding 25 years mortality in Italy did not differ greatly from that in France between 1877 and 1881.

There is no real equivalent to the Italian table for 1910–12 in which $_5q_0 = 0.238$. It lies half-way between the tables for France for 1877–81 ($_5q_0 = 0.270$), and 1898–1903 ($_5q_0 = 0.209$). In Fig. 3.8(*b*) we have compared the average values of these two tables with that for Italy. All the probabilities in the Italian table, except the first, are lower than the corresponding values for France, and the differences are largest between the ages of 25 and 50. At this level, mortality in infancy and childhood in Italy lagged

Table 3.3 Life tables for Italy 1862–1863 and France 1740–1749 and 1877–1881: Values of $_5q_x$ (per 1,000)

Age (x)	France 1740–49	Italy 1862–63	France 1877–81
0	474	467	270
5	107	59	33
10	49	31	21
15	50	36	31
20	60	55	40
25	69	52	47
30	72	50	49
35	82	59	51
40	103	60	55
45	117	71	63
50	136	85	81
55	168	121	107
60	225	168	156
65	315	234	213
70	410		329
75	533		449
80	660		615
85	785		

Table 3.4 Life tables for Italy 1910–1912; France 1877–1881, 1898–1903, and 1933–1938; and Sweden 1841–1855 and 1891–1900: Values of ${}_5q_x$

Age (x)	France 1877–81	France 1898–1903	Sweden 1841–55	Italy 1910–12	France 1933–38	Sweden 1891–1900
0	270	209	232	238	91	161
5	33	23	40	22	9	29
10	21	16	22	14	7	18
15	31	25	24	23	15	23
20	40	36	31	31	21	31
25	47	37	36	32	22	31
30	49	40	44	33	26	33
35	51	45	55	36	31	36
40	55	52	66	40	39	41
45	63	63	77	47	51	47
50	81	78	100	61	67	59
55	107	105	128	86	91	78
60	156	151	173	131	128	111
65	213	218	258	206	187	167
70	329	330	362	327	278	255
75	449	477	499	488	407	386
80	615	626	504	665	563	554
85				810	718	

behind that of France by about 20 years, and no longer by a full century. A good deal of the difference between the two countries, therefore, seems to have been made up. But the situation in Italy was even more favourable. At previous levels of child mortality, Italian adult mortality corresponded to that in France at the same time, but now it reached a level which French mortality was only to reach 25 years later. We must go to the French table for 1933–38 to find mortality levels at ages 35 years and over which correspond to those of the Italian table for 1910–12. It is, therefore, difficult to explain the difference between the French and the Italian patterns by the later start of the transition in Italy. Not only did Italian adults benefit from the reduction of mortality before Italian children did, their benefits have exceeded those of French adults since the beginning of the present century. It seems likely that these differences are the result of differences in lifestyles.

Comparisons with Sweden are more complex, and may lead to a slight modification of this conclusion. Mortality during the first five years of life in the Swedish table for 1841–55 was comparable to that in the Italian table for 1910–12 (Fig. 3.8(*b*)). Beyond the age of 30, the probabilities in the Swedish table are much higher than those in the Italian and even in the French table. However, Swedish and Italian mortality were about the same around the age of 20. Thus, whereas French and Italian patterns were fairly similar at ages in excess of five years, with some convexity in the curve between the ages of 10 and 30 years, the Swedish pattern is very different and follows an exponential law almost exactly after the age of 10.

However, the Swedish table in which adult mortality is similar to that of Italy in 1910–12, relates to 1891–1900. Thus, Italian adult mortality in 1910–12 lagged some ten years or more behind that of Sweden, because mortality of the elderly in Sweden was well below the figure shown in the Italian table. It is, therefore, not impossible to explain the difference in terms of a time lag. Moreover, between 1841–55 and 1891–1900 Swedish mortality during the first five years of life did not fall spectacularly (the value of ${}_5q_0$ decreased from 0.232 to 0.161).

In fact, the Swedish pattern of age-specific mortality changed radically. Towards the end of the previous century it approximated to that of France, but at a significantly lower level. Thus, the special feature of the Italian pattern of 1910–12, compared with that of France and Sweden in the 1890s, gave adults a double advantage (their level of mortality corresponded to that of Sweden in the 1890s and France in the 1930s) not only in relation to children, but also to the elderly (where mortality was at the level of France in the 1890s and of Sweden in the 1850s).

This very partial analysis of examples of countries in which the data are most complete does not make it possible to draw definite general conclusions. But it suggests that a difference between the Mediterranean pattern of age-specific mortality and that of northern and western Europe already existed during the first stage of the transition. It is also likely that at that time there was a difference between the western pattern (France) and the northern (England and Sweden), but that this difference tended to disappear towards the end of the nineteenth century.

2.4 Excess Mortality of Men

In pre-industrial Europe, differences between the mortality of men and women were never very important, though the quality of the data on this subject varies, and there may have been differential under-enumeration which could vitiate comparisons. We note, for instance, that in the seventeenth century the difference between the life expectancies of men and women in Geneva was less than one year in favour of men (26.2 years against 25.4).[20] During the eighteenth century, the difference may have been larger in Sweden, as calculations based on parish registers show a difference of 3.5 years in favour of women in 1751–55 (34.8 against 38.3 years).[21] But as the registration of deaths, particularly of deaths of young children, was

[20] A. Perrenoud, 'L'Inégalité devant la mort à Genève au XVIIe siècle', *Démographie historique* (*Population*, 30, special issue (1975)), pp. 221–43.

[21] J. Holmberg, 'A Study of Mortality among Cohorts born in the 18th and 19th Century', in A.M. Bolander (ed.), *Cohort Mortality of Sweden: Three Studies describing Past, Present and Future Trends in Mortality* (Stockholm, 1970), pp. 71–86.

probably still incomplete at the time, the deaths of girls may have been under-registered. Consider, therefore, the example of France.

In 1740–49 expectation of life at birth was 23.8 years for men and 25.7 for women, an advantage of 1.9 years in favour of women.[22] Does this mean that mortality during the eighteenth century was characterized by a relatively small excess mortality of men at the beginning of the period which declined with time? This is suggested by the Swedish figures also, as the difference between the life expectancies of men and women fell from 3.6 years in 1751–55 to 2.5 years in 1776–80. However, the figures must be interpreted with caution. Infant mortality was so high that slight differential under-enumeration of the deaths of children of one sex could vitiate any comparison. The figures for France are also liable to these errors, in spite of the attempts made to avoid them.

However, towards the end of the nineteenth century, the difference increased appreciably from 2.6 years in 1877–81 to 4.1 years on the eve of the First World War, and the increase continued without interruption until the beginnings of the 1980s and reached a value of 8.1 years in 1983–85 (Table 3.5). It is, therefore, only towards the end of our period that a change (the development of excess mortality of men) occurred that is typical of the present century. However, it is of some interest to look at the precursors of this development, and in Fig. 3.9 we show ratios of men's age-specific death rates in five-year groups to the corresponding rates for women at different points in time.

The curves for 1740–49 and 1820–29 are somewhat erratic, which suggests that there were some irregularities of observation. However, there was an excess mortality of women between the ages of 5 and 45, particularly for the period 1820–29, when the data were possibly of higher quality. They have already been analysed by Tabutin.[23] He attributes the excess mortality

Table 3.5 Life expectancy at birth in France at different periods by sex

Period	Life expectancy		
	Men	Women	Difference
1740–49	23.8	25.7	1.9
1780–89	27.5	28.1	0.6
1820–89	38.3	39.3	1.0
1877–81	40.8	43.4	2.6
1913	49.3	53.4	4.1
1983–85	71.0	79.2	8.2

[22] Blayo, op. cit. in n. 7.

[23] D. Tabutin, 'La Surmortalité féminine en Europe avant 1940', *Population*, 33(1) (1978), pp. 121–48.

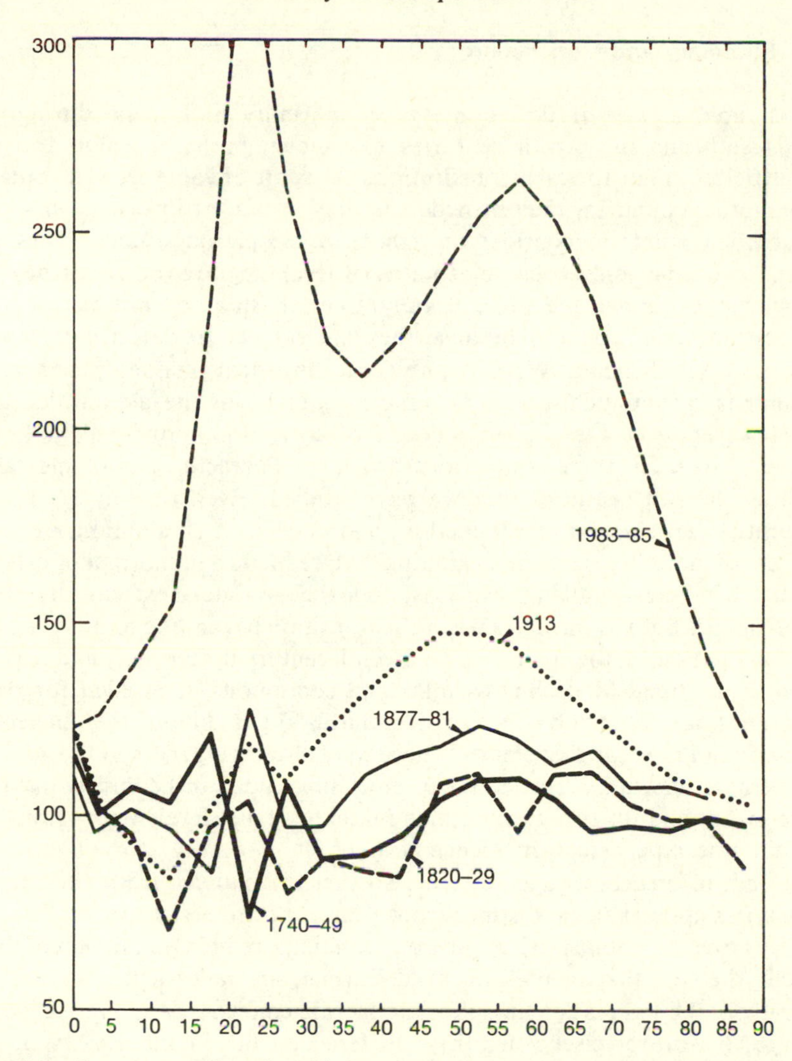

Fig. 3.9 Excess mortality of men in France by five-year age groups since 1740–1749

of women to the unfavourable conditions of women's lives, particularly during adolescence and motherhood. As sanitary conditions improved, this disadvantage was reduced. Moreover, during the period of industrialization, men's mortality tended to be more affected by some social factors, such as the excessive consumption of alcohol and tobacco, accidents at work, and traffic accidents. These all led to an increase in the excess mortality of men at adult ages. The trend had begun on the eve of the First World War, but can already be seen in the curve for 1877–81, and even more clearly in that for 1913.

3. Summary and Conclusion

This rapid survey of developments in mortality in Europe during the eighteenth and nineteenth centuries has shown both the value and the insufficiency of historical reconstitutions. They are of value because, outside the Nordic countries, they provide the only source of information which makes it possible to consider the whole of the period studied. They are insufficient, not only because at national level they are too rare (they are available for France and England only) to establish an overall picture on a European scale, but also because they are subject to defects that make comparisons difficult. We can only urge historical demographers in all countries to continue the work they have begun during the last few decades.

However, even the limited amount of data at our disposal makes it possible to reach some conclusions about the characteristics of mortality during the two centuries that we have studied. Even though the health transition has resulted in a reduction, and later in an elimination, of years of 'crisis' mortality, and the beginning of a reduction in 'normal' mortality everywhere, the overall impression is, none the less, one of extreme diversity. This applies both to the dates when the transition began (the mid-eighteenth century in France, the end of the nineteenth century in Germany and Russia) and to the trend of decline (regular and continuous in Sweden for three centuries, a long period of stagnation during the middle of the nineteenth century in France and England). There were also divergences in the age–sex patterns of mortality (reductions in mortality tended to be largest in those age groups and for the sex for which initial mortality levels were lower). In addition to a persistent difference between the mortality of the two sexes, we find differences in age patterns, so that the pattern in Mediterranean countries appears to be distinct from that in north-west Europe.

However, a number of important questions remain unanswered. Is it really the case that in pre-industrial Europe, mortality levels differed as greatly as the figures for England, the Nordic countries, and France would suggest? More precisely, are these differences due to the quality of the available data, or do they reflect real differences caused by climatic, cultural, or socio-economic differences? If the second alternative were the true explanation at the beginning of the eighteenth century, was this a permanent feature, or are we to assume that in countries like England, Norway, and Sweden there had been an earlier period of declining mortality?

Another interesting problem relates to the explanation of the differences between the age patterns of mortality in countries such as Italy and France. Is it really likely that adult mortality in Italy at the period when the transition is supposed to have begun was comparable to that in France, where the transition had already been under way for some time? Or did the transition in adult mortality in Italy begin earlier than has been thought?

More detailed studies are presented in other chapters in this volume, and some—particularly those concerned with cause-specific mortality—could provide answers to some of these questions. However, a definitive answer would require an improvement in the quality and reliability, as more extensive coverage, in the available statistics.

4 Health Transition and Cause-Specific Mortality

GRAZIELLA CASELLI *University of Rome 'La Sapienza'*

1. From Mortality Crises to the Modern Health Transition

At the beginning of the eighteenth century man had not yet succeeded in mastering the forces of nature, and life expectancy, which was short even in normal times, was affected by subsistence crises and famines which resulted in misery and extremely high death rates. The effects of these crises were often made worse by epidemics of plague and other fevers.[1]

This series of crises which lasted until the early decades of the nineteenth century, the most important of which affected the Baltic and Scandinavian regions and other areas in north-eastern Europe in 1708–09, was followed in most countries of central and northern Europe by a period when subsistence crises became rarer and affected mortality less. Epidemics, however, continued and typhus, smallpox, dysentery, and influenza were recorded throughout the eighteenth and a large part of the nineteenth centuries, but they were less lethal and less widespread than formerly. After the middle of the eighteenth century, the less serious nature of the crises was reflected by lower levels of mortality. Life expectancy began to increase in Sweden, Denmark, Norway, England, and France and had reached a figure of between 40 and 42 years by the early nineteenth century.[2]

In Mediterranean and eastern Europe, on the other hand, life expectancy remained low, and there was no indication that these countries would share in the progress achieved in northern and western Europe. Thus, in Italy, the combination of famine and plague made its reappearance with the famine and typhus epidemic of 1811–20, which was reminiscent of the demographic crises of the old regime.[3] By the beginning of the second half of the nine-

[1] K. Helleiner, 'La Population de l'Europe de la peste noire à la veille de la révolution démographique', in E. E. Rich and C. Wilson (eds.), *The Cambridge Economic History of Europe*, iv. *The Economy of Europe in the Sixteenth and Seventeenth Centuries* (Cambridge, 1987).

[2] M. Livi Bacci, *Popolazione e alimentazione: Saggio sulla storia demografica europea* (Bologna, 1987); E. A. Wrigley and R. S. Schofield, *The Population History of England 1541–1871* (London, 1981).

[3] E. Sori, 'Malattia e demografia', in F. Peruta (ed.), *Storia d'Italia, Annali 7: Malattia e medicina* (Turin, 1984).

teenth century life expectancy at birth in Italy was only about 30 years.[4]

The secular decline in mortality which in central and northern Europe had gone on for a century, began to differ in different parts of Europe between 1820 and 1830. Whereas the health revolution proceeded in Scandinavia where mortality continued to fall; in central and other parts of northern Europe mortality remained roughly constant until about 1870. It was only then that a second phase of decline began in those countries, at first hesitantly, but becoming more regular as time proceeded, and which resulted in what may be termed the modern health transition which only some years later extended to the Mediterranean countries. It was in the 1880s that mortality began to fall significantly in Italy, so that life expectancy at birth increased from 33 to 38 years within the ten years between 1881 and 1891.

The study of changes in mortality in European countries has led to the theory of demographic transition and has engaged the attention of scholars in many disciplines other than demography proper: economists, medical researchers, epidemiologists, and geneticists among them.[5] There is still considerable discussion about the reasons that underlie the decline of mortality (particularly during the eighteenth century), and many different views have been put forward.[6] It could hardly be otherwise, when mortality decline is studied by means of a single global indicator. It is seldom possible to study changes in sex and age-specific mortality, and rarer still to consider changes in causes of death before the beginning of the health transition. However, it is only by looking at changes in diseases which cause death that we shall be able to identify the external causes which have resulted in falling mortality. However, in the countries in which the decline in mortality started earliest, information about causes of death only became available once the health transition was already advanced.

Statistics on causes of death only began to be collected in the middle of the nineteenth century, and then only for some countries, and often only for their capitals or large cities. In England, a country in which the collection of statistical data on causes of death was pioneered, regular statistics only began in 1838, and only after 1848 were they presented in a form which made it possible to study changes in cause-specific mortality.[7]

The object of this chapter is to analyse the part played by changes in causes of death during the transition. This cannot be achieved for all countries or

[4] G. Caselli, 'Mortalità e soprovivenza in Italia dall'Unità agli anni '30', paper presented to the Conference on Spanish, Portuguese, and Italian Historical Demography, Barcelona, 22–25 Apr. 1987.

[5] T. McKeown, *The Modern Rise of Population* (London, 1976).

[6] McKeown, op. cit. in n. 5; Livi Bacci, op. cit. in n. 2; R. Rotberg and T. Rabb (eds.), *Hunger and History* (Cambridge, 1985); N.L. Tranter, *Population and Society 1750–1940: Contrast in Population Growth* (London and New York, 1985); J. Vallin, *Théorie(s) de la baisse de la mortalité et situation africaine* (Paris, 1987).

[7] T. McKeown and R. G. Record, 'Reasons for the Decline in Mortality in England and Wales During the Nineteenth Century', *Population Studies*, 16(2) (1962), pp. 94–122.

periods, because data are lacking. In countries such as Norway, where mortality declined continuously from the middle of the eighteenth century onwards, for instance, mortality by cause can only be studied during the later years of the transition. In countries, such as England, where the fall occurred early and was followed by stagnation and a later resumption of the decline, it is only possible to study the phase of stagnation and the second phase of decline (the modern transition). However, in countries such as Italy, where the decline began later, all the stages of the transition can be studied (Fig. 4.1).

By looking at cause-specific mortality and its changes in different

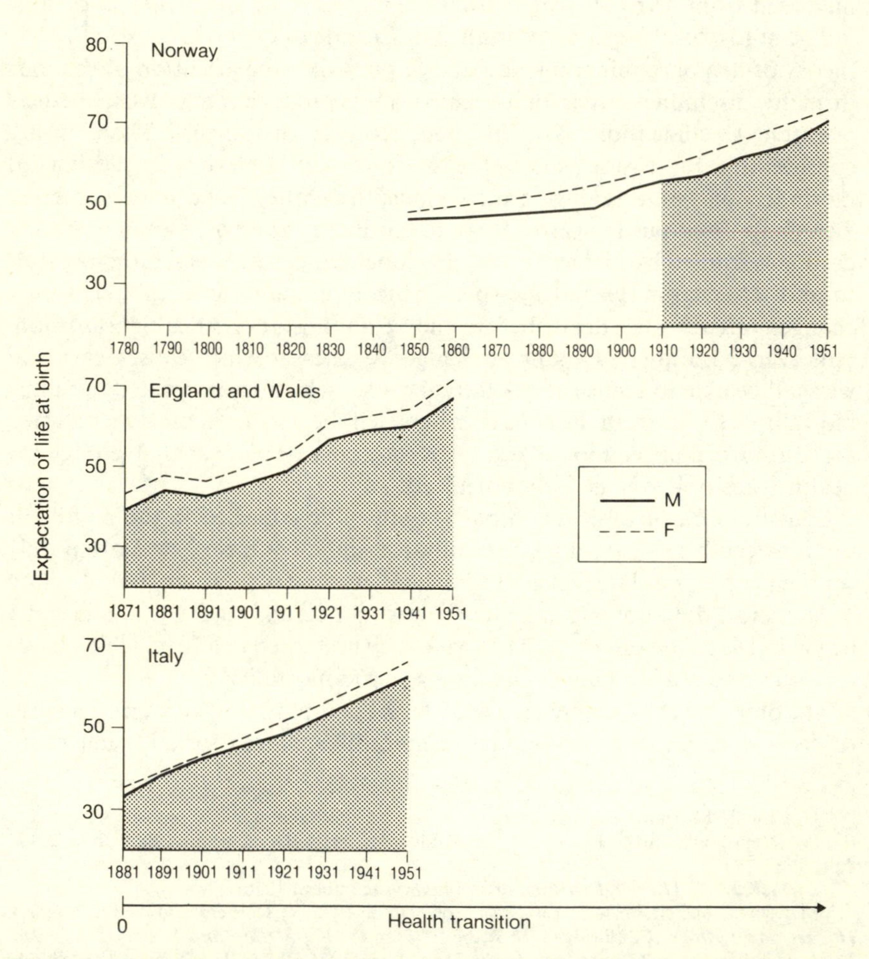

Fig. 4.1 The modern health transition: changes in life expectancy at birth in three countries representing the European transition: Norway, England and Wales, and Italy

countries it should be possible to arrive at a better understanding of the process of mortality change and to show how the transition resulted in a change from a situation in which infectious diseases and fevers predominated among causes of death to a more modern regime in which cardiovascular and malignant diseases are the most important causes of death.

Our analysis ends in 1951. It should be emphasized that this year has not been chosen because it marks an abrupt change in the transition. Mortality continued to decline after that date, and the decline is still continuing.

Our analysis will be based on statistics of causes of death for England and Wales between 1871 and 1951, and for Italy between 1881 and 1951. The Norwegian data which are available only for the later part of the transition (1910–51) will be used to complete our comparisons.

We shall take most of our data from the work by Preston, Keyfitz, and Schoen[8] which enables us to make both spatial and temporal comparisons. Their series have been adjusted and completed where necessary, using uniform criteria.[9] Clearly, however, in spite of attempts to make statistics of causes of death comparable between successive revisions of the International List of Diseases, registrations will have been affected by improvements in medical knowledge and diagnosis, as well as by differences in practice between different countries. However, by aggregating deaths from different causes we hope to have largely overcome these difficulties, and to have been able to point to the essential features of the situation in different areas and at different times.

2. Cause-Mortality Patterns at the Beginning of the Transition

Irrespective of whether figures are compared on a chronological basis or for the same stage of the transition, England and Wales lags behind Norway and Italy as far as mortality reduction is concerned. Even though differences between these countries have diminished they have not disappeared altogether. (See Fig. 4.1, and Table 4.1(*a*).)

An overall view of these differences will be affected by differences between mortality rates early in life. If we were to consider only life expectancy of males at their fifth birthday, we would find that in England and Wales and Italy, two countries for which comparisons are possible, the figures are often nearly the same.

The patterns of cause-specific mortality in the two countries were also

[8] S. H. Preston, N. Keyfitz, and R. Schoen, *Causes of Death: Life Tables for National Populations* (New York, 1972).

[9] All the Italian data on mortality by cause of death, including those for 1881 and 1891, relate to the whole of the national territory.

similar, at the beginning of the transition. Infectious diseases[10] caused about 30 per cent of all deaths; bronchitis, pneumonia and influenza about 15 per cent, whereas circulatory diseases (including cerebrovascular lesions) were only responsible for between 9 and 10 per cent of the deaths of men and 11 to 12 per cent of those of women (Table 4.2.). The comparison remains valid when age-standardized rates are used. These rates are shown in Table 4.5 and do not differ much from crude rates prevailing at the same time. There are, however, differences between the percentages of deaths from different causes. Diarrhoea and enteritis accounted for between 10 and 11 per cent of all Italian deaths, but for only 6 per cent of those in England and Wales. This difference can easily be explained in terms of the aetiology of these diseases which are closely linked to the environment and public health. The infrastructure of public health in Italy at the end of the nineteenth century was still relatively undeveloped, and intestinal diseases, often accompanied by typhoid fever, found fertile ground in the densely populated quarters of towns[11] and in the most impoverished and isolated rural regions of the country.[12] In Italy, climatic conditions were also particularly favourable for the development of these diseases during the hot season, and the number of infant deaths was at a maximum during the summer months. Towards the turn of the century this group of causes of death became the second most important.[13] (See Table 4.2 for the position in 1901.)

Another major difference between England and Wales and Italy relates to tuberculosis of the respiratory system; mortality from this cause was much heavier both absolutely and relatively in the former country. This difference cannot have been due solely to differences in medical practice or diagnostic conventions. It is true that towards the end of the previous century adequate means of diagnosing this disease were still lacking in a number of Italian regions, and that relatively less attention was paid to it than elsewhere in Europe, but more favourable climatic conditions and a later start and slower pace of urbanization could have acted as a check on tuberculosis, a disease which was more prevalent in northern and central Europe.

Apart from these differences, it would seem that at the beginning of the transition, mortality at ages exceeding five years was similar in the two countries in which social and economic conditions were very different. The

[10] These are deaths which are shown in the International Classification of Causes of Death as ch. 1, 'Infectious and Parasitic Diseases'. This group does not include all infectious diseases because some of them are classed as being diseases of the respiratory or the digestive system. Vallin and Meslé have shown that in France, ch. 1 of the classification only accounted for 20 per cent of all deaths from infectious diseases. See J. Vallin and F. Meslé, *Les Causes des décès en France de 1925 à 1978* (Paris, 1989).

[11] M. Livi Bacci, *La trasformazione demografica delle società europee* (Turin, 1977).

[12] L. Giglioli, *Malessere agrario ed alimentare in Italia* (Naples, 1903).

[13] Caselli, op. cit. in n. 4.

Table 4.1 Changes in the life expectancy at birth and fifth birthday in Norway, England and Wales, and Italy

Countries	Period[a]										
	1850	1861	1871	1881	1891	1901	1911	1921	1931	1940	1951
a e_0	Males										
Norway	45.5	46.0	47.4	48.6	49.1	54.0	56.4	57.8	62.6	–	70.8
England and Wales	39.9	40.5	39.2	44.3	42.0	45.0	49.4	55.9	58.2	59.4	65.9
Italy	–	–	–	33.3	38.4	42.5	45.9	49.3	53.8	–	63.9
	Females										
Norway	48.6	48.4	50.5	51.1	52.6	56.9	59.3	60.6	65.8	–	74.4
England and Wales	41.9	43.1	42.5	47.5	45.7	49.4	53.4	59.9	62.4	63.9	70.9
Italy	–	–	–	34.0	38.8	43.0	46.8	50.8	56.0	–	67.5
b e_5	Males										
Norway	52.1	53.5	53.3	54.5	53.8	56.6	57.8	58.4	61.9	–	68.4
England and Wales	49.7	51.2	49.2	52.1	51.3	54.5	56.9	59.3	59.9	60.0	63.8
Italy	–	–	–	50.3	53.2	54.6	56.4	57.4	59.7	–	64.5
	Females										
Norway	54.8	55.5	55.8	56.1	56.7	58.7	60.0	60.3	64.5	–	71.4
England and Wales	50.3	52.2	51.4	54.0	53.6	57.1	59.7	62.1	62.9	63.3	68.2
Italy	–	–	–	49.6	52.3	54.2	56.6	58.0	61.4	–	67.2

(–) Data not available.

[a] The exact periods for different countries are:
Norway 1846–50, 1861–65, 1871–75, 1881–85, 1891–95, 1901–05, 1910, 1920, 1930, 1951;
England and Wales 1848–52, 1861, 1871, 1881, 1891, 1901, 1911, 1921, 1931, 1940, 1951;
Italy 1881, 1891, 1901, 1910, 1921, 1931, 1950–53.

Sources: Jens Kristian Borgan, *Cohort Mortality in Norway 1846–1980* (Oslo, 1983); S. H. Preston, N. Keyfitz, and R. Schoen, *Causes of Death: Life Tables for National Populations* (New York, 1972); ISTAT, *Tavole di mortalità della popolazione italiana 1950–1953* (Rome, 1953).

Table 4.2 Percentage distribution of deaths by cause at the beginning of the second phase of the modern transition

Group of Causes of Death[a]	Males					Females				
	England and Wales			Italy		England and Wales			Italy	
	1871	1881	1901	1881	1901	1871	1881	1901	1881	1901
1. Infectious Diseases	29	25	20	29	14	30	25	18	29	15
Tuberculosis	14	14	11	7	8	13	14	9	9	7
(Tuberculosis of the respiratory system)	(10)	(10)	(8)	(6)	(5)	(11)	(10)	(7)	(8)	(6)
Measles, Scarlet Fever, Whooping Cough, Diphtheria	8	7	7	8	3	8	9	8	10	3
Typhus, Typhoid Fever	3	0	0	3	2	3	0	0	3	2
2. Bronchitis, Pneumonia, and Influenza	14	17	16	15	20	14	16	16	14	19
3. Diseases of the circulatory system	10	13	14	9	13	12	14	16	11	15
4. Diarrhoea and Enteritis	6	4	7	10	15	6	4	7	11	15
5. Diseases of infancy and early childhood	7	7	7	8	7	6	6	6	7	7
6. Accidents	5	5	5	3	3	2	2	2	1	1
7. Neoplasms	1	2	4	1	2	3	4	7	2	3
8. Others	28	27	27	25	26	27	29	28	25	25
All causes	100	100	100	100	100	100	100	100	100	100
Crude death rate (per 100,000)	2,394	1,999	1,811	2,813	2,246	2,133	1,781	1,579	2,706	2,151

[a] The reclassification of causes of death taken from the work by Preston, Keyfitz, and Schoen (see source to Table 4.1), was as follows (the numbers are those used in the International Classification of Diseases, 7th Revision)

1. Infectious diseases 001–138
   Tuberculosis 001–019 (Tuberculosis of the Respiratory System 001–008)
   Measles 085, Scarlet Fever 050, Whooping Cough 056, Diphtheria 055
   Typhus and Typhoid Fever 040–041, 100–108
2. Bronchitis, Pneumonia, and Influenza 480–502
3. Diseases of the circulatory system (incl. cerebrovascular disease) 330–334, 400–468
4. Diarrhoea and Enteritis 543, 571, 572
5. Diseases of infancy and early childhood 480–502
6. Accidents E800–E999
7. Neoplasms 140–239

Sources: Preston, Keyfitz, and Schoen, op. cit. in source to Table 4.1; General Register Office, *34th Annual Report of the Registrar General for the year 1871* (London, 1873); DIRSTAT, *Cause di morte 1881* (Rome, 1887).

process of mortality decline appears at first sight to have been independent of these differences. However, this conclusion runs counter to the rich literature of the contemporary as well as of the more recent period on the relation between mortality and economic conditions, and needs to be more closely examined.

We shall begin by examining the patterns of cause-specific mortality by age. A similar cause-of-death pattern for deaths at all ages may conceal very considerable differences between cause-specific mortality rates at different stages of life.

In order to avoid undue multiplicity of data, we have used a method which has recently been proposed by Pollard[14] which makes it possible to measure the contribution made by mortality from a specific cause to life expectancy. The results are shown in Table 4.3, in which the difference between the life expectancies in England and Wales and Italy at the beginning of the transition is broken down by age and cause of death.

The differences between mortality rates early in life clearly play an essential part in explaining differences in life expectancy. This is evident when we compare the values of the life expectancies at birth with those on the fifth birthday. The mortality of Italian males is higher than that of English males up to the age of 14, but the situation is reversed after that age. Causes of death which are responsible for the higher mortality of Italian young people are: infectious diseases (except tuberculosis of the respiratory system), the group consisting of bronchitis, pneumonia, and influenza (i.e. diseases of the respiratory system), and those diseases of the digestive system which are caused by infections (i.e. diarrhoea and enteritis), as well as diseases of infancy and early childhood (among which will be found other diseases of the respiratory and digestive systems, such as pneumonia of the newborn and infantile diarrhoea). Conversely, the death rates from almost all causes for adult and elderly Italian males are lower than the corresponding rates for English men, particularly death rates from diseases of the circulatory system, accidents and injuries, and tuberculosis of the respiratory system.

Thus, the life expectancy at birth of approximately 50 years which was recorded in England and Wales in 1871 and in Italy in 1881 (Table 4.1(*b*)) was the result of two different mortality regimes, which reflected different external factors. In England, where the process of industrialization was already advanced at the time, mortality was high particularly at working ages and from causes linked to poor living and working conditions (infectious diseases, particularly respiratory tuberculosis, diseases of the

[14] J. Pollard, 'Cause of Death and Expectation of Life: Some International Comparisons', in J. Vallin, S. D'Souza, and A. Palloni (eds.), *Comparative Studies of Mortality and Morbidity: Old and New Approaches to Measurement and Analysis* (Oxford, 1990). In order to use Pollard's model, we need to know the life-table probabilities of survival and cause-age specific death rates for the same period.

Table 4.3 Contribution of selected causes of death to the difference in life expectancy between England and Wales and Italy at the beginning of the modern phase of health transition by age group and sex

Group of causes of death	Total all ages years	%	0 years	1–4 years	5–14 years	15–39 years	40+ years
Males (e_0 England and Wales 39.17; Italy 33.26)							
1. Infectious Diseases	1.46	26	0.48	1.80	0.26	−0.95	−0.13
(Tuberculosis of the respiratory system)	(−0.82)	(−14)	(−0.01)	(0.11)	(0.03)	(−0.62)	(−0.33)
2. Bronchitis, Pneumonia, and Influenza	1.06	19	0.20	0.23	0.11	0.38	0.14
3. Diseases of the circulatory system	−0.26	−4	0.10	0.06	0.01	−0.27	−0.16
4. Diarrhoea and Enteritis	1.93	34	0.55	0.95	0.14	0.09	0.19
5. Diseases of infancy and early childhood	0.89	15	0.89	—	—	—	—
6. Accidents	−0.33	−6	0.10	−0.02	−0.06	−0.19	−0.16
7. Neoplasms	0.04	1	0.00	0.01	0.01	0.01	0.02
8. Other diseases	0.93	16	0.31	0.79	0.18	0.12	−0.48
Difference all causes[a]	5.72	100	2.64	3.81	0.65	−0.79	−0.59
All causes (per 100)		100	46	67	11	−14	−10
Females (e_0 England and Wales 42.26; Italy 33.99)							
1. Infectious Diseases	2.38	29	0.50	1.76	0.52	−0.50	0.11
(Tuberculosis of the respiratory system)	(−0.15)	(−2)	(−0.01)	(0.12)	(0.11)	(−0.31)	(−0.06)
2. Bronchitis, Pneumonia, and Influenza	1.11	13	0.28	0.30	0.11	0.31	0.11
3. Diseases of the Circulatory system	0.07	1	0.09	0.04	0.01	−0.18	0.11
4. Diarrhoea and Enteritis	2.25	27	0.68	1.03	0.19	0.11	0.23
5. Diseases of infancy and early childhood	0.80	10	0.80	—	—	—	—
6. Accidents	0.00	0	0.05	0.00	−0.03	−0.00	−0.02
7. Neoplasms	0.01	0	0.00	0.00	0.00	0.02	0.02
8. Other diseases	1.70	20	0.61	0.93	0.21	0.34	−0.40
Difference all causes[a]	8.32	100	3.01	4.07	1.02	0.09	0.13
All causes (per 100)		100	36	49	12	1	2

[a] Difference (all causes) may not always add to the total because of rounding.

circulatory system, and deaths from accidents). Italy suffered a disadvantage at younger ages, particularly in deaths from all infectious diseases (except respiratory tuberculosis).

Clearly, an analysis of cause–age specific mortality can show up differences in what at first sight appear to be similar regimes, and will lead to a proper assessment of the risks suffered by different populations at different periods. In England and Wales, the high death rate from accidents, particularly at working ages, was related to working conditions in mines and factories during a period of nascent capitalism. In 1868 William Farr stressed that of the 10,786 men and 2,423 women who died from accidental causes at ages exceeding five years:

> 797 people were killed on railways, and 1215 were killed in mines. Many men were poisoned by poisons unknown in the early age. In modern manufacturies many die of fatal accidents . . . At first sight it might appear that civilisation had augmented more than it had diminished the danger to mankind.[15]

Equally, the high mortality from tuberculosis at working ages leads us back to the description of the deplorable conditions of working-class housing in the towns: workers

> try, of course, to remain as near as possible to their workshops. The inhabitants do not go beyond the same or the next parish, parting their two-room tenements into single rooms and crowding even those.
>
> The result of this change is not only that the class of town people is enormously increased, but the old close-packed little towns are now centres, built round on every side, open nowhere to air, and being no longer agreeable to the rich, are abandoned by them for the pleasanter outskirts . . . and a population for which the houses were not intended and quite unfit, has been created, whose surroundings are truly degrading to the adults and ruinous to the children.[16]

These observations confirm those of many others to the effect that in the beginning industrial development in England was chaotic and uncontrolled.[17] This is also the reason why the health transition, which had begun relatively early in England, stopped for a while (unlike in other European countries, such as Norway) and that mortality ceased to fall for a period of nearly 50 years.

Infectious diseases of the digestive tract, on the other hand, which were a factor in the disadvantage of Italian mortality, particularly at young ages, were related to the fact that 6,404 (out of a total of 8,000 communes, accounting for 51 per cent of the population) in 1885 possessed no sewerage

[15] W. Farr, '*Letter to the Registrar General on the Causes of Death in England Year 1868*', *app. A to, 31st Annual Report of the Registrar General* (London, 1870).

[16] Public Health, *Eighth Report* (1865), cited by K. Marx, *Capital* ch. 23.

[17] McKeown and Record, op. cit. in n. 7.

system.[18] In addition, the water supply was poor not only in the towns, but also in the countryside, and at the time of weaning when children were particularly liable to infection they easily fell victim to gastro-intestinal diseases. At the end of the nineteenth century the small number of aqueducts in the kingdom dated back to Roman or medieval times. A single example will suffice to illustrate the deplorable condition of the drinking water: in Rome a number of wells were directly connected to the sewers and as their water was often preferred to that from aqueducts during the hot season because it was cooler; the population in fact drank diluted human excreta.[19]

Some of the observations relating to males also apply to females. However, the harmful effects of industrial development that affected the mortality of English adult men were less noticeable for women, who were not employed in the most dangerous occupations. Violent death was not a factor that caused the difference between the life expectancies of Italian and English women. The other diseases which led to an excess mortality of men in England were also less important for women, and differences were relatively small. Thus, the differences between the expectations of life for women in the two countries were larger (about 8 years) than those for men. Infant and child mortality of girls in Italy was higher than in England, but unlike in the case of men, the excess continued at older ages as well.

Lastly, the analysis of cause mortality suggests that in spite of the similarities which we noted at the outset, the modern phase of the transition began at different dates in the two countries and occurred under very different social and economic conditions. The differences in the pattern and level of mortality between England and Wales and Italy are related to the different conditions in the two countries in 1871 and 1881 respectively. Mortality in England, which had already experienced modernization, began to fall earlier than in Italy, and the pattern of cause mortality reflected this fact. In Italy, transition only began after the political unification of the country had been completed at a time when it was still relatively undeveloped economically, and the health situation reflected the pathological conditions of the past. It would be interesting to know whether these differences in development also led to differences in the nature of the health transition.

3. The Contribution of Different Causes of Death to Increased Life Expectancy

The progressive reduction of mortality led to a significant increase in the expectation of life, particularly at the beginning of the present century

[18] DIRSTAT, *Risultati dell'inchiesta sulle condizione igieniche e sanitarie dei comuni del regno: Relazione generale* (Rome, 1885), vol. ii, p. cxii.

[19] L. Faccini, 'Tifo, pensiero medico e infrastrutture igieniche nell'Italia liberale', in Peruta (ed.), op. cit. in n. 3.

(Table 4.1(*a*) and Fig. 4.2). Only the two world wars and the epidemic of Spanish influenza in 1918 interrupted this movement, without, however, affecting underlying trends.

We have used Pollard's method to estimate the contribution made by each cause of death to changes in the expectation of life in England from 1871, and in Italy between 1881 and 1951.[20] In Fig. 4.2, which is complemented by the data in Table 4.4, we show in the first place the extent of changes in life expectancy in the two countries separately for each sex. In England, its value increased by 27 years for men, from 39 to 66 years, and by 28 years for women, from 43 to 71 years. In Italy the gain for men amounted to 31 years (from 33 to 64 years) and 33 years for women (from 34 to 67 years).

The most important contribution to this increase was made by a reduction in the mortality from infectious diseases, particularly tuberculosis of the respiratory system, which accounted for some 40 per cent of the increase in life expectancy. Reduction in mortality from bronchitis, pneumonia, and influenza, and gastro-intestinal diseases (diarrhoea and enteritis) was the second most important factor. Taken together, these three groups of causes of death accounted for most of the reduction in mortality and explained nearly two-thirds of the gain in life expectancy.

In Fig. 4.2 we also show how the contribution to increased life expectancy due to changes in mortality from different causes has changed over time. In both countries, reductions in the mortality from bronchitis, pneumonia, and influenza, and the gastro-intestinal diseases only began to play an important part during the second decade of the twentieth century. Until 1910–11 the first group of diseases contributed relatively little, and the contribution of the second was, if anything, negative in both countries.[21]

By contrast, reductions in the mortality from infectious diseases occurred before 1920, and were responsible for increasing the length of life of men by 5.7 years in England and Wales and by 6.4 years in Italy; the corresponding figures for women were 7.0 and 7.4 years (see Table 4.4.)

It is interesting to note that during that period the gap between the mortality of Italy and that of England and Wales was somewhat reduced by a more rapid decline in the mortality from infectious diseases (other than tuberculosis) in the former country. A comparison of the two graphs in Fig. 4.2 bears witness to this. It would seem that the reduction of mortality from typhus and typhoid fever, measles, whooping cough, scarlet fever, diphtheria, and malaria[22] in Italy reproduced a situation which had occurred in England before the beginning of the transition.[23] This change

[20] Pollard, op. cit. in n. 14.

[21] For England and Wales, see McKeown, op. cit. in n. 5; for Italy, see Faccini, op. cit. in n. 19.

[22] Sori, op. cit. in n. 3.

[23] W. P. D. Logan, 'Mortality in England and Wales from 1848 to 1947', *Population Studies*, 4(2) (1950); G. B. Longstaff, 'The Recent Decline in the English Death Rate considered

Table 4.4 Contribution to gains in life expectancy resulting from the reduction of mortality from specific causes in England and Wales and Italy between 1871 or 1881 and 1951 by age group and sex

Group of causes of death	England and Wales 1871–1951								
	Total all ages		Total all ages						
	1871–1911	1911–1951	years	%	0 years	1–4 years	5–14 years	15–39 years	40+ years
Males									
1. Infectious Diseases	5.75	5.76	11.51	43	1.45	3.09	1.59	3.87	1.51
(Tuberculosis of the respiratory system)	(1.96)	(1.78)	(3.73)	(14)	(0.08)	(0.12)	(0.18)	(2.37)	(0.99)
2. Bronchitis, Pneumonia, and Influenza	0.89	2.58	3.47	13	1.22	1.09	0.12	0.35	0.70
3. Diseases of the circulatory system	0.56	−0.20	0.36	1	0.03	0.05	0.13	0.54	−0.40
4. Diarrhoea and Enteritis	−0.69	2.70	2.00	8	1.26	0.46	0.05	0.07	0.17
5. Diseases of infancy and early childhood	0.28	1.54	1.82	7	1.82	–	–	–	–
6. Accidents	0.47	0.61	1.08	4	0.06	0.15	0.16	0.38	0.32
7. Neoplasms	−0.53	−0.53	−1.06	−4	−0.01	−0.02	−0.03	−0.09	−0.90
8. Other diseases	3.53	3.90	7.43	28	2.37	1.54	0.45	0.88	2.19
Difference all causes[b]	10.26	16.36	26.62	100	8.22	6.35	2.47	5.99	3.59
All causes (per 100)				100	31	24	9	23	13
Females									
1. Infectious Diseases	6.39	5.74	12.13	43	1.45	3.43	1.81	3.98	1.44
(Tuberculosis of the respiratory system)	(2.44)	(1.70)	(4.14)	(15)	(0.07)	(0.13)	(0.28)	(2.70)	(0.97)
2. Bronchitis, Pneumonia, and Influenza	1.11	2.67	3.78	13	1.02	1.14	0.13	0.26	1.23
3. Diseases of the circulatory system	0.37	0.49	0.86	3	0.04	0.06	0.15	0.50	0.11
4. Diarrhoea and Enteritis	−0.59	2.60	2.01	7	1.16	0.49	0.05	0.08	0.23
5. Diseases of infancy and early childhood	0.33	1.44	1.77	6	1.77	–	–	–	–
6. Accidents	0.06	0.25	0.32	1	0.08	0.11	0.06	0.04	0.03
7. Neoplasms	−0.46	0.00	−0.46	−2	−0.01	−0.02	−0.02	−0.03	−0.38
8. Other diseases	3.68	4.39	8.07	28	1.90	1.52	0.44	1.38	2.85
Difference all causes[b]	10.90	17.57	28.47	100	7.40	6.74	2.61	6.21	5.51
All causes (per 100)				100	26	24	9	22	19

coincided with major public-health works in Italy (following the law of 27 December 1888), which affected the entire country towards the end of the nineteenth century,[24] and there were also improvements in nutrition and the general standard of living of the population, following on what has been

in Connection with the Cause of Death', *Journal of the Royal Statistical Society*, 97 (1884); McKeown and Record, op. cit. in n. 7; S. Phillips, 'A Review of Mortality Statistics during the Last Half Century', *Clinical Journal*, 33 (1908).

[24] L. Del Panta, *Evoluzione demografica e popolamento nell'Italia dell'Ottocento 1796–1914* (Bologna, 1984).

Table 4.4 (*Continued*)

Italy 1881–1951[a]								
Total all ages		Total all ages						
1881–1910	1910–1951	years	%	0 years	1–4 years	5–14 years	15–39 years	40+ years
Males								
7.23	4.85	12.08	40	1.88	4.92	1.76	2.26	1.27
(0.73)	(1.56)	(2.29)	(8)	(0.05)	(0.23)	(0.20)	(1.32)	(0.49)
0.72	4.02	4.75	16	1.06	1.13	0.16	0.84	1.56
0.15	0.37	0.52	2	0.16	0.11	0.11	0.13	0.01
−0.15	3.28	3.14	10	1.31	1.42	0.19	0.08	0.13
1.39	1.08	2.47	8	2.47	–	–	–	–
0.31	0.27	0.58	2	0.24	0.08	0.08	0.11	0.06
−0.17	−0.42	−0.59	−2	0.00	−0.01	−0.01	−0.04	−0.52
2.91	4.47	7.37	24	2.24	2.26	0.69	0.92	1.27
12.40	17.92	30.32	100	9.36	9.91	2.97	4.31	3.77
			100	31	33	10	14	12
Females								
7.60	5.69	13.29	40	1.87	5.07	2.19	2.76	1.40
(1.22)	(2.15)	(3.37)	(10)	(0.04)	(0.26)	(0.37)	(1.95)	(0.74)
0.55	4.09	4.64	14	0.97	1.28	0.24	0.64	1.51
0.22	0.85	1.07	3	0.15	0.10	0.11	0.15	0.56
−0.13	3.85	3.72	11	1.36	1.54	0.26	0.16	0.40
1.06	1.10	2.16	7	2.16	–	–	–	–
0.14	0.25	0.38	1	0.17	0.08	0.01	0.06	0.05
−0.06	−0.15	−0.21	−1	0.00	−0.01	−0.01	0.01	−0.20
3.25	4.83	8.08	24	2.14	2.31	0.63	1.59	1.41
12.64	20.50	33.14	100	8.82	10.37	3.43	5.38	5.13
			100	27	31	10	16	15

[a] *Sources*: ISTAT, *Annuario di demografia* (Rome, 1953); *Cause di morte 1887–1955* (Rome, 1958); A. Mineo and G. Giammanco, *La mortalità in Italia dal 1899 al 1961: Evoluzione e cause della mortalità differenziale nei due sessi* (Palermo, 1968).
[b] See Table 4.3.

called the 'Italian industrial revolution', a period which extended more or less from the 1890s to the First World War.[25]

When we consider the whole period beginning with the modern phase of the transition and ending in the middle of the present century and analyse

[25] Giglioli, op. cit. in n. 12.

the contributions to life expectancy resulting from the reductions in death rates in different age groups, we find both interesting similarities and differences in the contribution made by the three major groups of causes. (See Table 4.4 and for ages exceeding 5 years, Fig. 4.3.) In all cases, the major contributions to increased life expectancy were due to the reduction of mortality in the youngest age group, in which mortality from infectious disease and from bronchitis, pneumonia, and influenza fell by between 40 and 60 per cent, and mortality from gastro-intestinal disease by between 80 and 90 per cent. In the older age groups, reductions of mortality from respiratory diseases were well distributed, but the reduction of deaths from infectious disease, and particularly from tuberculosis, was concentrated at younger ages or in early middle life. Between 20 and 30 per cent of the gain due to the reduction of mortality from infectious disease, and between 60 and 65 per cent of that from tuberculosis were achieved in the age group 15–39 years.

Before turning to other causes of death, we will briefly refer to the residual category 'other causes' (mainly perinatal deaths and deaths from unknown causes). Reductions in mortality from diseases in this group, which contained different numbers of causes in different periods (30 per cent at the beginning of the period, compared with 14–16 per cent in England and 26–29 per cent in Italy in 1951) were responsible for an increase in life expectancy at birth of between 7 and 8 years (nearly 25 per cent) in both countries. In this case, too, the gain came largely from a reduction in infant mortality and mortality in middle age, but, interestingly enough, reductions in the mortality of women aged 50 and over were also not negligible. (See Fig. 4.3.)

The simple description of changes in causes of death which we have presented and which has included the principal causes of death in the past, and also during the mortality transition, illustrates the radical changes that have occurred in mortality patterns. Causes of death which are important in modern times (cardiovascular diseases and neoplasms) only played a marginal part in the transition. Changes in mortality from cardiovascular diseases served to increase life expectancy, whereas changes in mortality from neoplasms tended to shorten it, but the effects were limited for both causes. (Fig. 4.2 and Table 4.4.) It is the very stability of mortality from these causes during a period of otherwise declining mortality that gives them their importance in present-day mortality.

There are a number of interesting features relating to mortality from cardiovascular diseases. In the first place, there is a difference between death rates in middle age and among the elderly. Up to the age of 65 years (in England and Wales, 55–60 years for men), changes in death rates from these causes led to an increase in life expectancy; after that age, however, the effects were negative. This is particularly true of English males. Between 1911 and 1951 (Table 4.4), the life expectancy of English males was reduced by 0.2 years as a result of changes in cardiovascular mortality.

Malignant neoplasms are the only group of causes of death where changes in death rates have had a consistently negative effect on life expectancy in both countries and for both sexes (Fig. 4.2.). This was caused particularly by mortality at ages over 40. And, just as in the case of cardiovascular mortality, it was English men who were mainly affected, their expectation of life being reduced by a little more than one year.

Violent deaths merit special attention. Changes in mortality from this cause have, on the whole, resulted in an increase in life expectancy. We are still some way from the period when such deaths, particularly those from traffic accidents, increased sharply. At the end of the nineteenth century a large proportion of violent deaths was caused by accidents in the workplace, and—in England in particular—in the mines. Working conditions improved considerably during the twentieth century, and the numbers of deaths due to accidents at work diminished. The disadvantage suffered by men, and particularly by English working men, was much reduced (Table 4.2.).

Finally, we would mention the progressive increase in the difference between the expectations of life of men and women. This difference was negligible in England and Wales at the beginning of the period, and completely absent in Italy, but excess mortality of men has become one of the distinctive features of contemporary mortality patterns.

4. The New Pattern of Cause-Specific Mortality and the Reduction in Differences

By the end of the Second World War the health transition which began at different times and proceeded in different ways had resulted in a complete transformation in the pattern of cause-specific mortality. Although, life expectancy has continued to increase since then, the general pattern of cause-specific mortality has remained relatively unchanged. Nowadays, circulatory disease has become the principal cause of death for both sexes and, depending on the country, accounts for between one-third and one-half of all deaths. Neoplasms, the second most important cause of death, account for between 12 and 20 per cent.

Before the transition, the high mortality from infectious and acute diseases reflected the poor provisions made for health, and the relative lack of economic and social development of the period. Similarly, the emergence of the modern pattern of cause mortality is an indication of economic progress and improvements in the standard of living. New forms of treatment, better housing, public-health engineering, and health policies in the cities and in the countryside have, in combination, reduced the dangers of contamination and infection. It is, however, more difficult to struggle against the new causes of death which are rooted in the new lifestyles that

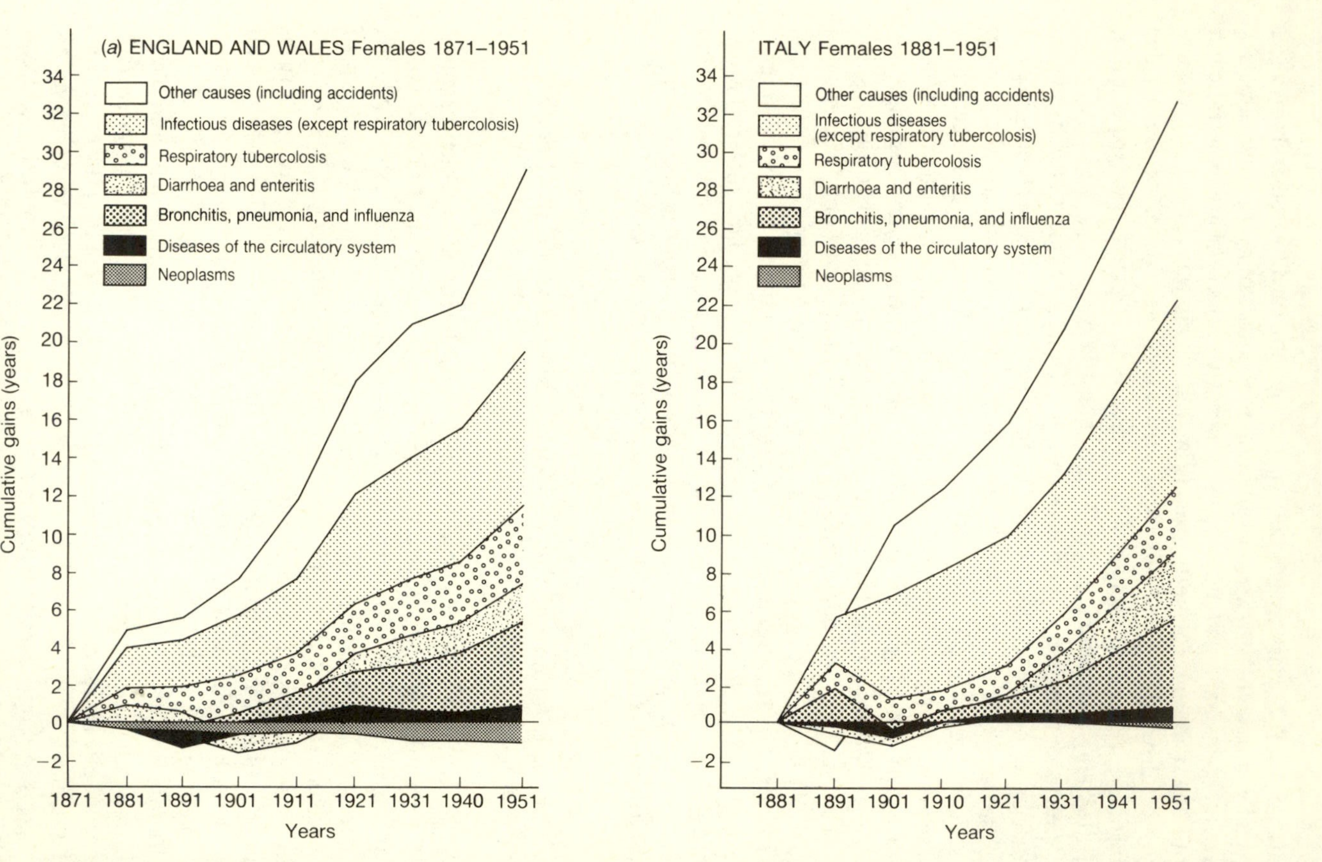

Fig. 4.2 Cumulative gains in life expectancy over ten-year periods resulting from the reduction of mortality from certain causes during

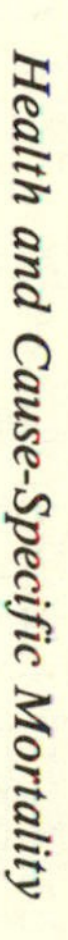

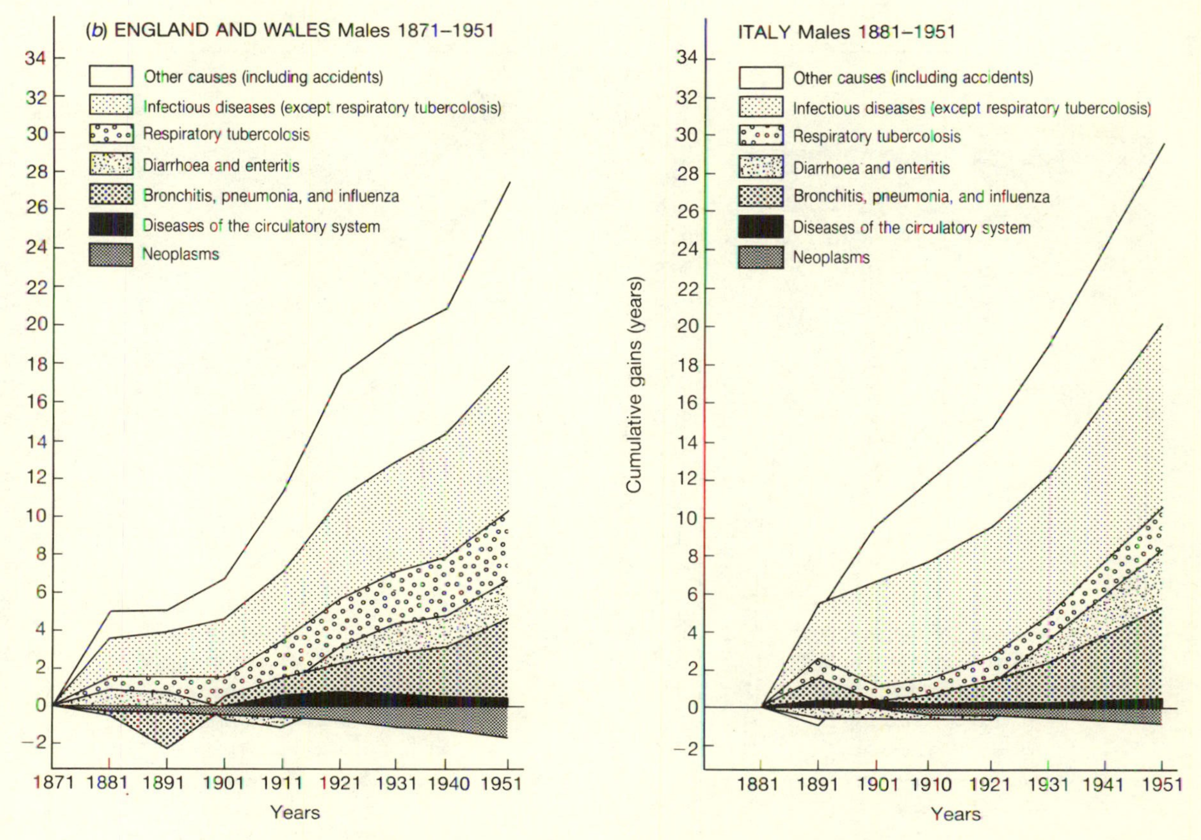
(b) ENGLAND AND WALES Males 1871–1951
Other causes (including accidents)
Infectious diseases (except respiratory tubercolosis)
Respiratory tubercolosis
Diarrhoea and enteritis
Bronchitis, pneumonia, and influenza
Diseases of the circulatory system
Neoplasms
Cumulative gains (years)
34
32
30
28
26
24
22
20
18
16
14
12
10
8
6
4
2
0
−2
1871 1881 1891 1901 1911 1921 1931 1940 1951
Years
ITALY Males 1881–1951
Other causes (including accidents)
Infectious diseases (except respiratory tubercolosis)
Respiratory tubercolosis
Diarrhoea and enteritis
Bronchitis, pneumonia, and influenza
Diseases of the circulatory system
Neoplasms
Cumulative gains (years)
34
32
30
28
26
24
22
20
18
16
14
12
10
8
6
4
2
0
−2
1881 1891 1901 1910 1921 1931 1941 1951
Years

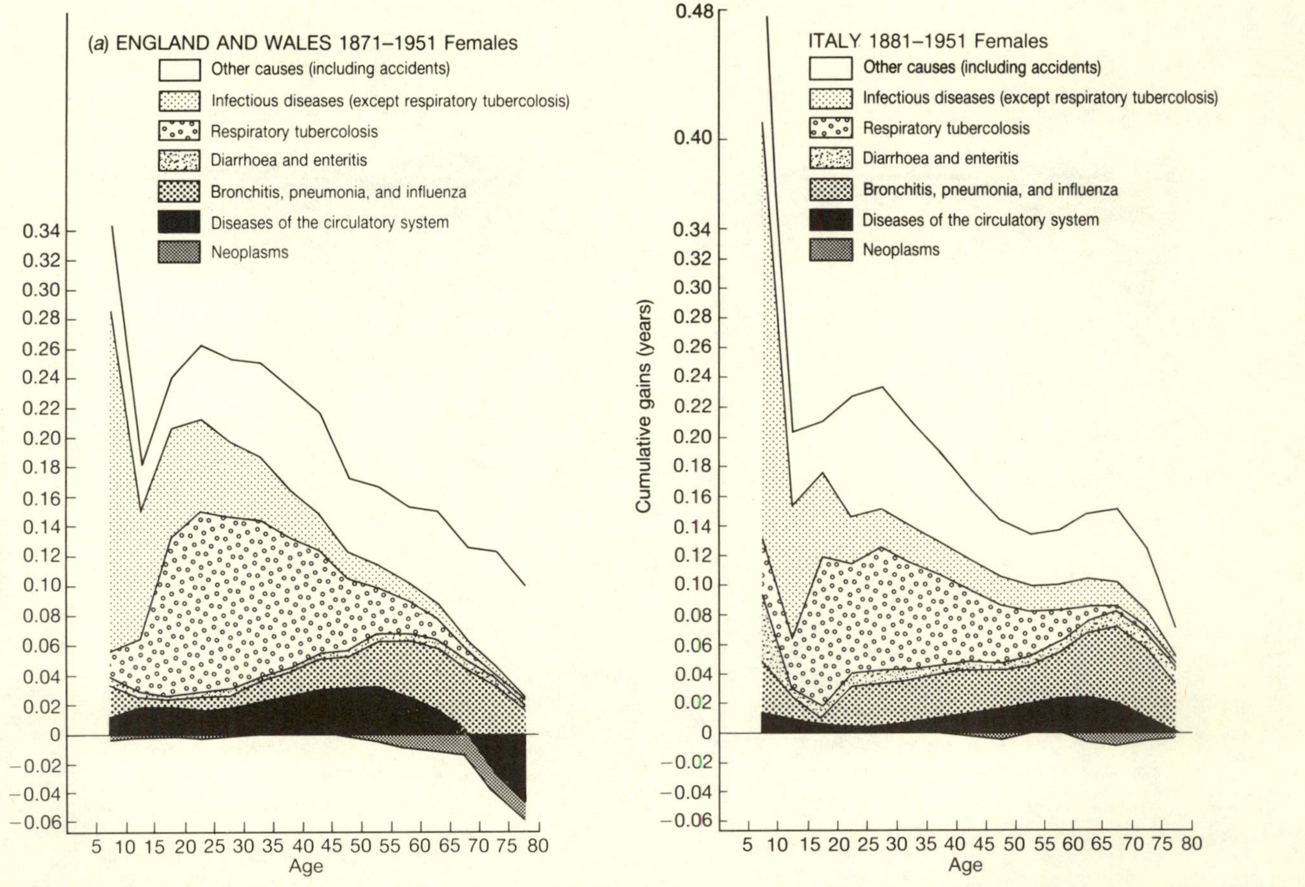

Fig. 4.3 Cumulative contribution by five-year age groups made by reduction in mortality from certain causes to increases in life expectancy: *(a)* females, *(b)* males

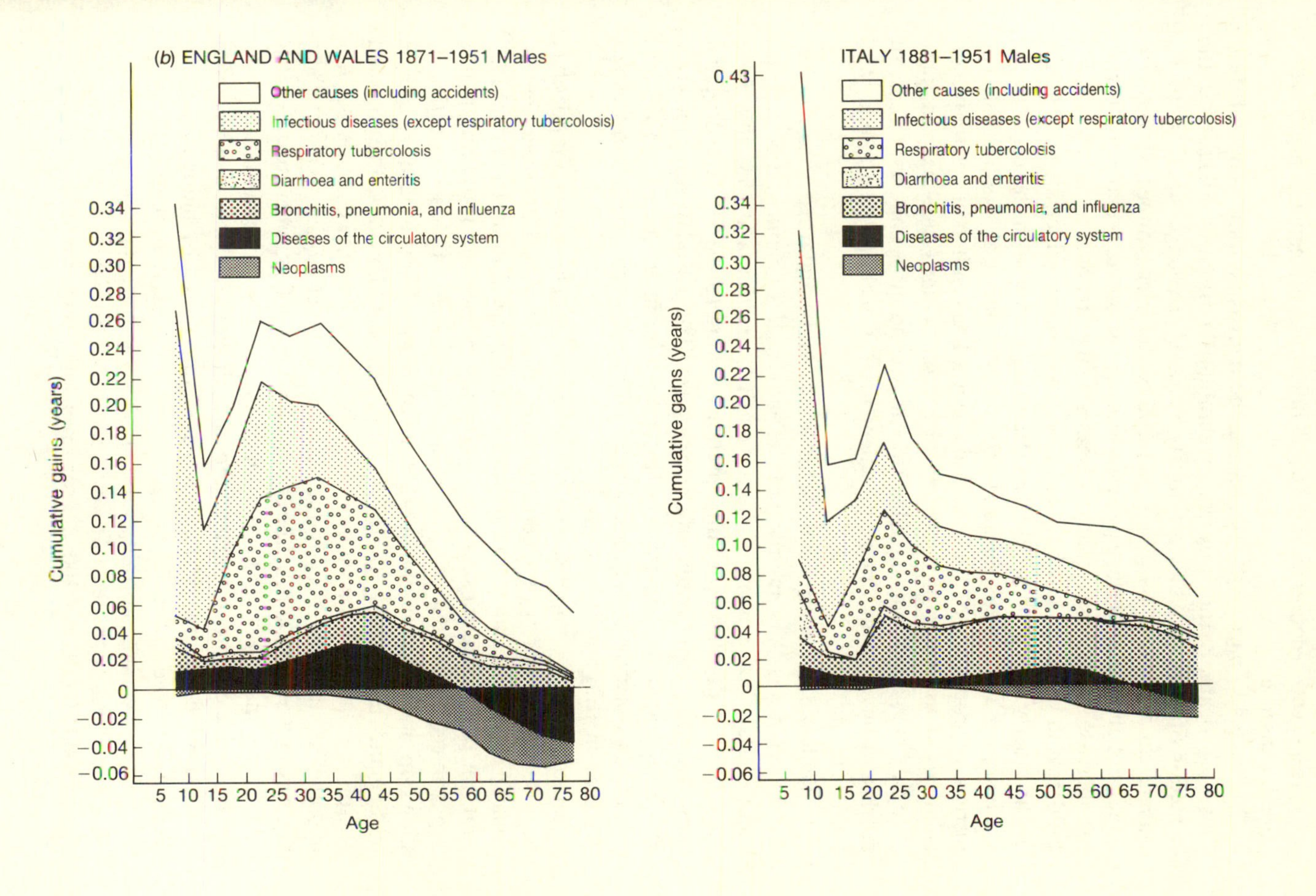
(b) ENGLAND AND WALES 1871–1951 Males
Other causes (including accidents)
Infectious diseases (except respiratory tubercolosis)
Respiratory tubercolosis
Diarrhoea and enteritis
Bronchitis, pneumonia, and influenza
Diseases of the circulatory system
Neoplasms
Cumulative gains (years)
0.34
0.32
0.30
0.28
0.26
0.24
0.22
0.20
0.18
0.16
0.14
0.12
0.10
0.08
0.06
0.04
0.02
0
−0.02
−0.04
−0.06
5 10 15 20 25 30 35 40 45 50 55 60 65 70 75 80
Age
ITALY 1881–1951 Males
Other causes (including accidents)
Infectious diseases (except respiratory tubercolosis)
Respiratory tubercolosis
Diarrhoea and enteritis
Bronchitis, pneumonia, and influenza
Diseases of the circulatory system
Neoplasms
Cumulative gains (years)
0.43
0.34
0.32
0.30
0.28
0.26
0.24
0.22
0.20
0.18
0.16
0.14
0.12
0.10
0.08
0.06
0.04
0.02
0
−0.02
−0.04
−0.06
5 10 15 20 25 30 35 40 45 50 55 60 65 70 75 80
Age

have come with economic and social development: cancers and cardiovascular disease.

Undoubtedly, part of the reason for the increasing importance of these causes of death is the progressive elimination of other risks, and the reduction of selection which previously operated at younger ages. However, changes in the cause pattern of mortality are also connected with the important changes in the age pattern of deaths which have come about with the increase in life expectancy: diseases which tended to attack mainly children and young people have given way to diseases which strike at adults or the elderly, and which have become more common in these groups.

Changes in the age distribution of the population are also important. The increasing proportion of adults and old people has resulted in greater weight being given to causes of death which are particularly prevalent in these groups. Thus, neoplasms have become the second most important cause of death and have become more prevalent than bronchitis, pneumonia, and influenza.

In Table 4.5, we show the patterns (crude and standardized for age) for the two countries. A comparison of the patterns in England and Wales with those of Italy between the beginning of the transition and 1951 illustrates the course of development. Information relating to the 1940s in England shows the progressive nature of these changes. The period of some ten years which separated the beginning of the transition in the two countries has remained stable: the situation reached in England during the 1940s was not achieved in Italy until ten years later.

Although a full comparison with the situation in Norway is not possible, because information for the period when the health transition began in that country is not available, the pattern of cause-specific mortality in 1951 confirms our conclusions about England and Wales and Italy, and makes it possible to point out the factors specific to each of these countries. It shows up, in particular, the importance of deaths from respiratory disease in England and Wales. In their study published in 1974 Preston and Nelson[26] explained this peculiarity in terms of the harsher climate, but this hypothesis is contradicted by the very low number of deaths from these diseases in Norway, and by the lower-than-expected number in Italy. It is more likely that this high proportion is the result of a combination of an unfavourable climate in England and air pollution. We are concerned with a period when English industrial towns were polluted by industrial smoke which led to the notorious smog, and this factor is probably sufficient to explain the high mortality from respiratory disease, and particularly from bronchitis. For men, the death rate from bronchitis in 1951 came to 49 per 100,000 (103 per 100,000 for bronchitis, pneumonia, and influenza

[26] S.H. Preston, and V.E. Nelson, 'Structure and Change in Causes of Death: An International Summary', *Population Studies*, 28(1) (1974), pp. 19–31.

Table 4.5 Changes in patterns of cause-specific mortality by major group of causes during the modern phase of the health transition

Group of causes of death	England and Wales						Italy				Norway	
	1871		1940		1951		1881		1951		1951	
	crude	stand.	crude	stand.	crude	stand.	crude	stand.	crude	stand.	crude	stand.
Males												
1. Infectious Diseases	29	30	8	10	4	6	29	30	6	7	5	7
2. Bronchitis, Pheumonia, and Influenza	14	14	16	17	15	14	15	15	10	11	5	6
3. Diseases of the circulatory system	10	9	34	23	45	35	9	8	34	23	37	25
4. Diarrhoea and Enteritis	6	6	1	2	0	1	10	11	4	6	0	1
6. Accidents	5	5	9	10	4	8	3	3	5	6	9	11
7. Neoplasms	1	1	12	9	16	15	1	1	12	9	19	16
8. Other diseases[a]	35	35	20	29	16	21	33	32	29	38	25	34
All causes	100	100	100	100	100	100	100	100	100	100	100	100
Crude and age-standardized rates (per 100,000)[b]	2,394	2,389	1,455	1,052	1,340	725	2,813	2,915	1,060	794	856	499

Table 4.5 (*Continued*)

Group of causes of death	England and Wales						Italy				Norway	
	1871		1940		1951		1881		1951		1951	
	crude	stand.	crude	stand.	crude	stand.	crude	stand.	crude	stand.	crude	stand.
Females												
1. Infectious Diseases	30	32	6	11	2	6	29	31	5	7	4	7
2. Bronchitis, Pneumonia, and Influenza	14	13	14	15	13	12	14	13	10	10	7	7
3. Diseases of the circulatory system	12	9	38	24	52	36	11	8	40	25	41	29
4. Diarrhoea and Enteritis	6	6	1	2	0	1	11	12	4	7	0	1
6. Accidents	2	2	7	9	3	3	1	1	2	2	4	4
7. Neoplasms	3	2	13	10	16	15	2	2	13	10	20	20
8. Other diseases[a]	33	36	21	29	14	27	32	33	26	39	24	32
All causes	100	100	100	100	100	100	100	100	100	100	100	100
Crude and age-standardized rates (per 100,000)[b]	2,133	2,098	1,286	799	1,176	493	2,706	2,851	938	651	828	375

[a] Including diseases of early childhood.

[b] Standardized rates calculated for the Model West Stable Population constructed by Coale and Demeny, with $e_0 = 45$ and $r = 0.02$ (A. J. Coale and P. Demeny, *Regional Model Life Tables and Stable Populations*, (Princeton, NJ, 1966).

combined) compared with 19 per 100,000 in Italy, and a rate for the group as a whole in Norway of 29 per 100,000.

Another peculiarity is the persistence of a relatively heavy mortality from gastro-intestinal diseases in Italy. This persistence, together with the backwardness of economic and social development by comparison with the two other countries, bears particularly heavily on mortality in early childhood. If the contribution made by different causes of death to the expectation of life in the three countries in 1951 is calculated (Tables 4.6 and 4.7), it is found that mortality from these diseases, which is heaviest in Italy and where the age distribution of persons who die from these diseases is concentrated at younger ages, reduces the life expectancy in that country by 2 years, compared with the situation in England and Wales and Norway. If deaths from other diseases of early childhood are added, the reduction increases to about 2.5 years.

The combined effects of the age and cause structure of mortality also show up some other differences. We have already commented on the high proportion of deaths from degenerative and circulatory diseases in England. This results in increasing differences between the mortality of men in the two countries, and a loss of two years of life expectancy in 1951 compared with Italy, caused almost exclusively by mortality after the fifteenth year of age. The factors which have led to a reduction in the difference between the expectations of life in the two countries from 6 years at the beginning of the transition to 2 years in 1951, have already been presented. Once the reasons for the remaining excess mortality in Italy (in mortality of early childhood and from infectious disease) have been overcome, the rank order of the two countries in the distribution of life expectancies was reversed, and this happened towards the end of the 1960s.[27] The comparison with Norwegian data once again shows the higher English mortality from diseases of the respiratory system and from neoplasms. In comparing English with Norwegian expectations of life (Table 4.7), these causes have contributed to the difference between the two expectations which amounted to seven years in 1910 and five years in 1951. The difference between the contributions made by these two groups of causes of death actually became larger, whereas that from other causes of death was reduced. At the same time, the disadvantage due to mortality from tuberculosis of the respiratory system from which Norway suffered was reversed. This is confirmed when Norwegian data are compared with those for Italy.

Most of the comparisons which have been presented for males apply to females. The transition has resulted in a gradual reduction in the differences between life expectancies, even though in 1951 the English and Norwegian figures exceeded the Italian by 4 and 7 years respectively.

[27] G. Caselli, and V. Egidi, *New Trends in European Mortality* (Council of Europe Population Studies, 5, Strasbourg, 1981).

Table 4.6 Contribution made by selected causes of death to the difference between the life expectancies of England and Wales and Italy by age group and sex

Group of causes of death	Beginning of the modern transition				1910–1911				1951			
	All ages	0–14 years	15–39 years	40+ years	All ages	0–14 years	15–39 years	40+ years	All ages	0–14 years	15–39 years	40+ years
Males												
Positive contributions												
1. Infectious diseases	1.46	2.54	−0.95	−0.13	−0.58	−0.69	0.41	−0.32	0.53	0.26	0.19	0.08
4. Diarrhoea and Enteritis	1.93	1.64	0.09	0.19	1.95	1.65	0.13	0.17	2.10	1.26	0.17	0.66
5. Diseases of infancy and early childhood	0.89	0.89	–	–	−0.23	−0.23	–	–	0.54	0.54	–	–
8. Other diseases	0.93	1.29	0.12	−0.48	1.47	1.44	0.21	−0.18	1.05	0.59	0.11	0.35
Negative contributions												
3. Diseases of the circulatory system	−0.26	0.17	−0.27	−0.16	−0.03	0.01	−0.02	−0.03	−1.23	0.06	0.04	−1.33
6. Accidents	−0.33	0.02	−0.19	−0.16	−0.30	−0.11	−0.06	−0.13	−0.05	−0.06	0.00	0.01
7. Neoplasms	0.04	0.02	0.01	0.02	−0.36	0.02	−0.00	−0.39	−0.76	−0.01	−0.06	−0.68
Contributions that have changed sign												
2. Bronchitis, Pneumonia, and Influenza	1.06	0.54	0.38	0.14	1.53	1.37	0.17	−0.01	−0.23	0.86	−0.01	−1.07
Difference[a]	5.72	7.10	−0.79	−0.59	3.44	3.45	0.85	−0.87	1.94	3.48	0.44	−1.99

Expectation of Life at Birth												
England and Wales	39.17				49.38				65.85			
Italy	33.26				45.89				63.75			
Females												
Positive contributions												
1. Infectious diseases	2.38	2.78	−0.50	0.11	0.27	−0.66	0.92	0.01	0.45	0.27	0.09	0.09
2. Bronchitis, Pneumonia, and Influenza	1.11	0.69	0.31	0.11	1.94	1.55	0.28	0.12	0.10	0.56	−0.02	−0.45
4. Diarrhoea and Enteritis	2.25	1.90	0.11	0.23	2.56	2.11	0.20	0.24	1.65	1.16	0.09	0.39
5. Diseases of infancy and early childhood	0.80	0.80	—	—	−0.09	−0.09	—	—	0.63	0.63	—	—
8. Other diseases	1.70	1.75	0.34	−0.4	1.90	1.71	0.30	−0.1	1.49	0.74	0.11	0.63
Contributions that have changed sign												
3. Diseases of the circulatory system	0.07	0.14	−0.18	0.11	0.29	−0.01	0.00	0.29	−0.23	0.06	0.08	−0.37
6. Accidents	0.00	0.02	0.00	−0.02	−0.11	−0.06	0.01	−0.06	−0.19	−0.04	−0.04	−0.11
7. Neoplasms	0.00	0.00	0.02	−0.02	−0.40	0.02	0.00	−0.44	−0.31	−0.01	−0.02	−0.27
Difference[a]	8.32	8.10	0.09	0.13	6.51	4.72	1.73	0.06	3.58	3.38	0.29	−0.09
Expectation of Life at Birth												
England and Wales	42.46				53.40				70.95			
Italy	33.99				46.79				67.25			

[a] See Table 4.3.

Table 4.7 Contribution made by selected causes of death to the difference between the life expectancies of Norway and England and Wales and between Norway and Italy by age group and sex

Group of causes of death		1910–1911		1951	
		Males all ages	Females all ages	Males all ages	Females all ages
Norway—England and Wales					
Positive contributions					
Other diseases[a b]		6.87	5.80	1.88	1.04
3. Diseases of circulatory system		1.20	1.39	2.54	1.99
7. Neoplasms		0.14	0.49	0.62	0.10
Negative contributions					
6. Accidents		−0.05	0.35	−0.41	0.07
Contributions that have changed sign					
Tuberculosis of the respiratory system		−1.26	−2.17	0.19	0.11
Difference[c]		6.90	5.86	4.82	3.31
Expectation of Life at Birth	Norway	56.41	59.32	70.85	74.38
	England and Wales	49.38	53.40	65.85	70.95
Norway—Italy					
Positive contributions					
Other diseases[b]		6.57	6.96	3.87	3.90
3. Diseases of the circulatory system		1.18	1.60	1.35	1.64
4. Diarrhoea and Enteritis		4.32	4.71	1.99	1.64
Negative contributions					
6. Accidents		−0.39	0.20	−0.45	−0.12
7. Neoplasms		−0.32	−0.03	−0.15	−0.22
Contributions that have changed sign					
Tuberculosis of the respiratory system		−1.04	−1.12	0.30	0.14
Difference[c]		10.31	12.33	6.91	6.98
Expectation of Life at Birth	Norway	56.41	59.32	70.85	74.38
	Italy	45.89	46.79	63.71	67.24

[a] Infectious diseases (except tuberculosis of the respiratory system); bronchitis, pneumonia, and influenza; diarrhoea and enteritis; diseases of infancy and early childhood.
[b] The same as [a]except diarrhoea and enteritis.
[c] See Table 4.3.

However, the English excess mortality from circulatory diseases and neoplasms began later for women, and was less marked than for men. There was practically no difference between the fates of women in England, Wales and Italy at the beginning of the modern phase of the transition and towards the end of the period, the English disadvantage amounted to only six months (compared with 2 years for men). This was the reason why the differences between the expectations of life of women in England and those of Italian women were higher than the corresponding figures for men—8 years at the beginning of the transition, and 3.5 years in 1951, compared with 6 and 2 years respectively.

5. The Three Stages of the Health Transition

In spite of the absence of data which would enable us to trace the beginnings and the path of the transition in different European countries, some general conclusions emerge from the analysis of available data.

In the first place, the relationship between the patterns of mortality of the transition and economic and social development and living standards explains the differences in the timing of the transition in different countries. Both changes in mortality patterns and social and economic development resulting from the industrial revolution, and the consequent improvement in living standards occurred later in southern Europe (represented here by Italy).

Equally, the specific pattern of the transition in some countries in which the industrial revolution began earliest (represented here by England and Wales) and which consisted of an early decline, followed by a period of constant mortality and a second period of decline, can be explained if we look at specific causes of death. The positive results which were achieved during the second half of the eighteenth and the beginning of the nineteenth centuries in reducing the mortality from traditional diseases[28] were cancelled by the rise in mortality from certain causes associated with the *laissez-faire* policies of the industrial revolution. Mortality from accidents, neoplasms, circulatory disease, and respiratory disease was higher in that country at the time when statistics of causes of death began to be collected, than previously. It was only through political intervention in the economic field (reduction of working hours, improvement of conditions at the workplace), social policy (housing), and public-health measures (improvements in water supply and sewerage, but also vaccination and new forms of treatment such as the isolation of tuberculosis patients) that these effects could be overcome, and a new and a more dynamic phase of the transition began. However, this stage has not resulted in overcoming the problems posed by cancer, or by diseases of the circulatory system in adult men.

Only in countries in which economic development began early, but proceeded slowly, did the risk of dying decline continuously, but again slowly. Even in those countries death rates from diseases of the circulatory

[28] McKeown, op. cit. in n. 5.

system and from neoplasms increased. For instance, in Norway where the expectation of life at birth increased by 14.5 years for men and by 15 years for women between 1910 and 1951, the effect of neoplasms and circulatory disease reduced this gain by about six months for each sex.

In spite of the differences in the beginning, development, and duration of the transition in different countries, some fundamental features are common to all: the major part played by the reduction of mortality from infectious and acute diseases, particularly among the young; the concentration of mortality on causes due to degenerative diseases, caused in part by heavier mortality from these diseases, but mainly by the reduction in deaths from other causes; the change in the age pattern of mortality caused by the success of the struggle against infant and childhood mortality, so that the importance of mortality at older ages increases.

The essential features of the transformation were complete by the time Europe had recovered from the ravages of the Second World War. By 1951 differences between life expectancies in the three countries had been much reduced and their mortality patterns were set. The beginnings of a new phase could be seen. This was characterized by the difficulties in containing the rise of mortality from neoplasms, achieving a fall in the mortality from diseases of the circulatory system, as well as an increase in mortality from traffic accidents. These were the main reasons which led to a reduction of the advantages which had been enjoyed for centuries by the peoples of west Europe in comparison with those of the south. Differences in expectations of life continued to diminish and, for men, reversed within less than 20 years, and the countries of southern Europe were in the van of the advance by the end of the 1960s.

5 Tuberculosis and the Decline of Mortality in Sweden

BI PURANEN *Institutet för Framtidsstudier, Stockholm*

During the last two centuries mortality has fallen substantially in all European countries. More than two-thirds of this decline is due to a reduction in deaths from infectious diseases, of which tuberculosis was by far the most important.[1] In this paper, we shall discuss the reasons for the decline in the importance of this disease. Has this change been caused by improvements in the standard of living, by medical interventions, or possibly by a change in virulence of the causative organism?

There are many problems in tracing movements in the death rate from tuberculosis over time and in different countries, or in undertaking longitudinal studies within one country. However, this type of study is possible for Sweden over the last 200 years.

1. Aims and Objects

Tuberculosis primarily attacks the lungs, but it can develop in all parts of the human body. Between 80 and 90 per cent of all known cases are pulmonary tuberculosis, because of the way in which this disease is transmitted. It is spread primarily by infection from person to person, by droplet infection, or indirectly through bacteria in the milk, dust, etc.[2] The degree

[1] There is considerable disagreement about the level, trend, and timing. See e.g. T. McKeown, *The Modern Rise of Population* (London, 1976), p. 64; id., R. G. Brown, and R. G. Record, 'An Interpretation of the Modern Rise of Population in Europe', *Population Studies*, 26(3) (1972), p. 348; T. McKeown and R. G. Record, 'Reasons for the Decline of Mortality in England and Wales during the Nineteenth Century', *Population Studies*, 16(2) (1962), p. 103; T. McKeown, R. G. Record, and R. D. Turner, 'An Interpretation of the Decline of Mortality in England and Wales during the Twentieth Century', *Population Studies*, 29(3) (1975), and the criticisms by Preston and others. S. H. Preston, *Mortality Patterns in National Populations with Special Reference to Recorded Causes of Death* (New York, 1976), pp. 20, 36, 46, 82; id., N. Keyfitz, and R. Schoen, *Causes of Death: Life Tables for National Populations* (New York, 1972); R. S. Schofield, 'Review of McKeown's Book', *Population Studies*, 31(1) (1977). For further references see B. Puranen, *Tuberculosis: Occurrence and Causes in Sweden 1750–1980* (Umeå Studies in Economic History, 7, 1984), esp. ch. 4.

[2] G. P. Youmans, *Tuberculosis* (Phil., 1979); K. Styblo, J. Meijer, and I. Sutherland, 'The Transmission of Tubercle Bacilli: Its Trend in Human Populations', *Bulletin of the International Union against Tuberculosis*, 1 (1969).

of overcrowding, and housing standards, are therefore important factors in its transmission. Well-nourished individuals are substantially more resistant to the disease than those suffering from malnutrition.

Like most other biological phenomena, tuberculosis occurs in waves. Changes in its incidence may be regarded as an immunological process, a natural selection due primarily to improved immunity.[3]
In this paper we shall discuss the following hypotheses:

1. the prevalence of tuberculosis in a given society is governed by immunological processes which result in epidemic waves;
2. variations in the death rate from tuberculosis can be explained by changes in the standard of living.

To treat these hypotheses adequately we shall need to examine:

(*a*) the possibility of measuring deaths from tuberculosis in the past;
(*b*) trends in mortality from tuberculosis;
(*c*) stability in the age and sex distribution of tuberculosis;
(*d*) possible changes in the virulence of the tubercle bacillus.

We shall discuss these problems in sections 2 to 5 of this chapter. In the following two sections we shall consider the principal explanations: the efficiency of acquired immunity and the standard of living. Finally, we shall deal with the role played by medical intervention, before reaching a conclusion.

2. Validity and Reliability

It is possible to make rough estimates of the changes in the death rate from tuberculosis in Sweden and Finland over the last 230 years by combining time-series from different sources. It will, of course, be necessary to make allowances for differences in the reliability of the sources and for the inevitable changes that have occurred in diagnostic practices over so long a period of time.[4]

[3] M. Turner, *Immunology of the Lung* (London, 1978); R. Y. Keers, *Pulmonary Tuberculosis* (London, 1978).

[4] There was an extensive discussion at the Royal Statistical Society in London about these problems. See G. B. Longstaff, 'The Recent Decline in the English Death Rate considered in Connection with the Causes of Death', *Journal of the Royal Statistical Society*, 97 (1884). This was followed by many others. See e.g. O. Dammer, *Handwörterbuch der öffentlichen und privaten Gesundheitspflege* (Stuttgart, 1891); S. Phillips, 'A Review of Mortality Statistics during the Last Half Century', *Clinical Journal*, 30 (1908); J. Brownlee, *An Investigation into the Epidemiology of Phthisis in Great Britain and Ireland* (Medical Research Committee: Special Report Series, London, 1918); F. Prinzing, *Handbuch der Medizinischen Statistik* (Jena, 1931); W. P. D. Logan, 'Mortality in England and Wales from 1848 to 1947', *Population Studies*, 4(2) (1950); I. Sutherland, 'John Graunt: A Tercentenary Tribute', *Journal of the Royal Statistical Society*, 126(4) (1963); D. V. Glass and D. E. C. Eversley, *Population in History* (London, 1965). See also B. Puranen, *Folksiukdomarna: Vägar till nuet 1800–1945* (Uppsala, 1984), and A. E. Imhof, *Aspekte der Bevölkerungsentwicklung in den Nordischen Ländern*

In the parish records, the clergy noted causes of death from around 1750. Clergymen were given training in pastoral medicine for this purpose. This was of a relatively high standard and was provided in the theological faculties. Moreover, the clergy acquired considerable empirical knowledge by meeting their parishioners regularly. The old medical treatises demonstrate how they recognized and classified different diseases, and it is possible to trace what books individual clergy had read.

Tuberculosis is a disease with relatively clear symptoms in its final stages. Its 'timetable' was well known, and the clergy could distinguish between its different phases. However, many different names were given to the disease. Pulmonary tuberculosis could be described as phthisis, consumption, haemorrhage from the lungs, pneumonia, and lung disease, among others. Only a few studies have been based on the nomenclature of the primary sources. Brugermann's book is an exception.[5] He wrote: 'chest disease is most often an early indication of tuberculosis and is therefore, distributed in a fashion which is more typical of tuberculosis, as will be discussed later.'

When mortality from pulmonary tuberculosis and other specific diseases of the chest increases, it is found that mortality from vaguer and less clearly specified diseases shows a corresponding decrease.[6] Other forms of tuberculosis, often secondary infections, were described as scrofula (inflammation and degeneration of the lymph nodes), tabes mesenterica (wasting), lupus vulgaris (infection of the skin), tubercular meningitis (brain fever), tubercular caries of the vertebrae, etc.[7] Atrophy and marasmus probably also included diseases which were of tubercular origin. In many unnamed children's diseases the tubercle bacillus contributed to the death; for instance 'convulsions' which were often given as a cause of death for children of tubercular mothers, 'water on the brain', 'hydrocephalus', etc. were probably often in reality cases of tubercular meningitis. Tuberculosis in the mother could lead to stillbirths or perinatal deaths. These connections between tuberculosis and other vaguer causes of death could be discovered only through an analysis of the family life-course.

Swedish statistics make it possible to compute comparatively accurate

1720–1750 (Berne, 1976); id., 'Die Todesursachen in Schweden und Finnland 1947–1973', in id., *Biologie des Menschen in der Geschichte* (Stuttgart, 1978), where the Scandinavian sources are discussed and compared with those in other European countries.

[5] J. Brugermann, *Der Blick des Arztes auf die Krankheit im Alltag 1779–1850* (Geschichtswissenschaften, Philosophische Fakultät der Freien Universität, Berlin, 1983), p. 263.

[6] B. Puranen, 'Dödlighet och dödsorsaker i Tuna 1805–1894, (Department of Economic History, University of Umeå, 1983); ead., 'Prästerskapets noteringar om dödsorsaker i sju socknar' (Department of Economic History, University of Umeå, 1984); also ead., op. cit. in n. 1.

[7] Scrofula and tabes mesenterica were largely diseases of the poor. See E. Lomax, 'Hereditary or Acquired Disease? Early Nineteenth-Century Debates on the Cause of Infantile Scrofula and Tuberculosis', *Journal of the History of Medicine and Allied Sciences*, 1 (1977); F. B. Smith, *The Retreat of Tuberculosis 1850–1950* (Sydney, 1988). It would be possible to use the scrofula rate as an index of deprivation.

rates of the incidence of tuberculosis, particularly of the pulmonary variety, by looking at the age distribution of deaths, the terms used by the certifying clergy, and the pattern of spread in different local areas. These primary sources can then be aggregated to reach conclusions at a wider level.[8]

3. Trends of Mortality from Tuberculosis in Sweden and Finland

The only international statistics about deaths from tuberculosis that are normally available relate to the later phases of the period, i.e. the time when the death rate from tuberculosis fell. This has led many writers to assume that the downward trend that is found in most European countries was a stable phenomenon, established in previous centuries. The figures were extrapolated backwards, to yield a relatively high estimate of the death rate from consumption during the eighteenth century.[9] However, Swedish and Finnish statistics suggest that death rates from tuberculosis during the eighteenth century were considerably lower, that the rates increased markedly during the first decades of the nineteenth century, reached a maximum, and subsequently declined. This 'rise and fall' pattern is found both in Sweden and in Finland. It raises the question whether this movement was caused by an 'epidemic wave', or by a substantial change in the standard of living of the majority of the population. In order to answer this question, it is necessary carefully to chronicle the course of events.[10]

In Finland the death rate from tuberculosis began to fall between 1861 and 1870, at first in the towns and somewhat later in the countryside. In Sweden the death rate began to fall in the towns between 1870 and 1875. Although the numbers of deaths from the disease have continued to fall in both countries since then, the rate of decline has not been even. The fall accelerated after the First World War and became even more marked after 1930. Finally, during the years after the Second World War and the introduction of chemotherapy, the number of deaths from tuberculosis fell drastically. These trends are true both of pulmonary tuberculosis and of other forms of the disease.

In Sweden mortality from tuberculosis increased slightly during the First World War and levelled out during the Second. In Finland, as in most other European countries, there was a substantial increase in mortality and morbidity from the disease during both world wars.

[8] Puranen, op. cit. in n. 1, ch. 2.

[9] McKeown, op. cit. in n. 1; R. Dubos and J. Dubos, *The White Plague: Tuberculosis, Man and Society* (London, 1953).

[10] G. Sundbärg, 'Dödligheten i lungtuberkulos i Sverige 1751–1830', *Statistisk Tidskrift*, 136 (1905).

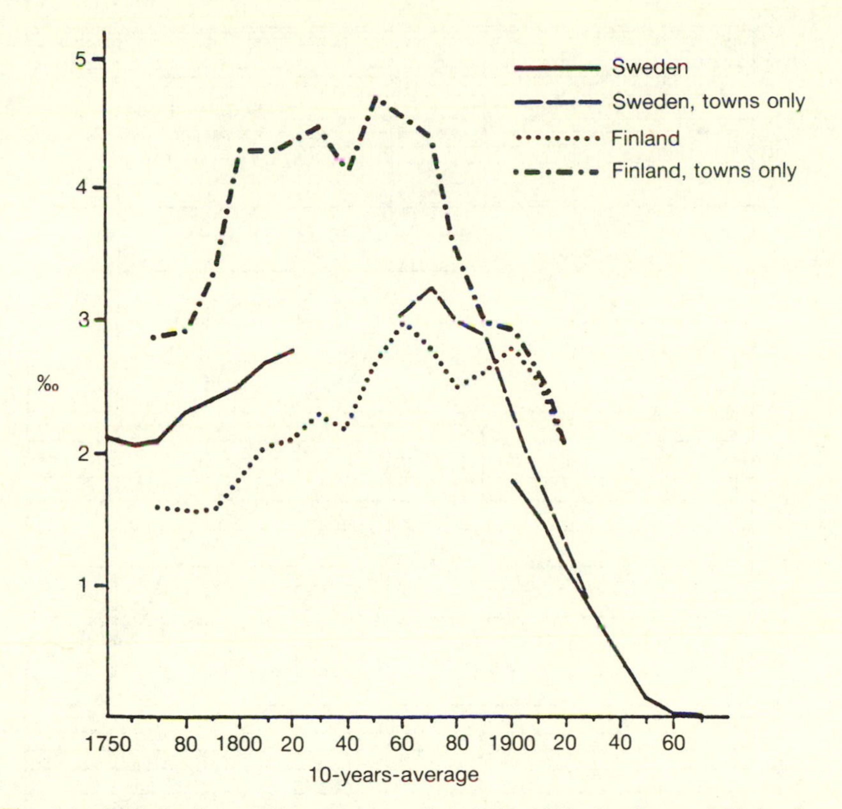

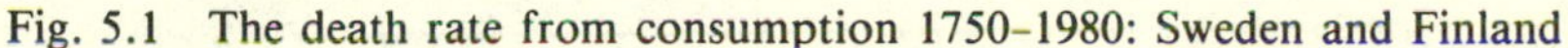

Fig. 5.1 The death rate from consumption 1750–1980: Sweden and Finland

Source: B. Puranen, 'Medicinens roll i kampen met tuberkulos och smittkoppor under tva arhundraden', *Hjärta-Kärl-Lungor*, 3 (1982), Fig. 2.

4. Mortality Differentials by Age and Sex

The question whether age and sex patterns of deaths from tuberculosis were stable over time is of vital importance for a comparison between the influence of social and immunological factors for mortality from tuberculosis.[11] In this study it is shown that the age structure of mortality

[11] In some studies based on period statistics it has been claimed that the incidence of tuberculosis had shifted to older ages. See J. Conybeare, 'The Effects on Mortality of Recent Advances in Treatment', *Journal of the Institute of Actuaries*, 73 (1947); W.P. Elderton, 'Merchant Seamen during the War', *Journal of the Institute of Actuaries*, 73 (1947); G. Dahlstrom and I. Sjögren, 'Tuberkulos', in B.G. Simonsson (ed.), *Lungsjukdomar* (Stockholm, 1967; 3rd edn., 1982). Others have claimed that there has been no such shift. See C.C. Spicer, 'The Generation Method of Analysis applied to Mortality from Respiratory Tuberculosis', *Journal of Hygiene*, 53(3) (1954); K.F. Andvord, 'What can we Learn by Studying by Generations?', *Norsk Magazin for Laegevidenskap*, 91 (1930); W.P.D. Logan and B. Benjamin, *Tuberculosis Statistics in England and Wales 1938–1955: An Analysis of Trends and Geographical Distribution* (General Register Office, London, 1957): W.H. Springett, 'An

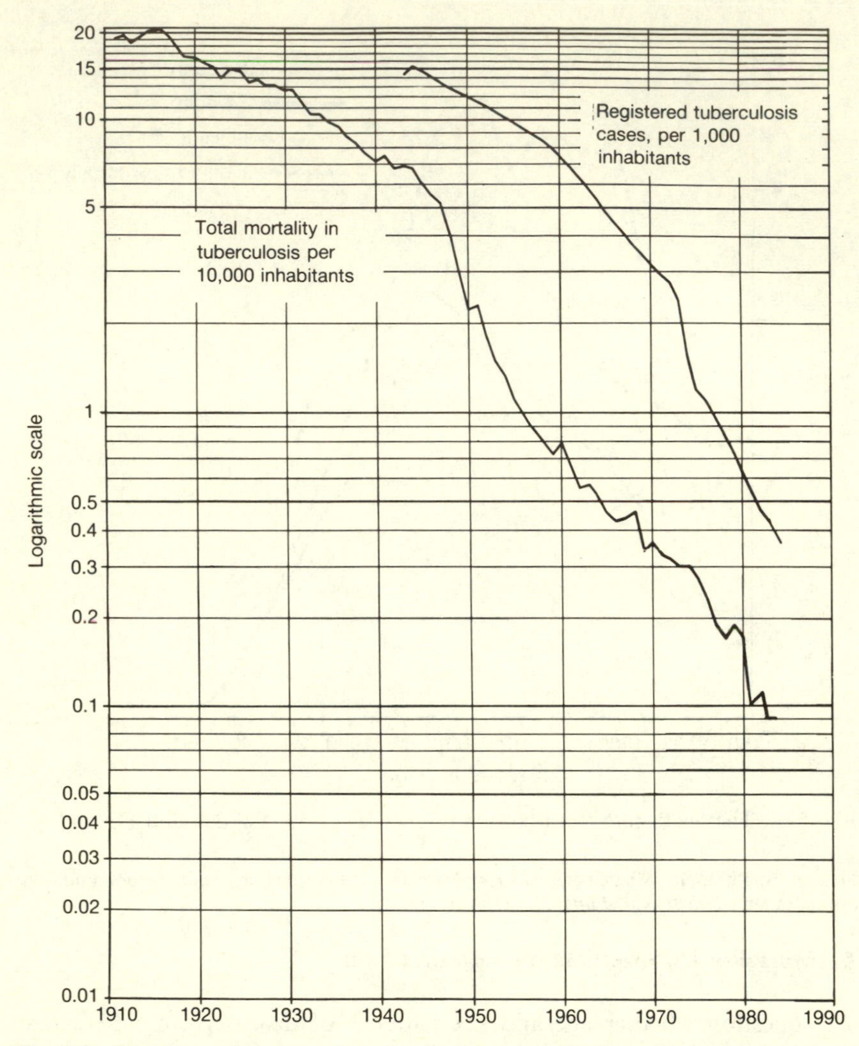

Fig. 5.2 Numbers of registered cases of tuberculosis and numbers of deaths from the disease in Sweden in relation to the whole population

from tuberculosis has been relatively constant, but that sex patterns of mortality from different kinds of tuberculosis have varied sharply. The age distribution of deaths in Sweden is one of high infant mortality, followed

Interpretation of Statistical Trends in Tuberculosis', *The Lancet* (1952) (i); R. H. Daw, 'The Trend of Mortality from Tuberculosis', *Journal of the Institute of Actuaries*, 76 (1950); W. H. Frost, 'The Age Selection of Mortality from Tuberculosis in Successive Decades', *American Journal of Hygiene*, 30 (1939); R. Malthete, 'A propos de l'âge phthisiogène', *Revue de la Tuberculose*, 10 (1946).

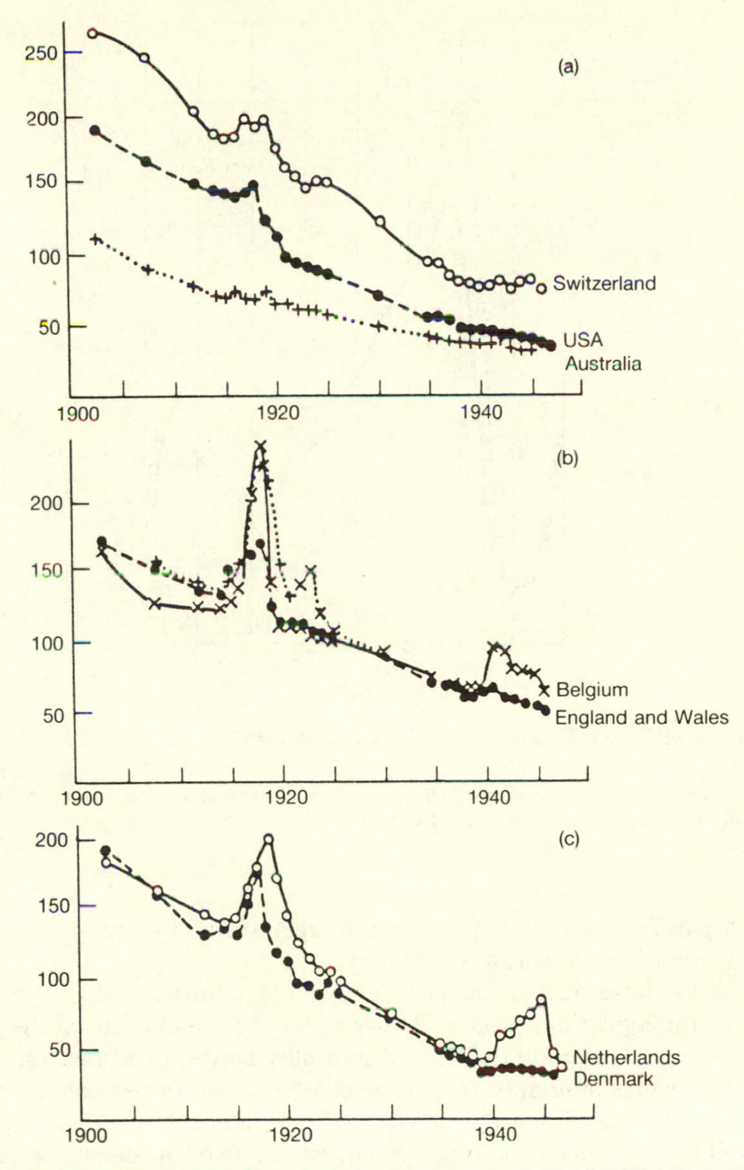

Fig. 5.3 Mortality from tuberculosis in different European countries per 100,000 population

Source: Dubos and Dubos, op. cit. in n. 9.

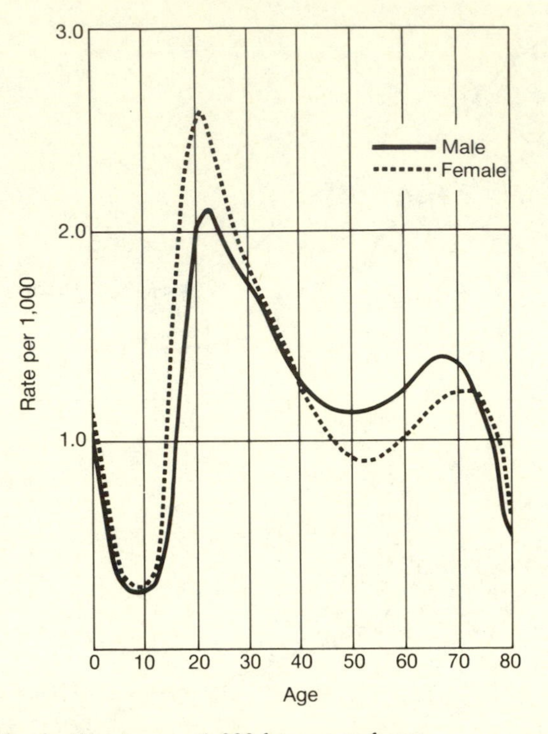

Fig. 5.4 Specific death rates per 1,000 by age and sex

Source: E. Nylen, 'Om tuberkulosdödligheten i Sverige under senare tid', *Svenska Nationalföreniugen mot tuberkulos*, 24 (1935).

by a sharp decline, particularly between the ages of 5 and 10, and succeeded by an increase in subsequent age groups.

During the latter part of the eighteenth century tuberculosis was widespread in the higher age groups. This was not due to changes in the age pattern, but to changes in the level of mortality between generations. The residual of higher mortality from tuberculosis in the earlier cohorts was larger than the peak of mortality at young ages in later cohorts. The peaking of mortality at young ages reflects the natural course of the disease. A large number of cases among the older age groups could, therefore, represent an increase in relapses caused by a general deterioration of health in these age groups.

Variations in age-specific death rates from tuberculosis are particularly pronounced for women, among whom the disease is concentrated in early youth and during their reproductive period.[12] Men predominate in the

[12] Pregnancy is a risk factor. The cell-mediated immunity is low as a result of production of corticosteroids. Cf. B. Larsen, 'Host Defensive Mechanisms in Obstetrics and Gynecology',

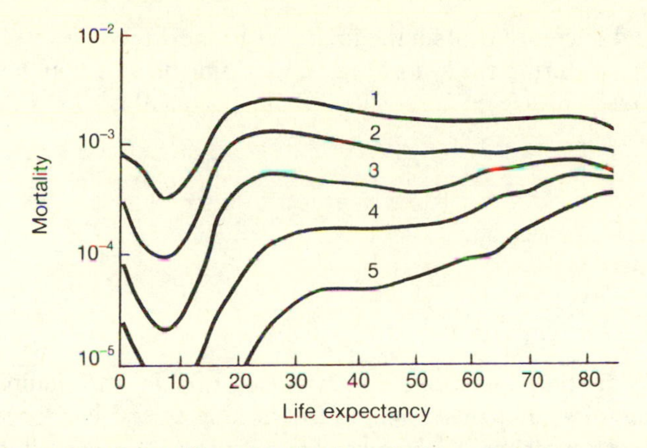

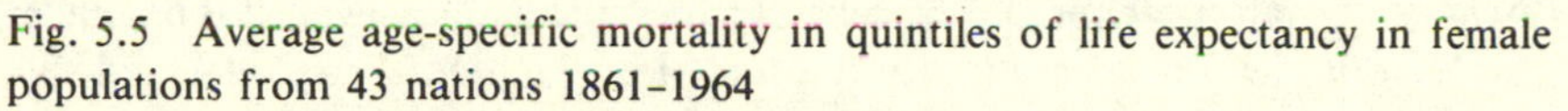

Fig. 5.5 Average age-specific mortality in quintiles of life expectancy in female populations from 43 nations 1861–1964

Note: 1st quintile: population with lowest life expectancies; 5th quintile: population with highest life expectancies.

Source: Preston, op. cit. in n. 1.

upper age groups, particularly in towns. There is also a strong correlation between life expectancy and age-specific death rates from tuberculosis. As is shown in Fig. 5.5, tuberculosis death rates among younger women are higher in populations in which life expectancy is low. In populations with high life expectancies, tuberculosis death rates seem to be higher in the older age groups.

5. Changes in Virulence

Changes in virulence have been put forward as an explanation of changes in the overall mortality rate.[13] No such changes in virulence of the tubercle bacillus have been demonstrated. The production of BCG vaccine from weakened bacilli of bovine tuberculosis, and resistance developed as a result of chemotherapy both suggest that the virulence of the tubercle bacillus has been very stable. Nor is it likely that changes in virulence should have occurred simultaneously throughout the Western world. Such a shift would

Clinics in Obstetrics and Gynecology, 10 (1983), pp. 39, 51 ff.; H. Alexander, 'Tuberkulose und Schwangerschaft', *Zeitschrift für Tuberkulose*, 83 (1939), p. 71; A. Grisolle, 'De l'influence que la grossesse et la phthisie pulmonaire exercent réciproquement l'une sur l'autre', *Archives générales de médecine*, 22 (1941), p. 41; E. Bovin, 'Om graviditet och lungtuberkulos', *Hygiea*, 95 (1933), p. 24.

[13] E.A. Wrigley and R.S. Schofield, *The Population History of England 1541–1871* (London, 1981), p. 46.

also make it difficult to explain the increases in mortality from tuberculosis which occurred during the wars (Fig. 5.3). Epidemics in populations that were previously protected also show that the bacillus can still be very virulent.[14]

6. Immunity

6.1 Acquired Immunity

Sufferers from some infectious diseases, e.g. measles or smallpox, enjoy lifelong immunity, and this explains the decline in the incidence of such diseases after an epidemic. In the case of tuberculosis, however, it is not clear how strong acquired immunity is and how patients are affected by immunizing measures.[15] The long-term effects of the new bacteriocidal chemotherapy are also unknown. In earlier generations, few Europeans escaped exposure to the disease. It is known from the reports of school medical officers, Mantoux tests, sputum tests, and X-rays that most children gave a positive reaction, before the introduction of BCG vaccination. The high incidence of tuberculosis in older age groups which can be documented over a period of 230 years in Sweden can be explained as being due to reinfections, i.e. cases in which the immunity that had been acquired did not last for very long.[16]

We find another interesting pattern if we look at new cases in Sweden broken down by age and nationality. New cases of tuberculosis in the younger age groups are found predominantly among immigrants, and there is a trend towards the higher age groups in the new cases diagnosed among Swedes. This phenomenon can be explained by differences between the incidence and prevalence of the disease in Sweden and in the immigrants' countries of origin.

The number of immune individuals in a society will depend on the number of occurrences of the disease in earlier generations and on the duration of acquired immunity. When a society is affected by tuberculosis for the first time, the course of the disease is acute and highly lethal. It takes at least a century for a disease such as tuberculosis to pass from an epidemic stage to an endemic one. The number of immune individuals is small. Many people are infected, but the course of the disease is slower and more chronic. Natural selection and child immunity are important at this stage.

[14] A.A. Rich, *The Pathogenesis of Tuberculosis* (Springfield, Ill., 1951), pp. 899 ff.

[15] M.B. Lurie, *Resistance to Tuberculosis: Experimental Studies in Native and Acquired Mechanisms* (Cambridge, Mass., 1964), ch. 2.

[16] Reinfection could be the result of an old infection (endogenous), or reinfection from an active case (exogenous). The proportions of these two types are unknown.

In most European countries, the second phase of the model was reached during the 1940s when effective chemotherapy was introduced. Populations had not yet reached the stage when acquired immunity predominated. The question arises whether such a stage would ever have been reached, if the natural history of the disease had been allowed to develop. The situation in many developing countries today suggests that acquired immunity to tuberculosis is neither sufficiently strong nor sufficiently long lasting.[17]

6.2 The 'Swedish Indians'—A Virgin Population?

During the latter part of the nineteenth and the beginning of the twentieth century, the death rate from tuberculosis increased substantially in the northernmost two-thirds of Sweden, known as Norrland. Around the turn of the century, that part of the country became rapidly industrialized, the principal industries were material-based, such as lumber and mining. Within a few decades Norrland changed from being a rather unimportant outpost into an area of substantial economic importance for the country. The situation was compared with that of the Klondyke, and parallels drawn with the position in North America.

One explanation of the high incidence of tuberculosis in that area is that the railway workers, miners, and workers in the sawmills who came to northern Sweden brought the disease with them, and spread it among the native population which was lacking immunity, in much the same way as happened with the American Indians, Eskimos, and other remote populations.[18]

This hypothesis can be confirmed or rejected by looking at the cause-of-death patterns for northern Sweden. A study of 54 parishes in northern Sweden shows that tuberculosis was endemic there from at least 1750, and that its incidence remained considerable 150 years later. The death rate from tuberculosis was between 3 and 3.5 per 1,000, and tuberculosis caused some 25 per cent of all deaths during the middle of the eighteenth century. Both the total death rate, and the death rate from tuberculosis then fell, but relative figures remained high.[19] The pattern of cause mortality in Norrland was very similar to that in the rest of the country, suggesting that the level of market integration was much higher than had been predicted and that there were unlikely to be many people who had not come into contact with the disease previously.

The incidence of tuberculosis and the high level of this disease among the elderly in the population suggest that changes in the standard of living,

[17] K. Styblo, 'The Number of Cases of Tuberculosis throughout the World', in WHO, *Defeat TB Now and For Ever* (Geneva, 1982).

[18] F. Henschen, *Sjukdormanas historia och geografi* (Stockholm, 1962), pp. 102 ff.; M.O. Burnet and D.O. White, *Natural History of Infectious Disease*. (4th edn. Cambridge, 1975) pp. 218 ff.; Imhof (1978), op. cit. in n. 4., p. 16.

[19] Puranen, op. cit. in n. 1., pp. 224 ff.

rather than immunological changes, were principally responsible for the changes in mortality from the disease.

6.3 Genetic Inheritance

Children of tubercular parents are not born with the disease; they are infected during their lifetime. It is possible, however, that they may have inherited a lower resistance to the disease.[20] It has been suggested that the decrease in the death rate from tuberculosis during the late nineteenth century was caused by an increased 'weeding out' of individuals with reduced resistance to the disease. In this way, total resistance in the population would gradually increase in successive generations. However, this theory suffers from a number of limitations.

Mortality from tuberculosis increases during times of famine and dearth. If the standard of living were to deteriorate in an area in which tuberculosis is endemic, then the death rate from the disease in the affected generation will be high. Natural selection will result in a larger proportion of the population in the succeeding generation being resistant, and the incidence of the disease will drop.

The theory also assumes that people who are infected with tuberculosis in a wartime generation will not reproduce, or that, if they did reproduce, their children would die from contagion. Such conditions may apply in some small groups, but we know that many of those infected did have children, and that even though the infant mortality of their children may have been high, a sufficient number of 'genetically affected' infants survived. Moreover, periods of crisis did not precede decreases in tuberculosis by some 30 years, as would have been expected had the theory been correct. This slow development of tuberculosis, added to the fact that large numbers of infected persons did manage to reproduce, makes a genetic explanation for the decrease seem highly improbable.

This should not be taken to mean that hereditary factors were of no importance in the course of the disease. Family reconstitution studies in seven Swedish parishes have shown that the hereditary element in the disease could not be ignored.[21] In retrospective studies it is not possible to separate the effects of heredity and environment. However, twin studies have shown that monozygotic twins suffered from a higher incidence of tuberculosis, even when they had been reared apart. These studies have proved that environment alone cannot be soley responsible for a poor prognosis.[22]

[20] Rich, op. cit. in n. 14; R.R. Puffer, *Familial Susceptibility to Tuberculosis* (Cambridge, Mass., 1944); Dubos and Dubos, op. cit. in n. 9.

[21] Puranen, op. cit. in n. 1, ch. 7; ead., 'Den vita döden – inte bara fattigfolkets sjukdom', *Historiärarnas Förenings Arsskrift* (1985), pp. 19 ff.

[22] G.W. Comstock, 'Tuberculosis in Twins: A Re-Analysis of the Prophit Survey', *American Review of Respiratory Disease*, 117 (1978), pp. 621 ff.

6.4 Bovine Immunization

Immunity need not necessarily have been acquired through infection by other humans. In areas in which bovine tuberculosis was widespread, the milk also contained tubercle bacilli. Differences between age-specific mortality rates from tuberculosis in parishes in which cattle were infected and those in which they were not, may have been due to this type of immunization. In parishes in which bovine tuberculosis was widespread, infant mortality from the disease was higher, but the overall death rates from the disease were lower than in others.[23] Bovine tuberculosis caused increased infant mortality from tuberculosis, but also provided some degree of protection against infection in later life to those who survived the primary infection.

7. The Effect of Changes in the Standard of Living

Differences in standard of living affect both exposure and resistance. Factors that increase exposure simultaneously reduce resistance. A high degree of overcrowding often went together with sub-standard housing, in which draughts and general lack of hygiene combined to affect the inhabitants' health and thus increased the risk of infection or relapse. Nutrition was another crucial factor.

7.1 The Relation between Pulmonary Tuberculosis and Poor Nutrition

People who enjoy a good diet are far more resistant to tuberculosis than those who suffer from malnutrition or whose diet is poor. Protein deficiency is particularly dangerous, especially a deficiency of animal proteins.[24] A reduction of nutritional intake would thus be expected to lead to an

[23] Puranen, op. cit. in n. 1, pp. 234 ff; I. Sjögren and I. Sutherland, 'Studies of Tuberculosis in Man in Relation to Infection in Cattle', *Tubercle*, 56 (1974), pp. 113 ff.

[24] See e.g. J. Marche and H. Grunelle, 'The Relation of Protein Scarcity and Modification of Blood Protein to Tuberculosis among Undernourished Subjects', *Milbank Memorial Fund Quarterly*, 28 (1950); I. Leitch, 'Diet and Tuberculosis', *Proceedings of the Nutrition Society* 3 (1945), p. 156; J. Downes, 'An Experiment in the Control of Tuberculosis among Negroes', *Milbank Memorial Fund Quarterly*, 28 (1950), p. 127; C.E. Palmer, S. Jablon, and P.Y. Edwards, 'Tuberculosis Morbidity of Young Men in Relation to Tuberculin Sensitivity and Body Build', *American Review of Tuberculosis*, 76 (1957), p. 517. As is shown in Fig. 5.3, the death rate from tuberculosis increased in both world wars. It doubled in Germany in 1946, when there was an acute shortage of food. W. W. Siebert, 'Beobachtungen über den jetztigen Verlauf der Tuberkulose', *Ärztliche Wochenschrift*, 1 (1946), p. 134; E. Grafe, 'Unternährung und Krankheit', *Deutsche Medizinische Wochenschrift*, 75 (1950), p. 44. The same phenomenon was noted in Denmark, when the Danes were forced to export their agricultural produce during the First World War. K. Faber, 'Tuberculosis and Nutrition', *Acta Tuberculosis Scandinavia*, 12 (1938), p. 289.

increased incidence of tuberculosis in societies in which the disease is endemic. A decrease in the incidence presupposes—at least for the period preceding modern chemotherapy and to some extent even later—higher nutritional standards.

The increase in the death rate from consumption coincided with a period when there was a high incidence of alcoholism. It has been established in modern studies that there is a clear relationship between the level of alcohol consumption and the incidence of tuberculosis, caused by poorer nutrition and a decline in general health.[25] The rise in the proportion of deaths from tuberculosis was striking; it increased from 7.2 per cent for the period 1717–80 to 11.7 per cent for 1821–30. In some areas deaths from tuberculosis amounted to between 40 and 50 per cent of all deaths. During this period, population in Sweden increased rapidly, particularly among the poorer agricultural classes. The growth of a landless proletariat was most marked in areas in which the tuberculosis rate was high, around Lake Mälaren and in southern Sweden. Later, when expansion moved to the north of the country, tuberculosis became more frequent there, whilst declining in southern and central Sweden.

7.2 The Exceptional Situation in Stockholm

Living conditions in the Swedish capital Stockholm were extremely poor. During the 80 years between 1750 and 1830, mortality rates from pulmonary tuberculosis exceeded 8 per 1,000, the highest known rate registered in any major city over so long a period. More than 20 per cent of the population died from consumption.[26] During the latter part of the nineteenth century, this extremely high death rate decreased.

The influence of the social environment can be studied by looking at the death rate from pulmonary tuberculosis in groups with extremely good and extremely poor living conditions. Three groups were studied: members

[25] See A. Hangren and B. Ohnell, 'Den soicialmedicinska bakgrunden vid aktiv tuberkulos', *Socialmedicinsk Tidskrift*, 4 (1969), p. 225; A. Hanngren and P. Reizenstein, 'Malnutrition och tuberkulos', *Klinisk Nutrition* (1968), pp. 220 ff.; M. Karvonen, 'Tuberkulooosin alueelliset piirteet Oulin läänissa', *Oulun Yliopisto* (1980), pp. 42 ff.

[26] In an epidemiological report carried out for the League for Nations in 1931 the figures for all European capitals were summarized for the preceding decades. In Budapest the death rate was also 0.008, and in another study it has been shown that the figures were equally high in Vienna during the 1860s. See S. Peller 'Mortality, Past, Present, and Future', *Population Studies*, 1 (1947–48), pp. 437 ff.; S. Peller, 'Zur Kenntnis der städtischen Mortalität im 18. Jahrhundert mit besonderer Berücksichtigung der Säuglings und Tuberkulosesterblichkeit', *Zeitschrift für Hygiene und Infektionskrankheiten* (1920), pp. 227 ff; see also P. Guillaume, *La Population de Bordeaux au XIXe siècle* (Paris, 1972), pp. 138 ff.; P. Pierrard, *La Vie ouvrière à Lille sous le second empire* (Paris, 1965), p. 138; J. Lehmann, *Dödeligheten af lungesvindsot i Kiöbenhavn* (Copenhagen, 1882), p. 8; L. Bollinger, 'Über Schwindsucht-sterblichkeit in verschiedenen Städten Deutschlands', *Münchener Medizinische Wochenschrift*, 42 (1895); G.H. Dovertie, 'Om lungsotens frekquens i Sveriges städer', *Hygiea*, 48 (1896), p. 393.

of the royal court, poor women inmates at Sabbatsberg Poorhouse, and prisoners at Norrmalms Women's Prison.[27]

All causes of death among members of the court between 1749 and 1860 were studied. Members of the court were divided into six social categories, so that members of the royal family were distinguished from courtiers, and these in turn from other groups of royal servants. Soldiers, the royal guards, and the king's artists were also assigned to special categories. Consumption was a common cause of death in all these categories, not excluding the royal family.[28] An examination of the court's expenditure on food shows that these highly placed individuals enjoyed a nutritionally good diet. In spite of this, members of the court were not able to resist the attacks of the tubercle bacillus. It would, therefore, appear that the part played by nutrition in relation to tuberculosis should not be exaggerated in a society where there is a high general risk of exposure to the disease. Nutrition was fairly good, even in the poorhouse and the prison. But both these institutions were badly overcrowded. Women in the poorhouse tended to be old and sick when they entered the institution, but the prisoners were often young and healthy women. But the prison journals show that their medical condition deteriorated after their reception into prison. A majority of them died before completing their sentences. The number of deaths from pulmonary tuberculosis and other deficiency diseases during the first half of the nineteenth century was very high—about 50 per cent.

During the period studied, there was a substantial improvement in nutrition, but all other conditions remained unchanged. There does not appear to have been a decisive change in the mortality from tuberculosis before and after the changes in nutrition occurred. The groups we studied were extremes. But the conclusion that exposure to the disease, rather than nutritional status, was the decisive factor that determined the mortality rate from tuberculosis may well hold true for larger populations. Pulmonary tuberculosis was the largest killer in all the poorer areas of Stockholm.

7.3 Urbanization

Another important factor that led to a high death rate from tuberculosis was rapid urbanization,[29] which considerably increased the risk of exposure.

[27] Puranen, op. cit. in n. 1, ch. 10.

[28] Mortality and esp. infant mortality were, however, lower among the aristocracy. See I. Elmorth, *För kung och fosterland: Studier i den svenska adelns demografi och öffentliga funktion 1600–1900* (Lund, 1981), pp. 130 ff.; Also compare the situation with that of the aristocracy in Britain, as shown by T.H. Hollingsworth, *The Demography of the British Peerage Population Studies*, 18, suppl. (1964), pp. 52 ff.

[29] Even though most towns were *villes rurales* (F. Braudel, *Civilisation matérielle et capitalisme* (Paris, 1967), p. 373; A.E. Imhof, 'Der agrare Charakter der Schwedischen und Finnischen Städte im 18. Jahrhundert im Vergleich zu Mittel und Westeuropa', *Akademie für Raumforschung und Landesplanung*, 88 (1974), p. 197), there were considerable differences between the death rates from tuberculosis. See also T. Shimao, 'Studies on Tuberculosis

However, the situation differed in different towns, the size of the town's population, the difference between the death rate from tuberculosis in the town and the surrounding countryside, and the proportion of the population employed in industry, were all important factors.

Mortality from tuberculosis was higher in a small town situated in an area in which tuberculosis was more frequent, than in a large town with a lower incidence of the disease. However, once the size of the town reaches a certain threshold (more than 50,000 inhabitants), size alone becomes the dominant factor. Until the mid-1930s tuberculosis rates were higher in the towns, but after 1936 the situation was reversed. Within ten years the tuberculosis rate was far lower in the towns than in rural areas.

There was a shift in other European countries as well, with rural rates beginning to exceed urban ones.[30] But there was no consistent pattern, though the degree of industrialization appears to have played a decisive part.[31]

7.4 The Level of Industrialization

In the course of half a century, an overwhelmingly agrarian country was transformed into an industrialized nation. The modernization of Sweden roughly coincides with the industrial breakthrough of the period 1870–1920. This was also a turning-point in the trend of tuberculosis, and mortality from the disease gradually declined over this period.

There are some obvious connections between tuberculosis and the level of industrialization. Thus, during the last decades of the nineteenth century, the highest proportions of workers employed in industry and the highest number of deaths from tuberculosis occurred in the iron and steel town of Eskilstuna. The neighbouring areas were also dominated by the same type of iron and steel industries, but tuberculosis rates were significantly lower.[32] This illustrates the fatal effects of a combination of certain kinds of industrial employment and urbanization.

Members of some occupations, such as metalworkers, smiths, and tailors were at higher risk than others. In the Eskilstuna study, morbidity from tuberculosis among grinders was five times as high as in other groups.[33]

Mortality in Sweden', *Acta Tuberculosis Scandinavia*, 32 (1956), Fig. 3, and also Fig. 5.1 in this vol.

[30] J.E. Backer, *Dödeligheten og dens arsaker i Norge 1856–1955* (Oslo, 1961), pp. 210 ff.; J.A. Verdoorn, *Volksgezondheid en sociale ontwikkeling: Beschouwingen over het gezondheitswesen te Amsterdam in de 19e eeuw* (Antwerp, 1982), pp. 52 ff.; L.J. Whitney, *Death Rates by Occupation based on Data of the US Census Bureau* (New York, 1930).

[31] G. Wolff, 'Tuberculosis Mortality and Industrialisation', *American Review of Tuberculosis*, 42 (1940), vols i, p. 26, and ii, *passim*.

[32] Puranen, op. cit. in n. 1.

[33] Ibid. pp. 282 ff. Cf. also contemporary studies in Germany, e.g. C.F. Favell, 'Grinders' Diseases', *Schmidts Jahrbuch*, 52 (1846), pp. 164 ff.; A. Oldendorff, 'Die Mortalitäts und Morbiditäts Verhältnisee der Metallschleifer in Solingen und Umgegend, sowie in Remscheid und Kronenberg' *Allgemeine Gesundheitspflege* (1882), pp. 230 ff.

There is also a clear relationship between tuberculosis, pneumoconiosis, and other diseases of the lung.[34] But alcoholism, housing standards, and nutrition were also important factors in Eskilstuna.

7.5 Housing

Overcrowding was serious, and not only in the towns. We know that the tubercle bacillus can survive in dust and dirt for a long time, so that overcrowding and poor hygiene are fatal factors in the disease.[35]

By studying the effects of the remodelling of an old mining village in Norrland into a modern town, we can measure the effect of changes in housing conditions. Before 1910 tuberculosis was widespread in the population of Kiruna, nutrition was poor, and working conditions bad. A thorough medical study was undertaken to show the exact situation relating to tuberculosis before the housing programme was begun. Another study in 1920 showed that there had been a significant change. Most of the children tested gave negative results, i.e. they had not been contaminated with the tubercle bacillus.[36]

In some coastal villages in northern Sweden, the disease was found in almost half the farms (48 per cent). The living conditions of the inhabitants and their general standard of health were investigated, and all the means to combat tuberculosis that were known at the time were then applied. The most important was to change the quality of housing. The old typical beds, with walls, a roof, and a little door to keep the cold out were demolished. The old habit of nailing up windows during the winter was abandoned. Attempts were made to prevent men from spitting on the floor and to educate the population in matters of hygiene. All these efforts resulted in a considerable drop in the morbidity from tuberculosis in the experimental area, compared with similar villages nearby.

8. Medical Intervention

Medical intervention has traditionally been treated separately when the decline in mortality is explained.[37] But we can regard improvements in

[34] A. Ahlmark, T. Bruce, and A. Nyström, *Silicosis and Other Pneumoconioses in Sweden* (Stockholm, 1960), ch. 2.

[35] Several investigations were carried out in Britain around the mid-19th cent. Cf. E. Chadwick, *Report on the Sanitary Condition of the Labouring Population of Great Britain* (London, 1842); L. Villerme, *Tableau de l'état physique et moral des ouvriers employés dans les manufactures du coton, de laine, et de soie* (Paris, 1840). See also P. Stocks, 'The Association between Mortality and Density of Housing', *Proceedings of the Royal Society of Medicine*, 2 (1934); L. Stein, 'Tuberculosis and the Social Complex in Glasgow', *British Journal of Social Medicine*, 6 (1952), and J. A. Burnett, *A Social History of Housing 1815–1870* (London, 1978) for further refs.

[36] G. Neander, *Tuberkulosens utbredning bland befolkningen i Kiruna* (Socialhygieniska studier och meddelarden, 1: Stockholm, 1910); G. Frank, *Kiruna 1900–1950* (Eskilstuna, 1950).

[37] T. McKeown and R.G. Brown, 'Medical Evidence relating to English Population

Table 5.1 Death rates from tuberculosis in the experimental area, compared with those in neighbouring areas, Norrbotten country, and Sweden

Area	Death rates from tuberculosis per 1,000		Percentage decrease
	1911–15	1921–25	
Experimental area	8.30	6.00	27.7
Neighbouring areas	3.99	3.97	0.5
Norrbotten county	3.29	2.93	10.9
Sweden	1.94	1.46	24.7

Source: G. Neander, *Anstalten Hälsan i Norrbottenoch studier över tuberkulosens utbredning i Sverige* (Stockholm, 1927), p. 98.

preventive care and therapy as improvements in the standard of living. If the issue is broadened to include attitudes towards public health and hygiene, the pattern becomes more complex. We shall consider direct medical intervention here. This took considerable resources for the provision of facilities and research. Private initiatives also played an important part, and we can identify three phases in the organization of tuberculosis therapy: traditional sanatorium therapy, surgical/instrumental treatment, and chemotherapy.

8.1 Sanatoriums

Towards the beginning of the century there existed only a very small number of specialized institutions for the care of tuberculosis patients. However, during the first decades of the twentieth century, the number of sanatoriums expanded rapidly. Treatment was based principally on fresh air, rest, and good nutrition.[38]

8.2 Surgical Measures

Treatment by pneumothorax became more widely used. This involved collapsing part or the whole of the diseased lung with the aid of nitrogen gas in order to allow the lung to rest, and so to facilitate the healing process. The method was later refined and combined with other surgical measures,

Changes in the Eighteenth Century', *Population Studies*, 9(2) (1955); T. McKeown, *Medicine in Modern Society* (London, 1965); id., *The Role of Medicine: Dream, Mirage or Nemesis?* (London, 1979); L. Thomas, *The Youngest Science* (New York, 1983); J. McKinley and S. McKinley, 'The Questionable Contribution of Medical Measures to the Decline of Mortality in the United States in the Twentieth Century', *Milbank Memorial Fund Quarterly* (1977); S. Mushkin *Biomedical Research: Cost and Benefit* (Cambridge, Mass., 1979).

[38] Smith, op. cit. in n. 7, ch. 4.

such as thoraco-plastic surgery, which involved the removal of a number of ribs. It also involved collapsing the affected lung to allow it to rest. It was not until 1950 that parts of the lung affected by tuberculosis were surgically removed. Earlier surgery often resulted in the disablement of the patients.

8.3 Preventive Measures

In addition to therapy, a wide range of preventive measures was applied.[39] Amongst them was the Calmette vaccine (BCG) which was introduced into Sweden in the 1920s, but its use was not widespread until the 1950s when more than 90 per cent of the population were covered by vaccination.[40]

Detection and diagnosis of the disease at public infirmaries was another preventive measure used in the struggle against tuberculosis. The use of mass X-rays which enabled large numbers of people to be screened also led to the more rapid detection of the disease, and, in addition, helped to limit its spread. Legislation making notification and treatment of the disease compulsory also played a decisive part.

8.4 Chemotherapy

A dramatic change occurred during the 1940s. For the first time in the long history of the disease, drugs were developed which were able to defeat the bacillus. At approximately the same time, two such drugs were discovered: PAS (para-amino-salicylic acid) and streptomycin. These discoveries by the Swede Jörgen Lehmann and the American Selman Waksman respectively were of historic importance.[41]

Ten years later, in 1952, a third drug INH (izoniazid) was discovered. Further advances have been made in this field, and a drug such as rifampicin not only limits the growth of the bacillus (bacteriostatic effect), but kills it

[39] The National Association against Tuberculosis initiated some hitherto untried preventive measures. Tuberculosis became a 'model disease': B. Puranen, 'Medicinens roll i kampen met tuberkulos och smittkoppor under tva arhundraden', *Hjärta-Kärl-Lungor*, 3 (1982); (also, ead., op. cit. in n. 1, ch. 10).

[40] A. Wallgren, 'Observations critiques sur la vaccination antituberculeuse de Calmette', *Acta Pediatrica*, 7 (1928), pp. 120 ff.; 'Le Rôle de la vaccination antituberculeuse dans la lutte contre la tuberculose infantile', *Acta Pediatrica*, 9 (1930), p. 410.

[41] There is some controversy about the timing and importance of these discoveries. See J. Comroe, 'Retrospectroscope, Pay Dirt: The Story of Streptomycin', *American Review of Respiratory Diseases*, 117 (1978), pp. 773 ff and 975 ff.; J. Lehmann, 'Determination of Pathogenicity of Tubercle Bacilli by their Intermediate Metabolism', *The Lancet* (1946) (i), p. 14; id., 'Twenty Years Afterwards: Historical Notes on the Discovery of the Antituberculosis Effect of Para-Amino-Salicylic Acid (PAS) and the First Clinical Trials', *American Review of Respiratory Diseases*, 90(6), (1964), p. 953; G. Birath, 'Introduction of Para-Amino-Salicylic Acid and Streptomycin in the Treatment of Tuberculosis', *Scandinavian Journal of Respiratory Disease*, 50 (1969), pp. 204 ff.; K. Toman, *Tuberculosis Case Finding and Chemotherapy* (WHO, Geneva, 1979), p. 75.

(bacteriocidal effect). By combining drugs that attack the disease in different ways, the emergence of bacterial resistance can be effectively avoided.[42]

8.5 The Effect of Medical Intervention

A classic argument in this field is that the decline in the incidence of different infectious diseases came much earlier than therapeutic measures, and that the latter, therefore, did not play a decisive part.[43] The problem with this view is that there are few good indicators that can be used.[44] In this context, studies of specific diseases can be of considerable value.[45]

A comparison between the decline in the number of deaths from tuberculosis in Sweden and the fall in the overall death rate shows an interesting pattern. Between 1875 and 1917 the relationship was almost constant, i.e. the death rate from tuberculosis and the proportion of all deaths from the disease declined at almost the same rate. The influenza pandemic of 1919 naturally caused a jump in the curve. But after 1919 the death rate from tuberculosis fell substantially more quickly than the proportion of all deaths from tuberculosis. This is a significant distinction which could be interpreted as follows.

Before 1917, declines in the death rate from tuberculosis were primarily due to improvements in the standard of living, whereas after 1919 specific measures against tuberculosis began to make their impact. The relatively late beginning of this breakthrough must be seen in the context of the First World War and the negative effects of the influenza pandemic.

[42] H.F. Dowling, *Fighting Infections: Conquests of the Twentieth Century* (Cambridge, Mass., 1977); K. Bartmann, 'Chemotherapie der Tuberkulose', *Deutsches Medizinisches Journal*, 19 (1968), p. 845; id., 'Die Entwicklung der Chemotherapie für Lungentuberkulose' *Praxis der Pneumologie*, 29 (1975), pp. 705 ff.; W. Fox, 'The Modern Management and Therapy of Pulmonary Tuberculosis'. *Proceedings of the Royal Society of Medicine*, 70 (1977), p. 4 ff.; O.E. Graessle and J.J. Piotrowski, 'The *in vitro* Effect of p-amino-salicylic acid (PAS) in preventing Acquired Resistance to Streptomycin by Myobacterium Tuberculosis', *Journal of Bacteriology*, 57 (1949), p. 459.

[43] McKeown, op. cit. in n. 1; R. Dubos, *Mirage of Health* (London, 1959); id., *Man, Medicine and Environment* (New York, 1968).

[44] Stewart used drinkable water and literacy as indicators: C.T. Stewart, 'Allocation of Resources to Health', *Journal of Human Resources*, 6 (1971), pp. 103 ff. See also W. McDermott, W. Deuschle, and A. Barnett, 'Health Care Experiment at Many Farms: A Technological Misfit of Health Care and Disease Pattern existed in this Navajo Community', *Science*, 175 (1972).

[45] B. Puranen, 'Tuberkulosens opgang och fall', *IHE Information*, 3 (1985); ead., 'Aids och samspillet mellem menneske, miljö og sygdom i historisk perspektiv', in Else-Marie Sejer Larsen (ed.), *Akilleshaelen* (Copenhagen, 1986); ead., 'Tidens sjukdomar är tidens själ', *Ottar*, 1 (1986); ead., 'Via Dolorosa – epidemiernes historie', *LTV: Helse og Sosialmagasin* (1987); ead., 'Risker och rötter: Sexualitet och riskbedömning i ett historisk perspektiv', *Socialmedicisnk Tidskrift*, 5–6 (1987).

9. Conclusion

Explanations in terms of immunological processes and standards of living have different time-horizons. A quarter of a millennium, the time-span of this study, is too short for a genetic or immunological perspective. The original epidemic waves (Fig. 5.4) are continually supplemented by waves of much lower amplitudes—mini-epidemics, that are the results of changes in the patterns of conduct and standards of living. The wave we have documented in this study can be identified as such a mini-epidemic (Fig. 5.1). Whereas immunological conditions affect the trend of overall mortality, the standard of living will affect short-term fluctuations.

The amount of exposure primarily reflects living conditions, especially standards of hygiene and population density, but the occupational structure and location also play an important part. The danger of exposure is much greater in towns than in the countryside, but regional differences, too, can have an effect. Awareness of the risk of contagion, and social measures, such as the availability of sanatorium care, which prevent patients from communicating the disease to others, also affect the degree of exposure to risk.

The outcome of a primary infection—cure, sickness, or death—will depend on virulence and immunity and on other factors that affect resistance, e.g. nutrition, the level of general health, the presence or absence of other diseases, psychological stress, age, alcoholism, and others. A society's immunological status is affected not only by earlier infections but also by vaccines (BCG). Virulence, on the other hand, is difficult to change, and in the case of the tubercle bacillus no change in virulence has been demonstrated.

In brief, it has been established that the principal components of the standard of living (particularly housing and occupation) markedly influence the risk of exposure, infection, and death. These socio-economic factors affect variations in tuberculosis directly, whereas virulence and immunity operate as factors that underlie the general level of morbidity and mortality from tuberculosis.

6 Cholera: A Victory for Medicine?

PATRICE BOURDELAIS *Centre de Recherches Historiques, Paris*

Among the great epidemics of the past, cholera appears today as one of the diseases which has been conquered by advances in medicine. However, for the last 20 years a seventh pandemic of cholera has been raging in an increasing number of countries, and medical men have been unable to check its spread. It is clear that medical progress cannot have been the sole explanation for the waxing and waning of epidemic diseases, and more generally for the decline in mortality. The study of cholera epidemics from their first appearance in Europe towards the end of the first third of the nineteenth century to the present day, makes it possible to estimate how much of the increasing decline in the number of cases and of victims of the disease can be attributed directly to progress in medical knowledge and techniques and the development of new methods of protection, and how much is due to social and cultural factors. Paradoxically, during recent years improvements in medical knowledge have not necessarily resulted in improvements in public health in the short run or even the medium-long run; indeed, they may have led to a relaxation in vigilance. Does this somewhat pessimistic point of view survive an analysis of long-run changes? If a seventh pandemic were, indeed, developing, it has not, up to now, reached the developed countries. Can an historical analysis provide the reason for this development?

For a long time the development of cholera pandemics appears to have been independent of the state of medical knowledge. During the first (1817–24) and the second (1829–37) pandemics, the progress of contagion was similar in areas in which Western medicine had little influence, and in Russia or in Europe.[1] For more than a year, in 1830–31, the newspapers regularly carried stories about the progress of the disease towards north-western Europe. However, the majority of articles were reassuring, particularly in France and in Great Britain. The geographical position of the Western European countries, their temperate climate, the richness of their agriculture and industry, the standard of education in hygiene among their inhabitants, and the development of medicine were all regarded as

[1] Patrice Bourdelais and Jean Yves Raulot, *Une peur bleue: Histoire du choléra en France* (Paris, 1987).

trump cards which suggested that this disease, which had originated in barbarian regions, would yield to the forces of civilization. This optimism of a dominant Europe soon had to give way to the facts. When the epidemic did spread to Western Europe, the shock was all the greater for the disappointment experienced. There were uprisings in many countries, and the popular mood varied from anger to extreme terror.[2]

Judgements about the ways in which the disease spread were developed from observation and studies in the field, but did not depend in any way on a correct medical understanding of the nature of the illness, nor of the mechanism by which it attacked the individual. The best example of this is provided by the empirical studies of Moreau de Jonnes, who was completely ignorant of the medical causes of cholera. However, basing himself on an accurate mapping of the progress of both the first and the beginning of the second pandemic of the disease, he pointed to the importance of man in the transmission of cholera over large distances through troop movements, pilgrimages, or—more mundanely—commercial contacts. In the bitter quarrel which had been raging since the beginning of the century between those who blamed contagion and those who accepted the miasmatic theory of disease, he placed himself squarely among the former, convinced that his epidemiological observations supported their case.

During the 1820s the disease spread through all European countries, and even to North America. It led to the imposition of quarantine regulations and *cordons sanitaires*, similar to those which had been imposed earlier to prevent the spread of the plague. But there were very large differences between the measures taken in different countries to place obstacles in the way of free movement. Within a period of months the dominant theory was replaced. Little by little, particularly as a result of observations first made in Russia, an increasing number of physicians regarded the contagion hypothesis as an exaggeration. In Moscow and St Petersburg it was found for the first time that the mortality of those who cared for cholera patients was no higher than in the population as a whole, that contagion seemed less certain than in the case of plague, and lastly that *cordons sanitaires* did not always prove effective in preventing the disease from spreading. Observers did not believe that contagion affected individuals exposed to risk unequally, which might have explained their observations, and the way was, therefore, opened for the rival theory. These observations were addressed to responsible authorities in Great Britain and France by physicians from these two countries who had been sent on a study mission, first to Russia and later to Poland, on account of their pre-eminence in their profession.

At the same time, during the first half of 1831, several papers by a Moscow physician, Dr Jachnichen, seemed to contradict the views put forward by

[2] For the violence of visual presentations, cf. Patrice Bourdelais and André Dodin, *Visages du choléra* (Paris, 1987).

Moreau de Jonnes and the contagionist school.[3] It was particularly Moreau de Jonnes's report made in 1824 to the Superior Council of Public Health on the cholera outbreak in Astrakhan which appears to have convinced governments and led them to adopt rigorous public-health measures, thus placing obstacles in the way of international commerce. This reaction upset Jachnichen, who did not hesitate to write: 'the gravest aspect is the interruption of trade when ships arriving at Marseille from Odessa are forced to remain in quarantine for 40 days; is not this one of the many misfortunes that have befallen traders as a result of certain reports about this pestilence?' This preoccupation with freedom of trade seemed to justify the efforts of the Moscow physician to prove that cholera was not a contagious disease, but a disease which 'penetrated' the organism through certain foci of infection.[4]

In England, in 1830–31, the Board of Health accepted the contagion theory and imposed a quarantine period of 14 days for all ships arriving from the Baltic, and enforced an inspection of cargo, particularly of raw materials destined for the textile industry (for example, flax). More than 3,000 vessels were delayed by this costly period of quarantine. The London businessmen and the Scottish merchants protested against the levels of health taxes and the loss of profit (as the restrictions meant that ships could only be used for one round trip during the season, instead of two), although others warned the authorities against the danger of importing the cholera through bales of flax.[5] The criticism of quarantine measures was directed first against the taxes that had to be paid, later (in November and December of that year), when it became clear that the measures were not effective, criticism turned to the measures themselves. From the moment when the disease reached London (on 13 February), voices were raised to the effect that it was undesirable to add famine and misery to the effects of the epidemic by the maintenance of quarantine. This argument was taken up in most European countries by all those who opposed these measures. In Great Britain, the public-health measures were, therefore lifted in March 1832.

During the last months of 1831 mainstream opinion moved against the contagionist thesis, on the basis of reports from the afflicted countries and the experience in Britain. When the epidemic arrived in France, therefore, the large majority of the medical profession and of those responsible for policy were convinced of the uselessness of quarantine or public-health measures. The reluctance of physicians to recognize the contagious character of this disease was in part due to the pleadings of merchants and to experience abroad. In addition, the first cases in Sunderland were not diagnosed,

[3] Alexandre Moreau de Jonnes, *Rapport au conseil supérieur de santé sur le choléra-morbus pestilentiel* (Paris, 1831).

[4] Dr Jachnichen, 'Mémoire sur le choléra-morbus qui règne en Russie, Addresse de Moscou à l'Académie des Sciences', *Gazette médicale* (5 Mar. 1831).

[5] R. J. Morris, *Cholera 1832: The Social Response to an Epidemic* (London, 1976).

and the nature of later cases was kept secret for several weeks. When in July 1832 Velpeau came out publicly in favour of the contagion theory, he explained a notice which had been inserted several months earlier in the newspapers in which the physicians at the Hôpital de la Pitié affirmed that cholera was not contagious. 'After long deliberations, this note should have been signed by all of us in order to reassure the public', Velpeau revealed, and added: 'As I was not convinced by the argument, it was pointed out to me that such an announcement being purely opportunistic would not have any scientific validity. I accepted this opinion and added my signature to those of my colleagues'.[6] As in Sunderland and in a number of other regions, attempts were made to reassure the population and to maintain a minimum of social cohesion during a politically troubled period. It was therefore economic, social, and cultural, rather than medical reasons which resulted both in the imposition, and later in the lifting, of quarantine measures and *cordons sanitaires*, and which affected the development of theories of contagion or non-contagion.

However, these factors did not always lead to a suppression of quarantine or public-health measures. In June 1832, when the first cases were noted in Quebec, quarantine measures were in force in Grosse Isle between Newfoundland and Prince Edward Island. Some vessels succeeded in passing through, out of range of the guns, and entered the St Lawrence river without stopping at Grosse Isle. In June the cholera reached Quebec, and showed that the public-health *cordon* could be pierced; however, quarantine measures were not lifted. The situation was, therefore, different from that found in Europe. French Canadians were frightened of the large numbers of English immigrants and accused them of having brought the cholera with them to Lower Canada in order to destroy the population of French origin.[7] In 1831 50,000 immigrants arrived in Canada, and at least 70,000 more were expected in 1832. English-speaking Canadians interpreted the maintenance of public-health and quarantine measures which had been lifted in Europe, together with publications which stressed the difficulties of life in Canada, as indications that French Canadians wished to put whatever obstacles they could into the path of English or Irish immigrants. Whereas in Europe economic and social pressure groups had managed to have quarantine measures lifted and to declare that cholera was not a contagious disease, the opposite was true in Canada, where quarantine was maintained and movement in the interior of the territory controlled. The principal cities thus tried to defend themselves against the importation of cholera. The primitive state of medical knowledge made it possible to hold these different attitudes. What happened once the organism responsible for the cholera was identified?

[6] Cited in Bourdelais and Raulot, op. cit. in n. 1, p. 75.

[7] Geoffrey Bilson, *A Darkened House: Cholera in Nineteenth Century Canada* (Toronto, 1980).

After Koch's discovery of the cholera vibrio in 1883–84 had put an end to uncertainty about the cause of the disease, diagnosis became more sure. From 1887 onwards, large-scale bacteriological tests among travellers coming from Europe made it possible to avoid the spread of the disease to New York. Proof that strict quarantine, helped by progress in medical knowledge was efficacious in prevention was overwhelming. Koch was obviously an advocate of public-health measures and of disinfection. He proved that the vibrio could be destroyed by boiling, a fact which Moreau de Jonnes had already established in his report of 1831, when he observed that some Russian peasants boiled their drinking water during cholera epidemics, and that they seemed to be less affected by the disease than other sections of the population. Koch also recognized that disinfection with carbolic, a product produced and recommended by Pierre Alexis Boboeuf at the beginning of the fourth pandemic could be helpful.[8]

However, in spite of progress in identifying the causative agent of the epidemic, preventive measures, and bacteriological diagnosis, the fifth pandemic, though much less widespread than preceding ones, did not spare all of north-west Europe. Hamburg was at the centre of the only European area which was really affected by the epidemic. The carriers were well known. They were Russian emigrants who were forced to leave their country because of the famine of 1891–92 and because of the expulsion of the Jews, and of whom nearly 100,000 embarked for the United States in the ports of Bremen and Hamburg.[9] They crossed Germany in sealed trains which only made technical stops. Difficulties, therefore, arose only when they reached the North Sea ports. But, whereas only six deaths were recorded in Bremen, in Hamburg the total number exceeded that in all previous outbreaks of the disease taken together. And this happened in spite of the fact that medical knowledge in these two towns which were not far from one another was exactly the same.

Though science offered the same weapons to each town, the response was different. Whereas the authorities in Hamburg gave relatively little power to the physicians, lest the commercial prosperity of the city be disturbed by too stringent medical measures, the councillors in Bremen took a completely different attitude. The attention given to public health was evident by the different equipment in the two cities and by completely different intellectual attitudes. In 1871–73 a central filtration plant for water had been constructed in Bremen, with water being filtered through sand, and members of the medical profession in the city followed Koch's discoveries with great interest. They were convinced that cholera was a contagious disease, and the authorities as well as the medical profession were also persuaded of the

[8] For illustrations, cf. Bourdelais and Dodin, op. cit. in n. 2.

[9] Richard J. Evans, *Death in Hamburg: Society and Politics in the Cholera Years 1830*–1910 (Oxford, 1987).

efficacity of quarantine and isolation. A hospital was, therefore, built at Bremerhaven, yellow flags were stocked, a disinfection plant was acquired, and arrangements were made for the isolation of suspects after medical examination. From the very outset of the danger, the authorities distributed instructions to the population on measures to protect themselves efficiently against the disease. They recommended that all water and milk be boiled, that the consumption of fresh fruit should be avoided, that people should wash and disinfect their hands frequently, and avoid crowds. As regards public health, Bremen aligned herself with Prussia, because the authorities considered that a full-scale epidemic would do more damage to the city than a temporary interruption of trade.

The authorities in Hamburg took a radically different view. Their liberal ideology was opposed to giving powers to the medical profession who might act against the commercial interests of the city. The behaviour of the Hamburg Senate remained the same throughout the nineteenth century; they kept silent when the first cases of the epidemic appeared, and gave no information about its spread until the number of cases was so large that they could no longer be concealed. In this way did the local authority hope to avoid public-health measures which might have interfered with trade. In spite of Koch's discoveries, the position taken by the authorities in 1892 favoured Pettenkofer's views, which were opposed to quarantine and the isolation of sick immigrants. The adoption of a somewhat old-fashioned medical theory therefore avoided a confrontation between public-health principles and the desire to maintain freedom of trade. The Chief Medical Officer in 1892 again chose the path of silence, so that there was an interval of eight days between the appearance of the first case and the official acknowledgement of the appearance of the disease. This attitude had consequences for the efficiency of the medical personnel employed by the city; the official responsible for the medical laboratories tried in vain to isolate the cholera vibrio for more than a week, whereas one of his colleagues who was familiar with Koch's methods managed to do so within a few hours. During this long period, no preventative measures were taken, and no advice was given to the population to boil their drinking water which was extracted directly from the river Elbe. The disease, therefore, spread with great rapidity, so that Koch when visiting the city was extremely surprised both by the lackadaisical attitude of the authorities and by the deplorable sanitary and social conditions in some of the poorer quarters. He managed to persuade the authorities to distribute boiled water by using the vans of a local brewery, to close schools and public baths, and to provide instructions relating to preventative measures which the population was invited to observe. The Senate accepted Koch's instructions without great enthusiasm. It remained unconvinced of the cause of the disease which Koch had isolated eight years earlier and of the efficacity of the measures which he suggested. A vaccine had been available since 1885, and was purified by Haffkin at the

Institut Pasteur in Paris in 1892. In Hamburg, medical progress was not sufficient to convince local politicians, nor was it efficacious in preventing the spread of the disease.

After this last almost incredible episode, no further serious outbreaks of cholera have been recorded in developed countries. The First World War did not lead to a recrudescence of the sixth pandemic, probably as a result of preventive vaccination by the Germans of their troops, and of the adoption of chlorination of water by the French. Between 1920 and 1935 it seemed as if epidemic cholera had been defeated. Then, at a time when the knowledge of the carriers of the vibrio and of conditions which favoured an epidemic was more widespread than ever, after a half-century of quiescence, a seventh pandemic began during the early 1960s and spread throughout the African continent during the following decade. This new and unexpected outbreak can be explained primarily by the revolution in transport. Aircraft could now travel from centres in which the disease was prevalent in less than a day. The large number of passengers—several hundred per aircraft—linked with the speed of travel, makes this new method of diffusion extremely dangerous. Moreover, persons who regularly use air transport make it more difficult to maintain sanitary control at national frontiers. Free movement of the cholera vibrio is assured, particularly as many governments in affected countries do not declare its existence to WHO. However, international organizations are now able to trace the paths of transmission by looking at the annual number of cases and at the number of affected countries (Fig. 6.1). It is true that these are minimum figures, but in spite of frequent failures to report the disease, the astonishing progress of the pandemic can be followed and it is highly probable that the number of cases has been under-reported by governments. The cholera vibrio now welcomes the traveller who crosses the Mediterranean, or who visits African countries. The African continent has become a second ecological cradle of the disease, in addition to the ecological niche in Lower Bengal which has existed for several centuries. However, in spite of many links with Europe, only a relatively small number of cases have been reported there, e.g. 35 during 1986 in France.[10] How can this weak diffusion of the disease be explained without returning to regional or local factors which affect the epidemiology of cholera?

Ever since the first pandemic, researchers have wondered why the disease affected a particular region or part of a town, or took its toll of members of certain occupations while sparing others. Every aspect of economic, social, cultural, and biological life was investigated in order to answer this question. In this large field of suspect factors, we shall try and isolate those

[10] André Dodin, 'Actualités du choléra d'importation en France', *Médecine et Hygiène* (March 1987).

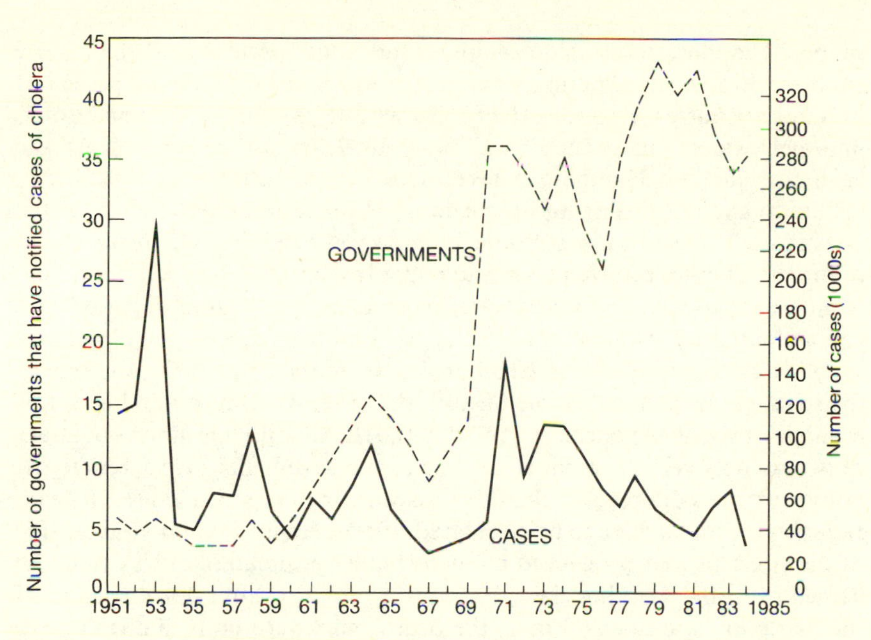

Fig. 6.1 Incidence of cholera and numbers of governments that have notified the disease according to WHO

which seem capable of enabling us to understand the reasons why the disease appears to be limited to the less developed countries.

For nearly a century specialists have regarded water contamination as a method of transmitting cholera. Ever since 1831–32 researchers have stressed the relations which appeared to exist between water courses and the geographical diffusion of the disease. In 1848–49, and even more definitely in 1854, John Snow showed empirically that the closure of the pump in one of the most affected areas of London resulted in a considerable reduction in the number of new cases during the following days.[11] His success led to a concentration of epidemiological researches dealing with the part played by water, to the detriment of other factors. But there was a positive aspect to this as well; it encouraged towns to speed up the construction of systems of water distribution and to use sand filtration, and this practice resulted in a reduction of the number of cases of typhoid as well as of cholera.[12] As regards the latter disease, until recently specialists have tried to show that mortality from the disease depended directly on the quality of the water

[11] Cf. Bourdelais and Dodin, op. cit. in n. 2, pp. 73–79, for further discussion of this point.
[12] Jean Pierre Goubert, *La Conquête de l'eau* (Paris, 1896). For a more precise investigation cf. Evans, op. cit. in n. 9.

supply. The most celebrated example, after Snow's removal of the handle from the Broad Street pump, was the extraordinary mortality experienced in Hamburg during the outbreak of 1892. The neighbouring town of Altona, in which water had been filtered since 1859, hardly suffered from the epidemic, whereas Hamburg, where there was no filtration, paid a heavy tribute to cholera throughout the century.[13] More recently, a study of the atlas of the Prefect of Paris, Poubelle, has shown that in 1832 the two sides of the rue Chaillot received their water supply from different sources. Even-numbered houses received their water from the canal d'Ourcq which was not contaminated by *cholera vibrio* whereas the other side of the street was supplied by the fire-pump at Chaillot, i.e. from the Seine.[14] On one side of the road, cholera claimed 5 victims, on the other 41. But in looking at this example, it should be borne in mind that the rue Chaillot lay at the boundary of two socially very different areas; one of the pavements gave access to the houses of the bourgeoisie, the other to working-class dwellings. If death rates from cholera were to be calculated, the 5 deaths on the bourgeois side of the street probably relate to a much smaller population at risk than the 41 deaths in the working class. Without wanting to hold that the ratio of the two populations was 8 to 1, the death rates were more similar to one another than would appear from the raw figures of deaths.

In the light of recent researches which stress the decisive importance of human contacts in the transmission of the disease we may even ask whether John Snow's observations cannot be explained by the removal of the pump handle resulting in a diminution of transmission from hand to hand, and to a reduction of human contacts at what was a popular meeting-place. However, the importance of water as a factor in the transmission of the disease must not be underestimated, and Hamburg provides the most spectacular example of this. The principal reason why the most recent pandemic has not reached developed countries is probably the existence of a system of supplying filtered and treated water in these countries; this prevents 'long' cycles from beginning and developing. The existence of a proper system of sewerage and refuse disposal, as well as general developments in public health, must also be taken into account.

Another question which has often been raised relates to the effect of the general standard of health of the population on individuals' resistance to cholera. Simple logic may suggest that such a relationship exists, but it is difficult to obtain definitive proof of this. We have been able to show that during the French cholera epidemic of 1854 the two *départements* which were most affected were also those in which the population had been subjected to the greatest hardships and shortages during the two preceding years.[15] Malnutrition probably aggravates the effects of cholera, the more

[13] Evans, op. cit. in n. 9, pp. 290–93.

[14] Bourdelais and Dodin, op. cit. in n. 2, pp. 76–77.

[15] Bourdelais and Raulot, op. cit. in n. 1, pp. 91–95.

so as malnourished individuals are likely to pay less attention to the quality of the food that they consume. Hunger drives them to a point where they eat whatever is available, hastily, and without circumspection or prudence.

It has often been stated that casualty rates in an epidemic are higher in the lower social groups than in the population as a whole. This statement may even be regarded as applying to the present pandemic, the effects of which are restricted to the poorest countries. However, we must draw attention to an important point of method. We have been able to show by calculating life tables for deaths from cholera, that age is an important factor which influences the probability of dying from that disease. Thus, in the *département* of Ariège in 1854, the risks of dying from cholera were six times as high in some age groups as in others. Before concluding that there is an excess mortality of between 20 and 30 per cent in a particular social group, it would be necessary to calculate standardized death rates. It is difficult to find another variable (e.g. occupation) which has as large an effect on cholera mortality as has age.

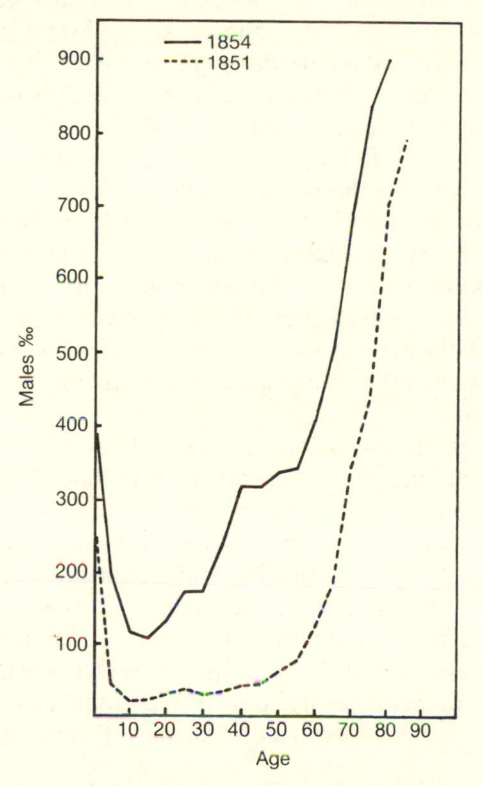

Fig. 6.2 Probabilities of dying (all causes) in Ariège 1854

Source: Bourdelais and Raulot, op. cit. in n. 1, p. 275.

However, even allowing for this factor, we cannot rule out the existence of a social gradient in cholera mortality. Thus, in 1854 in the *arrondissement* of Vervins, where there are detailed data which enable us to consider this point, the fatality rate appears to have been higher among the poor than among farmers, even though members of the former group were generally younger than those of the latter.[16] If older people have lower resistance to the ravages of cholera, the poor who have been weakened by long nutritional privations react even more strongly. Moreover, as the importance of human contacts has been proven, we must also remember the greater crowding of persons both in urban and in rural slums as a factor favouring the spread of the disease. Before returning to problems of personal hygiene, however, we shall recall briefly, giving dates, the arrangements for medical care that have led to a reduction in the fatality of cholera.

In 1832 and in 1854 there were few methods of treating the disease effectively, but of those that were used, some were less damaging than others. However, it is unlikely that the quality of these treatments would have resulted in a social gradient in mortality. Among the innovations which may have saved the lives of some individuals we must mention rehydration. Russian and English physicians, followed by some of their French colleagues, realized the need to replenish the liquids lost by cholera patients. Several contemporary accounts attest that they prescribed enormous quantities of water for their patients. Their methods achieved some success, though they made no attempt to inject a solution of water and mineral salts directly into the patients' bloodstream.

The technique of perfusion had not yet been perfected, and patients would die of phlebitis or septicaemia instead of being killed by cholera. The technique only began to be successfully used at the beginning of the present century. But the decisive improvement in the medical management of the disease dates from the mastery of the techniques of rehydration and the use of sulphonamides and other drugs which have become available during the last 20 years.

Thus, the defeat of cholera did not owe anything to the efficacity of treatment until the end of the Second World War. Protective measures designed to prevent the entry of the disease and bacteriological tests, following the discovery of the vibrio, have made it possible to contain its spread to the less developed countries. Individual protection based on the advice not to drink unboiled water, eat fresh fruit, wash one's hands, and to disinfect soiled areas gradually began to have an effect towards the end of the nineteenth century. It is reasonable to ask whether it was not the development of personal hygiene, rather than advances in medical knowledge, that has let to the erection of an efficient barrier against the cholera.

Nor can it be argued that these practices were adopted as a deliberate

[16] Ibid., pp. 119–23.

measure resulting from a better scientific and empirical understanding relating to the prevention of disease. Such a view would merely be a retrospective projection of contemporary ideas. Norbert Elias has maintained that there was no relation whatever between rules of hygiene and changes in social behaviour.[17] The majority of behavioural constraints which people imposed upon themselves in intercourse with others were the result of the development of 'delicacy and sensibility' and not of attempts to safeguard health. These new forms of behaviour (e.g. washing one's hands before sitting down to a meal, rather than simply at its end) were later legitimated by medical knowledge and considered as being 'good hygiene'. To regard hygiene as a cause of changing social behaviour is a rationalization a posteriori of changes in behaviour for which other social factors were responsible. Considerations of hygiene, which appear to be so clear and convincing today, did not become manifest before the nineteenth century, but, even so, they antedate the first menaces of cholera in Europe. Since the end of the eighteenth and the beginning of the nineteenth century, factors which could affect the quality of the atmosphere have been watched, e.g. proximity of cemeteries to villages or towns, and the activities of artisans, and later of industry, which led to pollution. One of the obstacles to the bourgeois order in the cities, which was most actively resented by the new élites, was the filthiness of the slums and the lack of cleanliness of those who lived in them. They were dreaded as dirty places swarming with people, and their inhabitants became more numerous as the towns grew. The working classes were seen as dangerous because they were regarded as a threat to public order, and also because their conditions of life brought about a miasma of stench and damaged the centre of towns permanently. As part of the public-health movement, campaigns were mounted to improve this situation and to reduce the dangers for the population as a whole. Throughout the July monarchy and until the end of the century, the French authorities believed that the problems raised by epidemics were purely technical and could be solved by a combination of administrative and technical measures.[18] By the end of the nineteenth century it appeared that cholera had been defeated by these technical measures. But the study of reactions to leprosy, plague, syphilis, and cholera shows that these depended not only on the nature of the disease, but also on the social structure, scientific knowledge, and the affective relations between individuals in each epoch. Clearly, the public-health movement of the nineteenth century was given an impetus by the arrival of the cholera, but measures designed to safeguard public health had already been in operation previously and originated in the public's dislike of smells and dirt, and in the arrival of a group of engineers and administrators which resulted in a first attempt at a technical

[17] Norbert Elias, *La Civilisation des moeurs* (Paris, 1973); id. *La Dynamique de l'Occident* (Paris, 1975).

[18] Johan Goudsblom, 'Les Grandes épidémies et la civilisation des moeurs', *Actes de recherche en Sciences Sociales* (1987).

infrastructure. Even without cholera, public-health reforms would have been introduced in Europe, though the delay might have been longer. The fear of cholera speeded up the process, but it was certainly not the only motivating force.

These differences in the reaction to the epidemic of 1831–32 in Britain, Canada, and France, and in 1892 in Hamburg, show how progress in medical knowledge was translated into different policies by the authorities. Until the end of the nineteenth century at least, each town or region chose that medical theory which fitted in best with its own economic, social, or ethnic interests. Thus, after more than eight years, the Hamburg authorities appear to have denied the validity of Koch's discoveries. However, little by little the new medical knowledge came to be accepted by all. It is only the application and mastery of medical treatment which can explain the remarkable reduction in the fatality rate from cholera, during the present pandemic, compared with the past. The difficulties that the authorities face today are different. Whilst a good proportion of those afflicted can now be treated and cured, it has become impossible to prevent the spread of cholera to other regions, because neither quarantine measures nor *cordons sanitaires* commend themselves in present-day conditions. Yet, such measures can be very efficient, as is proved by the success of the authorities in the USSR in isolating the outbreak that occurred in the Astrakhan region in 1970. All that is needed is that governments should be prepared to use such measures and that there should be an administrative apparatus which is capable of enforcing them. These conditions are not met in the countries which have been affected or threatened by the disease during recent years. They are generally too poor even to be able to organize mass vaccination when the disease strikes.

In developed countries, on the other hand, the disease has not struck, even though no measures were taken to contain it. Clearly, the good physical condition of the population, surveillance and bacteriological testing of drinking water, and proper treatment of sewage have all contributed to the efficiency with which the disease has been prevented. They are reinforced by changes in social habits, which, as we have seen, have resulted from an increased cultural sensibility, rather than from being forced on the population by experience of the disease. If this situation were also to apply in the less developed countries which are today threatened by the cholera, action by the medical profession and by WHO will not be sufficient to contain the disease. Public health and personal hygiene which were so efficient in the battle against a number of epidemic diseases, among them cholera, only developed with changes in outlook that followed changes in the social structure (the disappearance of extreme want and of malnutrition). This is bound to be a slow process. For the time being, the cholera vibrio can look forward to a reasonably secure future.

7 Nutrition, Immunity and Infection

PETER G. LUNN *MRC Dunn Nutritional Laboratory, Cambridge*

In attempting to define the cause of the decline in premature mortality which has occurred during the past 200 years in countries which are now developed, one clear direction of investigation is to draw comparisons with parts of the world which remain underprivileged. If we understand which environmental factors are responsible for the continued high levels of early mortality in such countries, it should be possible to identify which aspects of socio-economic development have helped to reduce the problem.

Clearly, one of the major differences between the developed and developing world is in nutrition and nutritional status. Food availability for the majority of people in developing countries is at best marginal, and chronic undernutrition throughout life is often the norm.

In addition, health workers in such communities are aware of a synergistic interaction between malnutrition and infection. The problem is seen most dramatically in children of pre-school age among whom growth rates are at their highest, and where fluctuations in food availability consequently have their maximum effect. However, coupled with the often uncertain supply of food are a host of other poverty-related factors, e.g. inadequate and overcrowded housing, poor water supply and sanitation, etc. which combine to make the environment hazardous in terms of exposure to bacterial, viral, and parasitological infections. In the midst of these many interacting constraints on healthy growth, what exactly is the relationship between nutrition and infection? How does infection affect nutrition and nutritional status, and what physiological mechanisms are involved in these interactions? These are the questions which I hope to consider in this review.

Infant mortality differs greatly between the developed and developing nations of the world, and in many parts of the latter, up to 50 per cent of children never live to see their fifth birthday. One of the most consistent relationships seen in children throughout the world is that between mortality and birthweight.[1] Babies whose birthweights are between 2.0 and 2.5 kg. are eight times more likely to die during the neonatal period, and their mortality during the post-neonatal period is four times that of those with

[1] WHO, 'The Incidence of Low Birthweight: A Critical Review of Available Information', *World Health Statistics*, 33 (1980), p. 197.

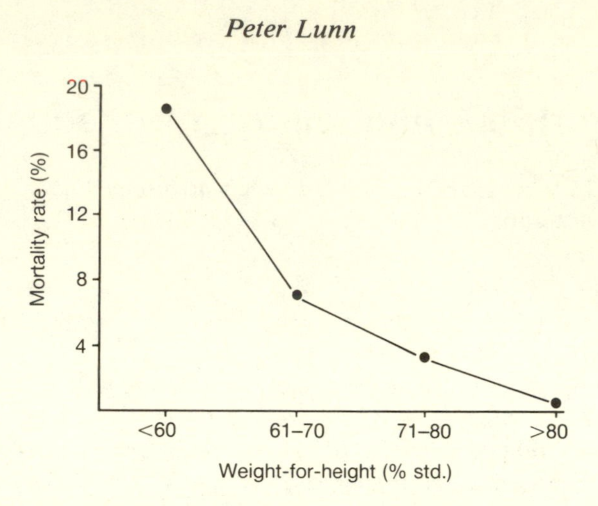

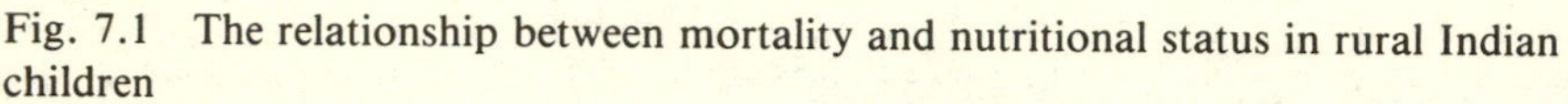

Fig. 7.1 The relationship between mortality and nutritional status in rural Indian children

Source: Chandra and Chandra, op. cit. in n. 3.

birthweights above 3.0 kg.[2] The relationship between mortality and weight deficit (a measure of nutritional status), however, extends well beyond birthweights. Fig. 7.1 shows how the likelihood of death varies with the percentage of expected weight-for-height in a group of rural Indian children aged between 1 and 24 months.[3] Below a weight-for-height of 60 per cent of normal, which represents severe wasting, the risk of death was almost twenty times greater than in infants whose weight-for-height indices exceeded 80 per cent of normal. Studies of mortality such as these, however, reflect only the tip of the iceberg, and most investigations into nutrition-infection interactions are concerned with morbidity.

1. Aetiology of Malnutrition

Before going further, it is important to understand how a healthy child at birth can become so dangerously malnourished. Fig. 7.2 shows the typical growth chart of a rural Gambian child.[4] The infant's birthweight was just below 3 kg., but for the first four months of his life he grew well and in fact

[2] A. Ashworth and R.G. Feacham, 'Interventions for the Control of Diarrhoeal Diseases among Young Children. Prevention of Low Birthweight', *Bulletin of the WHO*, 64 (1985), p. 165.

[3] S. Chandra and R.K. Chandra, 'Nutrition, Immune Response and Outcome', *Progress in Food and Nutritional Science*, 10 (1986), p. 1.

[4] J.A. McGregor, A.K. Rahman, A.M. Thomson, W.Z. Billewicz, and B. Thompson, 'The Health of Young Children in a West African (Gambian) Village', *Transactions of the Royal Society of Tropical Medicine and Hygiene*, 64 (1970), p. 48.

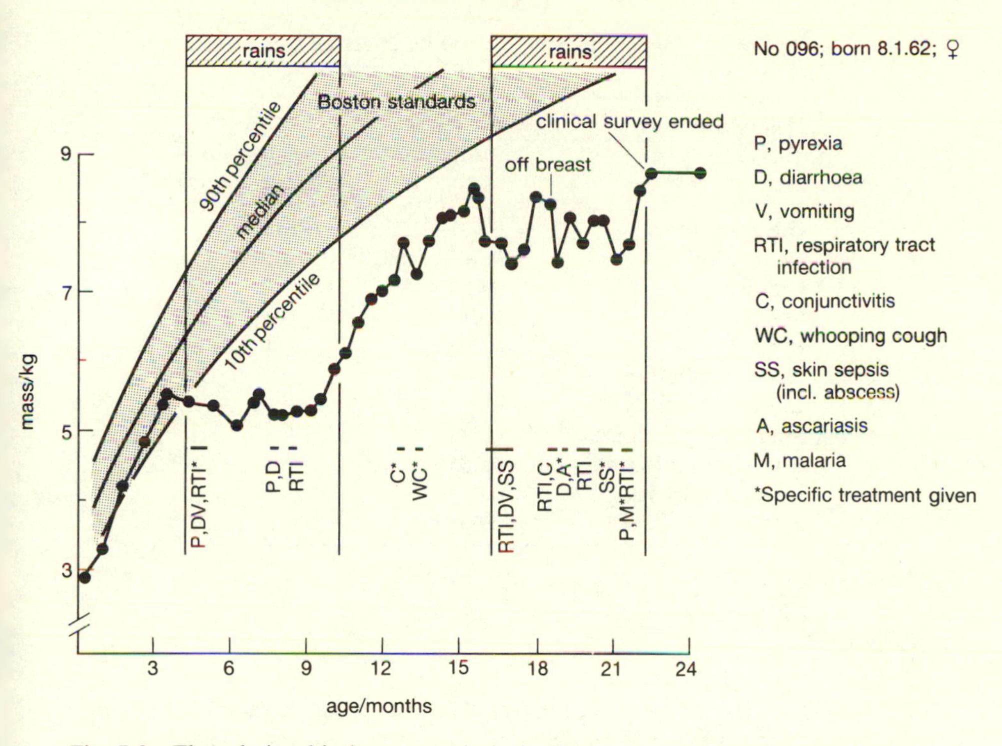

Fig. 7.2 The relationship between gain in body mass and the pattern of infection in a rural Gambian infant

Source: McGregor *et al.*, op. cit. in n. 4.

was catching up to the mean expected value. Shortly after four months, however, something obviously went very wrong and during the next six months the child's weight remained static. Growth then resumed at about ten months of age and for six months achieved a rate which paralleled the standard, but there was no catch-up, so the weight deficit remained constant. Thus, when a second period of zero growth occurred at sixteen months, the child was already nutritionally compromised, and his weight status fell to an even lower level.

The causes of these marked reductions in growth performance are very clear; they occurred during the rainy season of the year and were associated with a battery of illnesses, particularly repeated attacks of gastro-enteritis. It was known that food availability also decreased at about this time, but subsequent regression analysis showed that only during two months of the year (July and August) was it severe enough to impair growth.[5] For the rest of the year supplies were adequate for a near-normal growth rate. This type

[5] M. G. M. Rowland, T. J. Cole, and R. G. Whitehead, 'A Quantitative Study into the Role of Infection in determining Nutritional Status in Gambian Village Children', *British Journal of Nutrition*, 37 (1977), p. 441.

Table 7.1 Disease prevalence and its effect on weight gain of rural Gambian children aged 3–36 months

Disease category	Prevalence (proportion of time ill)	Effect on weight gain (g per month)
Gastro-enteritis	0.131	−101[a]
Helminths	0.003	+1
Giardiasis	0.038	−7[b]
Malaria	0.010	−8[c]
Pyrexia MO	0.006	−4
Upper respiratory	0.099	−10
Lower respiratory	0.045	+1
Mild skin infections	0.044	0
Severe skin infections	0.065	−1
Infectious disorders	0.011	+1
Non-specific disorders	0.004	+2[b]

[a] $p < 0.001$
[b] $p < 0.01$
[c] $p < 0.05$

of analysis further showed that diarrhoeal disease had a far greater impact on growth than other infections suffered by the children.[6] (Table 7.1.) On average, a rural Gambian child suffered from gastro-enteritis for 13.1 per cent of the time, i.e. on about one day in eight, and this resulted in an average decrease in weight gain of 101 g. per month over the whole year. However, as diarrhoeal problems occurred mainly during the six months of the rainy season, the effect on growth at this time could be almost double this figure, and almost negate the average growth rate of 240 g. per month for normal children of this age. More-frequently ill children must therefore be expected to lose weight. Of the other illnesses, only malaria had a significant effect on growth, but its impact was only about 10 per cent that of diarrhoea. Although this information comes from a single country, data from other parts of the developing world confirm diarrhoeal disease to be the most important cause of child morbidity and mortality.[7] Other illnesses which have been implicated are infectious diseases such as measles and whooping cough, and lower respiratory tract infections.[8]

[6] T. J. Cole and J. M. Parkin, 'Infection and its Effect on the Growth of Young Children: A Comparison of the Gambia and Uganda', *Transactions of the Royal Society of Tropical Medicine and Hygiene*, 71 (1977), p. 196.

[7] R. Martorell, J.-P. Habicht, C. Yarborough, A. Lechtig, R. E. Klein, and D. Western, 'Acute Morbidity and Physical Growth in Rural Guatemalan Children', *American Journal of Diseases of Children*, 129 (1975), p. 1296; R. Martorell and T. J. Ho, 'Malnutrition, Morbidity and Mortality', *Population and Development Review*, 10, Suppl. (1984), p. 75.

[8] R. Martorell, 'Child Growth Retardation: A Study of its Causes and its Relationship to

2. Mechanisms of Weight-Faltering during Illness

2.1 Decreased Food Supply

Virtually all infections are associated with some degree of anorexia and this is particularly marked in children. Episodes of pain, vomiting, abdominal distension, fever, and general malaise undoubtedly decrease the appetite. Exacerbating the anorexia, however, is the widespread tendency for normal foods to be withdrawn during episodes of illness and replaced by a more liquid diet with diluted levels of most nutrients. In developing countries this is frequently the result of cultural beliefs and taboos, but it can still be seen in the Western world. Whilst short-term treatment of this type may be justified, particularly in diarrhoeal disorders, prolonged use of diluted foods will inevitably lower the nutritional status of the patient.[9]

2.2 Malabsorption

Even when food is consumed it may not be effectively absorbed. Diarrhoeal disease of virtually any origin is associated with decreased absorption of all three major nutrients, i.e. carbohydrate, fat, and protein, and a number of trace elements and vitamins.[10] Reasons for this include a reduced intestinal transit time, allowing less time for absorption, and pathogen-induced damage to the structure and function of the intestinal mucosa. The scale of the malabsorption is difficult to assess, but one study in Guatemala indicated an energy loss of 500–600 kcals/day in young children, a value approaching half the normal total daily consumption.[11]

2.3 Metabolic Changes: The Acute-Phase Response

Inflammation occurring in response to any infective organism, even the mild challenge imposed by vaccination, initiates a series of biochemical reactions within the body known collectively as the acute-phase response. This is the process by which the body mobilizes tissues and reserves to provide energy and substrates to fuel the response to the infection. Skeletal muscle in particular is depleted as protein is broken down and used to produce both energy and amino acids for the synthesis of antibodies, other immune processes, and the repair of damaged tissue. Nitrogen released during

Health', in K. Baxter and J.C. Waterlow (eds.), *Nutritional Adaptation in Man* (London, 1985), p. 13; L.J. Mata, *The Children of Santa Maria Cauque: A Prospective Field Study of Health and Growth* (Cambridge, Mass., 1978).

[9] N. S. Scrimshaw, 'Effect of Infection on Nutrient Requirements', *American Journal of Clinical Nutrition*, 30 (1977), p. 1536.

[10] N. S. Scrimshaw, 'Significance of the Interactions of Nutrition and Infection in Children', in R.M. Suskind (ed.), *Textbook of Pediatric Nutrition* (New York, 1981), p. 229.

[11] I.H. Rosenberg and N.S. Scrimshaw, 'Malabsorption and Nutrition', *American Journal of Clinical Nutrition*, 25 (1972), p. 1046.

gluconeogenesis is excreted mainly as urea in the urine, and total body nitrogen losses greatly exceed the amount that would be predicted from reduced consumption alone. Powander[12] has calculated an average loss of 0.6 g. of protein/kg/day during most illnesses, but this rises to 0.9 g./kg./day with diarrhoea. At this rate of loss it is easy to understand that when diarrhoea occurs chronically over several weeks or even months, children can become irredeemably wasted. Other nutrients are also lost from the body, often precipitating symptoms of vitamin deficiency.[13]

2.4 Catch-Up Growth

During illness energy stores of glycogen and fat are used up, but the major cause of weight loss and the most difficult to replace post-infection is the loss of protein from skeletal muscle. Following an infection, a well-nourished child markedly raises his food consumption and can quickly make up the nutrient losses suffered during the illness. Rates of catch-up growth up to twenty times normal growth rate have been recorded.[14] However, for the child who lives in an area with limited food supply the substantial increase in intake required i.e. 15 per cent more energy and 40 per cent more protein is simply not available, and the rate at which catch-up occurs depends very heavily on food supply. Thus, in areas where infections are frequent this restriction will mean that individuals are unlikely to recover their pre-infection weight before becoming ill again. In such countries, growth-faltering with each episode of illness becomes cumulative and results in a gradual downward spiral in nutritional status.

3. Impact of Nutritional Status on Susceptibility to Infectious Disease

Whatever the cause of the deterioration in nutritional status, it has become generally accepted that malnutrition predisposes an individual to infectious diseases. Moreover, when illness does strike, it is likely to be more severe, prolonged, and carries an increased risk of death or permanent damage. However, not all infections are affected in the same way; some respond far more than others. Table 7.2 shows the extent to which various illnesses are reported to be influenced by a reduced nutritional status.[15]

[12] M.C. Powander, 'Changes in Body Balances of Nitrogen and Other Key Nutrients: Description and Underlying Mechanisms', *American Journal of Clinical Nutrition*, 30 (1977), p. 1254.

[13] Scrimshaw, op. cit. in n. 10.

[14] A. Ashworth, R. Bell, W.P.T. James, and J. Waterlow, 'Calorie Requirements of Children recovering from Protein-Calorie Malnutrition', *The Lancet* (1968) (ii), p. 600.

[15] R.K. Chandra, 'Nutrition, Immunity and Infection: Present Knowledge and Future Directions', *The Lancet* (1983) (i), p. 688.

Table 7.2 Infectious diseases influenced by nutritional status

Disease category	Influence		
	Definite	Variable	Slight
Bacterial	Tuberculosis Bacterial diarrhoea Cholera Leprosy Pertussis Respiratory infections	Diphtheria Staphylococcus Streptococcus	Typhoid Plague Tetanus Bacterial toxins
Viral	Measles Rotavirus diarrhoea Respiratory infections Herpes	Influenza	Smallpox Yellow fever ARBO[a] Encephalitis
Parasitic	Pneumocystis carinii Intestinal parasites Trypanosomiasis Leishmaniasis Schistosomiasis	Giardia Filariasis	Malaria
Fungal	Candida Aspergillus	Mould toxins	
Other		Syphilis Typhus	

[a] arthropod-borne virus

In order to consider the interaction between malnutrition and disease in more detail, Tomkins,[16] has defined four states during an infective illness when nutritional status may exert an effect.

3.1 Incidence

The first possible point of interaction is in the incidence of the illness, i.e. the number of new cases of infection per head of population that occur within a specified time. In essence, the incidence depends on whether the host's immune response can overcome the rate of replication and spread of the invading organism. Early data from Europe during the two world wars[17] indicated a substantial increase in the incidence of tuberculosis

[16] A.M. Tomkins, 'Protein-Energy Malnutrition and Risk of Infection', *Proceedings of the Nutrition Society*, 45 (1986), p. 289.

[17] K. Faber, 'Tuberculosis and Nutrition', *Acta Tuberculosa Scandinavica*, 12 (1938), p. 287; C.E. Palmer, S. Jablon, and P.Y. Edwards, 'Tuberculosis Morbidity of Young Men in Relation to Tuberculin Sensitivity and Body Build', *American Review of Tuberculosis*, 76 (1957), p. 517.

in severely malnourished populations; Gordon *et al.*[18] have reported an increased incidence of typhus, respiratory, and diarrhoeal disease in poorly nourished areas of the developing world. However, more recent data have not confirmed these results and in several studies carried out in Bangladesh,[19] Costa Rica,[20] Guatemala,[21] and Indonesia[22] it was found that the relationship between measurements of weight deficit and the incidence of diarrhoeal-disease episodes in children was minimal or absent. Similarly, respiratory-tract infections could not be related to nutritional status in studies in Costa Rica,[23] Indonesia[24] and The Gambia.[25] On the other hand, it is well documented that malnourished surgical patients in developed countries do have a greater risk of developing post-operative sepsis, and experimental work with animals invariably demonstrates such a relationship.[26] In addition, in one recent field-study in Nigeria the author did report a more than doubled incidence of diarrhoeal disease in wasted children with an expected weight-for-height below 80 per cent.[27] There are, however, many possible explanations for these discrepant results. For example, the severity of the malnutrition may be important, since severely depleted patients show the relationship, whilst those with mild to moderate malnutrition do not. Alternatively, other environmental factors in the developing world, for example the frequency of exposure to disease organisms may be so great as to override any relationship between disease incidence and nutritional state.

3.2 Severity

A more certain relationship exists between host nutritional status and the severity of disease. Infections regarded as simply troublesome in the

[18] J.E. Gordon, M.A. Guzman, W. Ascoli, and N.S. Scrimshaw, 'Acute Diarrhoeal Disease in Less Developed Countries', *Bulletin of the WHO*, 31 (1964), p. 9.

[19] R.E. Black, K.H. Brown, and S. Becker, 'Malnutrition is a Determining Factor in Diarrhoea Duration but not Incidence among Young Children in a Longitudinal Study in Rural Bangladesh', *American Journal of Clinical Nutrition*, 39 (1984), p. 87; L. C., Chen, A. K. M. A. Chowdhury, and L.S. Huffman, 'Anthropometric Assessment of Energy-Protein Malnutrition and Subsequent Risk of Mortality among Pre-School-Aged Children', *American Journal of Clinical Nutrition*, 33 (1980), p. 1836.

[20] J.W. James, 'Longitudinal Study of the Mortality of Diarrhoeal and Respiratory Infection in Malnourished Children', *American Journal of Clinical Nutrition*, 25 (1972), p. 690.

[21] H.S. Delgado, V. Valverde, J.M. Belizan, and R.E. Klein, 'Diarrhoeal Diseases, Nutritional Status and Health Care: Analysis of their Interrelationships', *Ecology of Food and Nutrition*, 12 (1983), p. 229.

[22] A. Sommer, J. Katz, and I. Tarwotjo, 'Increased Risk of Respiratory Disease and Diarrhoea in Children with Pre-Existing Mild Vitamin A Deficiency', *American Journal of Clinical Nutrition*, 40 (1984), p. 1090.

[23] James, op. cit. in n. 20.

[24] Sommer *et al.*, op. cit. in n. 22.

[25] A.M. Tomkins, D. Dunn, and R. Hayes, 'Nutrient Intake during Diarrhoea in Young Children', in T.G. Taylor (ed.) *Proceedings of the XIII International Congress of Nutrition* (London, 1986), p. 110.

[26] Chandra, op. cit. in n. 15.

[27] A.M. Tomkins 'Tropical Malabsorption: Recent Concepts in Pathogenesis and Nutritional Significance', *Clinical Science*, 60 (1981), p. 131.

developed world change their character and become potential killers in the Third World. Thus, mild respiratory illness tends to develop into bronchitis and pneumonia. Measles is associated with very severe symptoms and is invariably followed by complications such as pneumonia, septicaemia, encephalitis, and diarrhoea, and is consequently associated with a high mortality. In Nigeria and The Gambia respectively, the case fatality rates quoted for this disease are 7 per cent and 14 per cent respectively, compared to less than 0.1 per cent in Europe and North America.[28] Measles severity, however, does vary from country to country even in similarly malnourished groups, and other factors, particularly house overcrowding, seem to be important.[29]

Diarrhoeal disease can quickly result in life-threatening dehydration because of severe loss of water and minerals.[30] Intestinal parasites are also more prevalent in malnourished children, they harbour greater numbers of *ascaris*, *giardia lambia*, and *strongyloides stercoralis*, with the latter causing particularly extensive damage in the nutritionally depleted intestine.[31] Skin diseases such as *herpes simplex* tend to spread well beyond their normal limits of the mucocutaneous junctions.[32]

3.3 Duration

The duration of an illness in malnourished individuals in the developing world is often difficult to define because of the almost invarible complications and secondary infections that follow closely behind the initial disease. In practice, the more severe the illness, the longer it lasts and the longer the time taken to recover from it. Repair of tissue damages is, like catch-up growth, strictly limited by food supply and when this cannot be adequately increased reparative processes will progress more slowly.[33] Perhaps the best insight into the complexity of the situation can be obtained by considering the impact of diarrhoeal disease. It is generally agreed that episodes of diarrhoeal disease last longer in malnourished individuals and Martorell[34] has described a graded duration of illness with various

[28] S.D. Foster, 'Immunizable and Respiratory Diseases and Child Mortality', *Population and Development Review*, 10, suppl. (1984), p. 119.

[29] H.M. Coovadia, A. Wesley, and P. Brian, 'Immunological Events in Acute Measles influencing Outcome', *Archives of Diseases in Childhood*, 53 (1978), p. 861.

[30] D.L. Palmer, F.T. Koster, A.K.J. Alam, and R. Islam, 'Nutritional Status: A Determinant of Severity of Diarrhoea in Patients with Cholera', *Journal of Infectious Diseases*, 134 (1976), p. 8.

[31] V.M. Duncombe, T.D. Bolin, A.E. Davis, and J.D. Kelly, 'The Effect of Iron and Protein Deficiency on the Development of Acquired Resistance to Reinfection with *Nippostrongylus brasiliensis* in Rats', *American Journal of Clinical Nutrition*, 32 (1979), p. 553.

[32] R.K. Chandra, 'Influence of Nutritional Status on Susceptibility to Infection', in H.H. Draper (ed.), *Advances in Nutritional Research*, vol. ii (New York, 1979), p. 57.

[33] J.D. Butzner, D.G. Butler, O.P. Miniats, and J.R. Hamilton, 'Impact of Chronic Protein Caloni Malnutrition on Small Intestinal Repair after Acute Viral Enteritis: A Study in Gnotobiotic Piglets', *Pediatric Research*, 19 (1985), p. 476.

[34] Martorell, op. cit. in n. 8.

measurements of nutritional status. Some episodes of diarrhoeal illness can last for months, but it is probable that the cause of the symptoms changes during the course of the illness. Although it is likely that expulsion of the infective organisms may be delayed by poor nutrition, there are, in addition, a series of possible complications which can result in diarrhoea persisting long after the infective agent has been eliminated.[35]

The sequence of events seems to be that initially the small intestinal mucosa are damaged by a pathogenic organism. This immediately reduces their ability to absorb nutrients at a normal rate and also results in the loss of several digestive enzymes, e.g. the dissacharidases, particularly lactase, which is found as the most exposed part of the villi. Following elimination of the pathogenic organism, the lack of an increased food consumption, exacerbated by nutrient malabsorption, markedly impedes the rate of intestinal mucosal repair. Thus, the damage persists for longer, and during this time the tissue is more open to attack by further pathogens but in addition can be more easily penetrated by food-protein antigens leading to acquired food-allergy syndromes.[36] For example, prolonged diarrhoea in many malnourished children in Indonesia is caused by cow's-milk protein intolerance and symptoms persist until the offending food is withdrawn.[37] Invasion of the small bowel by colonic bacteria frequently occurs and this may partially explain the observation that malabsorption of nutrients and dissacharidase deficiency seem to become persistent and self-generating.[38] All the complications will tend to lower nutritional status further, thus creating a vicious circle which must be broken if the child is to survive.

3.4 Outcome

The final phase of an illness is either death, full recovery, or recovery with persistent or even permanent damage. The relationship between nutritional status and mortality has been discussed above, and there is little doubt that a wasted child is at a greater risk of death. Stunting, however, seems to be less important in this respect.[39] Full catch-up in height and weight, even in developed countries, can take many years but in the developing world a permanent stunting of growth following each infection is the norm.[40]

Even without recurring complications it can be many months before a

[35] A.S. McNeish, 'The Interrelationship between Chronic Diarrhoea and Malnutrition', in J.A. Walker-Smith and A.S. McNeish (eds.), *Diarrhoea and Malnutrition in Childhood* (London, 1986), p. 1.

[36] J.A. Walker-Smith, 'Temporary Syndrome of Food Intolerance. Pathology and Mechanisms of Food Allergy', in Walker-Smith and McNeish (eds.), op. cit. in n. 35, p. 185.

[37] P.D. Manuel, 'The Role of Cow's Milk Protein Intolerance in Chronic Diarrhoea in a Developing Country', in Walker-Smith and McNeish (eds.), op. cit. in n. 35, p. 193.

[38] M. Gracey, M., 'Bacterial Overgrowth in the Small Intestine. Causes and Consequences', in Walker-Smith and McNeish, op. cit. in n. 35, p. 40.

[39] Martorell and Ho, op. cit. in n. 7.

[40] Scrimshaw, op. cit. in n. 10.

damaged gastro-intestinal tract returns to normal, but some illnesses, notably measles, also leave a legacy of a markedly disrupted immune system. In The Gambia, 10 per cent of children who survived an episode of measles died during the nine months following this illness, a figure far greater than the 1 per cent frequency of death in children who had not contracted the disease.[41] Such observations clearly raise questions about the state of the immune system in malnourished individuals and the role it plays in preventing and limiting invasion by pathogenic organisms.

4. Nutrition and the Immune System

An association between malnutrition and depressed host resistance to infection has been recognized for centuries. Only in recent times, however, has it become clear that tissues associated with the immune system, such as the thymus gland and lymphoid tissues, are more sensitive to nutritional deficits than many other organs of the body. In protein-energy malnutrition (PEM), histomorphological abnormalities occur in the thymus including a reduction in size and weight, depletion of lymphocyte numbers, and loss of cortico-medullary corpuscles. Similar degenerative changes are seen in the lymphoid areas of the spleen and lymph nodes. The tonsils are also much reduced in size. These observations have in recent years led to a series of investigations into the precise way in which the immune system becomes compromised by malnutrition.[42]

The various components of the immune system can be grouped into three main categories: the cell-mediated immune system, the humoral or antibody system, and non-specific mechanisms.

4.1 Cell-Mediated Immunity

The normal operation of this system depends heavily on the thymus-dependent T-lymphocytes. When such cells are exposed to antigens, metabolic changes including cell division occur, resulting in the formation of a clone of cells which carry on their cell-surface a receptor which is specific for the sensitizing antigen. On re-exposure to the same antigen, these transformed cells secrete lymphokines which initiate the inflammatory mechanism.

In about 15 per cent of children with protein-energy malnutrition the total lymphocyte count is reduced, but closer examination reveals .that this reduction is mainly due to the much larger fall in the number of

[41] H.F. Hull, P.J. Williams, and F. Oldfield, 'Measles Mortality and Vaccine Efficacy in Rural West Africa', *The Lancet* (1983) (i), p.972.
[42] R.K. Chandra, *Immunology and Nutritional Disorders* (London, 1980).

T-lymphocytes.[43] Even more specifically, within the T-cell sub-classes, it is the T_4 helper lymphocytes which are most severely affected with a smaller reduction in the T_8 component.[44] As it is necessary for these lymphocytes to complete their maturation and differentiation within the thymus gland, their reduction in the malnourished child might be expected. Coupled with the fall in T-cell numbers is an increase in the so called 'null' lymphocytes. These are now thought to be incompletely differentiated pre-T-lymphocytes which because of the thymic atrophy, or perhaps more specifically the much-reduced levels of thymic hormone, have failed to complete their development. Refeeding of the individual, or even *in vitro* incubation of such cells with thymic hormone, results in their conversion to mature T-lymphocytes. It, therefore, seems clear that the reduced levels of thymic hormone observed during protein-energy malnutrition do result in a faulty production of T-lymphocytes.[45] Other changes in cell-mediated immunity have been described in malnourished children. There is a reduction in the migration of lymphocytes into the gastro-intestinal tract. Lymphoid aggregates in the intestine are small and the number of epithelial lymphocytes and submucosal plasma cells is lowered.[46] The blood of such subjects has been reported to contain inhibitors of the lymphocyte response to antigen stimulation and also has high concentrations of cortisol which is reported to cause lympholysis. Interferon secretion also seems to be reduced.[47]

That the cell-mediated immune system has become compromised can be demonstrated in a number of ways, but the test of delayed cutaneous hypersensitivity is perhaps most frequently used. These tests have shown that the ability to mount a primary response to a subcutaneously applied antigen is reduced, but more importantly, malnourished children frequently do not become sensitized by exposure to antigens. Even when sensitization does occur, the ability to recall and respond to a secondary challenge is much impaired. In studies in East Africa for example, fewer than half the children tested showed a positive Mantoux test following vaccinations with BCG, and in one severely malnourished group, no positive tests at all were observed.[48]

[43] Id., 'Lymphocyte Subpopulation in Human Malnutrition. Cytotoxic and Suppressor Cells', *Pediatrics*, 59 (1977), p. 423.

[44] Id., S., Gupta, and H. Singh, 'Inducer and Suppressor T-Cell Subsets in Protein-Energy Malnutrition: Analysis by Monoclonal Antibodies', *Nutrition Research*, 2 (1982), p. 21.

[45] J. W. Olusi, G. B. Thurman, and A. L. Goldstein, 'Effect of Thymosin on T-Lymphocyte Rosette Formation in Children with Kwashiorkor', *Clinical Immunology and Immunopathology*, 15 (1980), p. 687; S. Zaman and T. Jackson, 'The *in vitro* Effect of the Thymic Factor Thymopoietin on the Subpopulation of Lymphocytes from Severely Malnourished Children', *Clinical and Experimental Immunology*, 39 (1980), p. 717.

[46] M. Shiner, 'Immune Mechanisms in the Small Bowel Mucosa of Children with Malnutrition', in *Frontiers of Gastrointestinal Research*, xiii (Basle, 1986), p. 172.

[47] M. E. Gershwin, R. S. Beach, and L. S. Harley, *Nutrition and Immunity* (New York and London, 1985), p. 60.

[48] R. M. Suskind, 'Malnutrition and the Immune Response', in *Textbook of Pediatric Nutrition* (New York and London, 1981), p. 241.

Similar evidence of marked malfunction of the system have been obtained by other methods of assessment, e.g. circulating T-lymphocyte numbers or by *in vitro* stimulation of lymphocytes using a mitogen such as phyto-haemaglutamin or concanavelin A. Abnormalities in these measurements become greater with the severity of malnutrition, and it has been suggested that these indices of cell-mediated immune competence could be used as an index of nutritional status.[49]

4.2 Humoral Immunity

This immune system which involves the B-lymphocyte and antibody production seems in general to be little affected by even severe malnutrition, but there are some important exceptions to this rule. The number of B-lymphocytes in the blood is not reduced in protein-energy malnutrition and the concentrations of the antibody immunoglobulins IgG, IgM, and IgA tend to be higher than normal. This elevation is particularly seen in IgA values, an effect which is believed to be due to the constant exposure of the small intestine to pathogenic organisms.[50] Similarly, blood IgE concentrations can become greatly raised in response to helminthic parasite invasion of the gut. Despite the already high levels, immunoglobulin production is capable of responding to infection, and the increase elicited by many antigens, e.g. tetanus and polio, is quite normal. However, the response to other diseases, including diphtheria, typhoid, and yellow fever, is impaired.[51] Also reduced is the production of those antibodies which require the presence of the thymus-derived helper T-lymphocytes.[52]

Perhaps of greater significance than these changes is the effect malnutrition has on secretory IgA. These antibodies are synthesized in cells in the exposed mucosal areas of the body and released on to the surface and are particularly important in combating invading organisms in the nasopharynx and gastro-intestinal tract. The concentration of secretory IgA is reported to be generally low in malnourished children, but more importantly, the response to challenge with polio or measles vaccines is very much reduced.[53] Whether this is due to a reduced rate of production of the antibodies, or occurs because of fewer secretory cells in the submucosal layers, or both, is not known. However, it seems likely that a deficiency of secretory IgA in the nasopharynx removes an important barrier to measles infection and may at least partially explain the particular susceptibility of nutritionally

[49] Chandra, op. cit. in n. 15.

[50] Gershwin, *et al.*, op. cit. in n. 47.

[51] Ibid.

[52] R. K. Chandra, 'The Nutrition-Immunity Infection Nexus: The Enumeration and Functional Assessment of Lymphocyte Subsets in Nutritional Deficiency', *Nutrition Research*, 3 (1983), p. 605.

[53] Id., 'Reduced Secretory Antibody Response to Live Attenuated Measles and Polio Virus Vaccines in Malnourished Children', *British Medical Journal* (1975) (ii), p. 583.

deprived children to this disease. A similarly impaired response would reduce the immunocompetence of the intestinal mucosa and allow the abnormal bacterial colonization of the small bowel which is a very common finding in malnourished infants with diarrhoeal problems.

Finally, if an individual becomes malnourished during the development of the humoral immune system, i.e. during late gestation or early post-partum, the whole mechanism can be compromised. Thus full-term infants with a birthweight below 2,500 g. frequently exhibit low levels of immuno-globulin with much reduced antigen-induced response. These deficiencies can be very persistent and, in the absence of a good diet, may last for years, or become permanent. Thus, small-for-date babies constitute a separate and very vulnerable group in terms of susceptibility to infection, and this deficiency is reflected in the much increased mortality of such children.[54]

4.3 Other Immune Mechanisms

The opsonizing ability of the blood is reduced in severe protein-energy malnutrition, at least partially, as a result of a reduction in some parts of the compliment system. The total haemolytic component is lowered and specific deficiencies in the levels of the C_1, C_2, C_3 and C_5 components have been described. The concentration of factor B may also be decreased. However, there is disagreement over whether these changes occur in mild to moderate protein-energy malnutrition, but when present they are undoubtedly associated with increased susceptibility to bacterial diseases in particular.[55]

Phagocytic cell function has also been examined in malnourished infants. The number of circulating leucocytes and neutrophils appears unchanged, but alterations in function were noted. Chemotactic migration tended to be delayed and during infection was clearly reduced.[56] Ingestion of organisms appeared to be normal, but intracellular killing of both bacteria and fungi was impaired. However, like the changes in the complement system, it seems that these alterations in function are seen mainly in severe malnutrition, or could perhaps be dependent on some specific micronutrient deficiency.[57]

Other factors not normally thought of as barriers to infection can also be affected. For example, hydrochloric-acid production by the stomach is reduced when nutritional status is poor, and the resulting higher-than-normal pH in the gastro-intestinal tract allows diarrhoea-causing pathogens better access to their target organ. It is possible that cholera vibrio organisms are able to enter the gut in very high numbers as a result of this deficiency.[58]

[54] Id., 'Fetal Malnutrition and Post-Natal Immunocompetence', *American Journal of Diseases of Children*, 129 (1975), p. 450; Gershwin *et al.*, op. cit. in n. 47.

[55] Suskind, op. cit. in n. 48.

[56] Chandra and Chandra, op. cit. in n. 3.

[57] Suskind, op. cit. in n. 48.

[58] Gershwin *et al.*, op. cit. in n. 47.

5. Significance of Changes in Immune Processes

There can be little doubt that the changes described in the preceding paragraphs will result in an impaired level of immuno-competence, and thus an increased susceptibility to infectious diseases. However, the picture is far from clear. Most of the investigations have involved severely malnourished children, and the question relating to the stage of malnutrition when particular components of the immune system become compromised cannot be fully answered. Some deficiencies, particularly those in the cell-mediated immune system, do appear to be affected at an early stage of undernutrition, but how severe such changes need to be before immune status is affected can only be answered in part. From observations made on subjects with specific immune deficiencies it appears that the T-lymphocytes number needs to fall below 40 per cent of normal before there is an increased risk of infection.[59] Similarly, the concentration of complement component C_3 can fall to 20 per cent before the system becomes defective. However, the number of variables is vast; different parts of the immune systems will respond differently to different infections and may be dependent on specific nutrient requirements. The term malnutrition has been used very loosely in this discussion to mean food inadequacy in general, but it is now well known that specific vitamins and minerals as well as the macronutrients are essential for a normal immune response. Nevertheless, it seems probable that where reductions in the immune components described are found, there will be an overall increased susceptibility to infectious disease.

6. Conclusion

Nutrition, infection, and immunity are closely interrelated and changes in one component will inevitably cease alterations in the other two. Malnutrition is associated with a lowering of immuno-competence in individuals and this will be expressed as a greater susceptibility to infectious disease. Infection will clearly result in a more malnourished subject and complete the vicious circle. However, it must be accepted that other environmental factors play perhaps very important roles in the relationship between nutrition and infection. Just as immuno-competence may be regarded as an indicator of nutritional status, so could nutritional status be used as an indicator of other poverty-related conditions such as poor housing, hygiene, and sanitation, etc., as well as food availability. Thus although nutrition plays a major part, the extent to which other socio-economic variables contribute to disease prevalence and mortality remains to be assessed.

[59] Chandra, op. cit. in n. 52.

8 Medicine and the Decline of Mortality: Indicators of Nutritional Status

RODERICK FLOUD *City of London Polytechnic*

1. Introduction

It is now almost ten years since the beginnings of a concerted effort to use anthropometric indicators of nutritional status in the service of demographic and economic history. Before that time, anthropometry had been largely the preserve of human biologists, nutritionists, and anthropologists, although Le Roy Ladurie had used measurements of French conscripts as part of his description of French society at the end of the Napoleonic period.[1] This is not to say that anthropometry had not been used by historians; from the earliest days of the study of the subject, there has been considerable interest in the heights, weights and growth of people during the past, and calculations of change over time have commonly been made.[2] Moreover, the concept of the 'secular trend' in growth in height and weight had entered all textbooks of human biology as one element of the changes which had been observed in developed countries and could now be observed in developing countries.[3] But the aim of such calculations and concepts was

[1] E.R. Ladurie, *Le Territoire de l'historien* (Paris, 1973); J.-P. Aron, P. Dumont, and E. R. Ladurie, *Anthropologie du conscrit français d'après les comptes numériques et sommaires du recrutement de l'armée 1819–1826*. (Paris and The Hague, 1972).

[2] J. Beddoe, 'On the Stature and Bulk of Man in the British Isles', *Memoirs of the Anthropological Society of London*, 3 (1870), pp. 384–573; British Association for the Advancement of Science, *Final Report of the Anthropometric Committee* (London, 1883); E.M.B. Clements, 'Changes in the Stature and Weight of British Children over the Past 70 Years', *British Medical Journal*, 24 (1953) (ii), pp. 897–902; S. Rosenbaum, '100 Years of Heights and Weights', *Journal of the Royal Statistical Society*, A151 (1988), pp. 276–309; J.M. Tanner, *Growth at Adolescence*, (2nd ed., Oxford, 1962); *Foetus into Man: Physical Growth from Conception to Maturity* (London, 1978); *A History of the Study of Human Growth* (Cambridge, 1981).

[3] H. Bakwin, 'The Secular Trend in Growth and Development', *Acta Paediatrica*, 53 (1964), pp. 79–89; A. W. Boyne and I. Leitch, 'Secular Change in the Height of British Adults', *Nutrition Abstracts and Reviews*, 24 (1954), pp. 255–69; A.W. Boyne, F.C. Aitken, and I. Leitch, 'Secular Changes in the Height and Weight of British Children, including an Analysis of Measurements of English Children in Primary Schools 1911–1953', *Nutrition Abstracts and Reviews*, 27 (1957), pp. 1–18; N. Cameron, 'The Growth of London Schoolchildren 1904–1966: An Analysis of Secular Trends and Intercounty Variation', *Annals of Human Biology*, 6 (1979), pp. 505–25; S. Chinn and R.J. Rona, 'The Secular Trends in the Heights of Primary Schoolchildren in England and Scotland from 1972 to 1980', *Annals of Human Biology*, 11 (1984), pp. 1–16; T.K. Landauer, 'Infantile Vaccination and the Secular Trend in Stature', *Ethos*, 1

to use historical evidence to aid an understanding of human growth; only during the past ten years, with the notable exception of the work of Chamla, Olivier, and their colleagues,[4] has human growth been used to aid an understanding of recent history.

The aim of this short chapter, therefore, is to survey the progress that has been made in the use and understanding by historians, economists, and demographers of indicators of nutritional status and to suggest directions for future research, with particular reference to the causes of the European mortality decline between 1700 and 1914. Partly to save space and partly because almost all the studies which I shall discuss have been based on the measurement of height as the primary anthropometric indicator of nutritional status, I shall refer throughout to heights as the main subject of study. This does not imply either that height is the only appropriate indicator, or that it is anything more than a convenient index of nutritional status, which is itself a net measure of a whole complex of environmental influences on the human body which determine its health, growth, and strength.

2. The Main Findings

It is illuminating to recall the state of knowledge which existed ten years ago among the historians and economists who then tentatively set out to explore the use of height measurements in history; most at that time were associated with a research programme on the decline of mortality in North America. They sought a measure which would illuminate the health before migration of those men and women who were later to encounter the environment of North America and whose experience was to be included in the mortality statistics of that region. Most of those historians and economists received with incredulity the idea that height might provide such an indicator;

(1973), pp. 499–503; B. O. Ljung, A. Bergsten-Brucefors, and G. Lindgren, 'The Secular Trend in Physical Growth in Sweden', *Annals of Human Biology*, 1 (1974), pp. 245–66; H. V. Meredith, 'Findings from Asia, Australia, Europe and North America on Secular Change in Mean Height of Children, Youths and Young Adults', *American Journal of Physical Anthropology*, 44 (1976), pp. 313–26; G. M. Morant, 'Secular Changes in the Height of the British People', *Proceedings of the Royal Society*, B137 (1950), pp. 443–52; J. C. Van Wieringen, 'Secular Growth Changes', in F. Falkner and J. M. Tanner (eds.), *Human Growth* (New York, 1978); N. Wolanski, 'Secular Trend in Man: Evidence and Factors', *Colloquia in Anthropology*, 2 (1978), pp. 69–86.

[4] M. C. Chamla, 'L'Accroissement de la stature en France de 1880 à 1960: Comparaisons avec les pays d'Europe occidentale', *Bulletin et mémoires de la société d'anthropologie de Paris*,[40] 6 (1964), pp. 201–78; G. Olivier, 'Anthropologie de la France', *Bulletin et mémoires de la société d'anthropologie de Paris*[12], 6 (1970), pp. 109–87; G. Olivier, L. Chamla, G. Devigne, A. Jacquard, and E. W. R. Iagolnitzer, 'L'Accroissement de la stature en France, 1. L'Accélération du phénomène, 2. Les Causes du phénomène: Analyse univariée', *Bulletin et mémoires de la société d'anthropologie de Paris*[13], 4 (1977), pp. 197–214.

although, like most of their contemporaries, they had become used to the idea that heights were increasing in European societies, this increase was attributed either—among those particularly ignorant of genetics—to genetic change or, at least, to contingent events related to food intake such as the rationing of food supplies during the Second World War and the provision of free milk and orange juice.

While a rapid reading of textbooks in human biology soon made it clear that possible causes of changing height were more complex and that increases in height had already begun during the nineteenth century, the stress in such textbooks on the secular trend led to the initial belief that all that was needed was to estimate the slope of that trend in various European countries, to discover when the upward trend had begun—since it was immediately evident that the Romans had not been 1 m. tall, and to compare European trends with those in North America. While it became clear very quickly that it would be worthwhile to investigate past differences in the heights of members of different socio-economic groups, this was seen as an adjunct to the main study of trends which, it was assumed, could be estimated by taking a series of snapshots of average heights at widely spaced intervals. It was also thought that there would be little difficulty in estimating those average heights, and that their main value would be for comparisons between Europe and America.

In the event, almost all these initial beliefs proved to be fallacious. The concept of the secular trend was quickly discarded, the importance of estimating the heights of geographical and socio-economic groups was enhanced, and the problems of estimation were soon found to be formidable. In addition, the focus of attention shifted away from the mortality decline in North America. What, then, are the main findings that have emerged from this painful process of discovery?

First, we look at the long-term movement of heights. Studies of long-term changes in the United States,[5] Britain,[6] Austria-Hungary,[7] and in ten other European countries[8] have shown that a variety of patterns of growth may

[5] L. Sokoloff and G.C. Villaflor, 'The Early Achievement of Modern Stature in America', *Social Science History*, 6 (1982), pp. 453–81; R.W. Fogel, 'Nutrition and the Decline in Mortality since 1700: Some Preliminary Findings', in S.L. Engerman and R.E. Gallman (eds.), *Long-Term Factors in American Economic Growth* (Conference on Research in Income and Wealth, 41, Chicago, Ill., 1986).

[6] R.C. Floud, K.W. Wachter, and A.S. Gregory, *Height, Health and History: Nutritional Status in Britain 1750–1980* (Cambridge, 1990).

[7] J. Komlos, 'Stature and Nutrition in the Habsburg Monarchy: The Standard of Living and Economic Development in the Eighteenth Century', *American Historical Review*, 90 (1985), pp. 1149–61; id., 'Patterns of Children's Growth in East Central Europe in the Eighteenth Century', *Annals of Human Biology*, 13 (1986), pp. 33–48.

[8] R.C. Floud, *The Heights of Europeans since 1750: A New Source for European Economic History* (NBER Working Paper, 1318), also published as 'Wirtschaftliche und soziale Einflüsse auf die Körpergrössen von Europäern seit 1750', *Jahrbuch für Wirtschaftsgeschichte* (1985), pp. 93ff.; *Measuring the Transformation of European Economies* (CEPR

be observed. Heights in the United States reached modern standards during the eighteenth century, but there was a sustained period of declining heights during the middle of the nineteenth century; this decline can also be found in Britain, where it applies to men born between approximately 1830 and 1860. It was preceded there by slow growth during the late eighteenth century and was succeeded by a period of rapid growth in heights during the twentieth century. In other European countries, too, heights increased relatively slowly during the nineteenth century and their populations were almost always shorter than equivalent groups in the Americas and in Britain, but in all there was rapid growth during the twentieth century, although at different rates and from different starting-points and with pauses, although not actual retrogression, which seem to have been most commonly associated with the world wars. Very broadly, these different levels and patterns appear to be associated with levels of income and of mortality,[9] but many features remain unexplained.

National averages are, in fact, often a frustrating source of information, since it has become increasingly clear that so many of the factors which influence changes in height operate at small-group or even individual levels, and that aggregation to national levels makes it more, rather than less, difficult to explain the changes that are observed. Researchers in both America and Britain have, therefore, increasingly examined deviation from a national average, although the nature of the conscription records which form the main source of information on continental Europe has made it difficult to extend this mode of analysis to that area. In both Britain and America, however, it has been possible to examine the relative heights of both socio-economic and geographical groups.

In Britain, for example, two kinds of source make this possible. First, comparison of the records of the Marine Society, which took boys from the London slums, with the records of the Royal Military College at Sandhurst, which recruited the sons of the upper classes, revealed two main findings: first, the children of the Marine Society were extremely short by modern standards, well below the first centile of modern height distributions and equivalent in height and pattern of growth only to some deprived children in parts of the developing world.[10] The Sandhurst boys, by contrast, were some 10 in. (25 cm.) taller early in the nineteenth century, so much taller that the Marine Society and Sandhurst distributions hardly overlap. It is of

---

Discussion Paper, 33; London, 1985); id., 'Anthropometric Measures of Nutritional Status in Industrial Societies: Europe and North America since 1750', in A. Sen and S. Osmani (eds.), *Undernutrition and Living Standards* (Oxford, 1990).

[9] R. H. Steckel, 'Heights and *per capita* Income', *Historical Methods*, 16 (1983), pp. 1–7.

[10] R. C. Floud and K. W. Wachter, 'Poverty and Physical Stature', *Social Science History*, 6 (1982), pp. 422–52; P. B. Eveleth and J. M. Tanner, *Worldwide Variations in Human Growth* (Cambridge, 1976); J. M. Tanner, R. H. Whitehouse, and M. Takaishi, 'Standards from Birth to Maturity for Height, Weight, Height Velocity and Weight Velocity: British Children 1965', *Archives of Diseases in Childhood*, 41 (1966), pp. 454–71, 613–35.

particular interest, however, that the Sandhurst children were approximately at the fiftieth centile of the modern standard, still much shorter than modern upper-class children. Since it is difficult to believe that the Sandhurst children were nutritionally deprived (although we know too little of child feeding practices), the use of modern studies from the developing world suggests that their relative shortness may be attributed to the overall disease environment from which even their wealth could not protect them.[11]

The value of the examination of differences in height is not confined to such extreme examples. Studies of the relative heights of the English and Scots reveal that during the eighteenth and early nineteenth centuries the Scots, both from urban and rural areas, were consistently taller than the English, a pattern that is now entirely reversed. In both England and Scotland, town dwellers were shorter than the inhabitants of rural areas, with Londoners always at the bottom; again, these relationships have largely been overturned, although Londoners are still slightly shorter than the inhabitants of the prosperous areas around the capital.[12] While most of these movements correspond with what we know about movements in relative income levels, the Scottish advantage in earlier years does not; either the 'good Scots diet' of oatmeal, or the relative freedom from the worst urban diseases before the middle of the nineteenth century, or both, may be behind the finding.

Height data also allow us to discriminate between the experience of different social and occupational classes. The contrast between the Marine Society and Sandhurst is an extreme example, but the evidence of British and American military recruits during the eighteenth and nineteenth centuries shows the extent of differences in nutritional status even within the working class from which almost all the soldiers and marines were drawn. Thus, in Britain, white-collar workers were taller than the skilled and semi-skilled industrial workers, who were in turn taller than most labourers, while domestic servants appear to have been the shortest of all. However, these differences changed over time. They have also apparently persisted, although the recent survey of heights and weights used only a fivefold division of social class, rather than the much more complex stratification which is possible with historical data.

The extent and nature of inequality in a society and its reflection in anthropometric measures is particularly interesting. In all European societies, with the possible exception of Sweden, class differences in height continue to be found; comparison with historical data shows that those differences have narrowed substantially, but they are still highly significant, both statistically and in terms of the persistence of differences in income and

[11] J.N. Rea, 'Social and Economic Influences on the Growth of Pre-School Children in Lagos', *Human Biology*, 43 (1971), pp. 46–63.

[12] Floud, Wachter, and Gregory, op. cit. in n. 6; T. Knight and J. Eldridge, *The Heights and Weights of Adults in Great Britain* (London, 1984).

lifestyle. It remains puzzling, however, that the substantial increases in income among the working classes of Europe during the twentieth century have not removed class differences, and this suggests once again that factors other than income deserve attention.

One last finding is worth notice. It has been a central feature of height studies, most of which have been based on military data, that height was used by military recruiters as a means of discriminating between those who were fit enough for a military life and those whose health or physique was not good enough. Height was thus a crude means of quality control. It was usually, however, supplemented by a medical examination, and some sources of evidence thus contain information on both the height and the medical condition of potential recruits; Fogel *et al.* used the records of the Union Army in the Civil War to examine the relationship between height and the likelihood that a recruit would be rejected on medical grounds.[13] They found a clear inverse relationship which closely parallels in shape the results of modern studies on the relationship between height and mortality, and which suggests a common optimum height, within these two very different societies, of 188 cm.[14]

3. Problems of Method and Interpretation

In the preceding section we gave an extremely brief survey of a large volume of literature; in this section we describe the major problems which have been encountered during the course of the research, together with some issues of interpretation which still require to be resolved.

There is no doubt that the main difficulties of the research stem, as indeed they should, from the complexities of the relationship between the environment and human nutritional status as reflected in height. A particularly difficult set of issues surrounds the ages at which nutritional status exerts influence on growth in height; it does not do so, of course, after growth has ceased in the late teenage years or in the early twenties, but most of the data which are available relate to young men at those or later ages. Two problems in particular arise: first, if we are to identify factors causing change in height, we need to know whether it is likely that those factors operated most strongly shortly after birth, in childhood, at the adolescent growth spurt, or thereafter. Matters are complicated by the fact that there are few studies of teenagers in the developing world, but a brief summary of a complex

[13] R.W. Fogel, C.L. Pope, N. Scrimshaw, P. Temin, and L.T. Wimmer, 'The Aging of Union Army Men: A Longitudinal Study' (Mimeo, University of Chicago, Center for Population Studies, 1986).

[14] H.T. Waaler, *Height, Weight and Mortality: The Norwegian Experience* (Oslo, 1984); M.G. Marmot, M.J. Shipley, and G. Rose, 'Inequalities in Death. Specific Explanations of a General Pattern', *The Lancet* (1984), pp. 1003–06.

literature would be that the most crucial period of interaction between the environment and growth occurs in infancy, between weaning and about the age of three. If deprivation is acute and prolonged at those ages, then height will be permanently affected.[15] Only in very unusual circumstances, such as the command economy of the slave plantations studied by Steckel,[16] will catching up of growth be possible.

The second problem arises because both cross-sectional and historical studies have shown that improving environmental circumstances will increase both the tempo of growth and the absolute height; as an example, members of wealthier communities typically are not only taller but also reach the adolescent growth spurt earlier than do those in poorer communities. It follows that height alone—either during growth or as final height—does not fully reflect the benefits of an improving environment; instead, both absolute height and tempo of growth should be combined in a single measure, which has not yet been devised. It remains true, however, that improvement in absolute height can be regarded as a lower bound.

The major statistical issue in height studies stems directly from the nature of the sources which must be used. Almost all historical evidence of height is based on military records, and nearly all these show some evidence of the exclusion of some short recruits. In some cases, as with many of the records of European conscripts or with those of the Union Army, the numbers excluded on the grounds of height are so small that they can be ignored. In others, as with the British army which excluded up to half of a particular age group from measurement or recruitment, the problem is acute. It is for this reason that so much time and effort has gone into the invention of statistical methods which exploit the normality of height distributions and allow for the estimation of both average height and deviations from it.[17]

Problems of method are, however, of less importance than problems of interpretation. If we are to make use of height evidence, we must know what it means. In one sense, this is a problem not for historians or economists, but for human biologists who seek to explain the physical and endocrinological processes of growth; much still needs to be understood in this field, but research there needs to be accompanied by investigation of the environmental correlates of height growth, to which social scientists can

[15] F. Falkner and J.M. Tanner, *Human Growth* (2nd edn., New York, 1986); FAO/WHO/UNU, *Energy and Protein Requirements* (WHO Technical Report Series, 725, Geneva, 1985); R. Martorell and J.-P. Habicht, 'Growth in Early Childhood in Developing Countries', in Falkner and Tanner (eds.), op. cit. in this note, vol. iii, pp. 241–59.

[16] R.H. Steckel, 'Growth, Depression and Recovery: The Remarkable Case of American Slaves', *Annals of Human Biology*, 14 (1987), pp. 111–32.

[17] K.W. Wachter, 'Graphical Estimation of Military Heights', *Historical Methods*, 14 (1981), pp. 31–42; K.W. Wachter, and J. Trussell, 'Estimating Historical Heights', *Journal of the American Statistical Association*, 77 (1982), pp. 279–303; J. Trussell and K.W. Wachter, *Estimating the Covariates of Historical Heights* (NBER Working Paper, 1455, New York, 1984); Floud, Wachter, and Gregory, op. cit. in n. 6.

contribute. In summarizing studies made before 1974, Eveleth and Tanner identified, among environmental influences, nutrition and disease, socio-economic level, urbanization, seasonal and climatic variation, psycho-social stress, and the secular trend, for which 'factors such as improved nutrition, control of infectious disease through immunisations and sanitation, more widespread health and medical care, and population mobility, (both geographically to urban areas and socially upward) appear to be responsible'.[18] Since 1974, further research has added variables such as income per head and the level of inequality, education, and 'health behaviour',[19] while, as I have argued above, reducing the value of the concept of the secular trend.

In one sense, this long list of correlates of height growth merely emphasizes that height, or nutritional status, sums up all the many aspects of what can alternatively be called the 'standard of living' of a population. Since this is so, and since the findings which are reported above anchor height so firmly into the economy and society of the past, anthropometric studies represent a considerable advance on past methods of studying living standards, which have often been confined to the calculation of series of real income and real wage statistics. On the other hand, the very diversity of environmental factors which can affect height, and the fact that these determinants have not so far been integrated into a satisfactory causal model, leads to frustration. It would be good to know why a particular increase in height occurred, whether it sprang, for example, from an increase in income or from a decrease in work intensity; at the moment, we can rarely or ever make such a statement with any confidence.

It is clear, however, that height is both a sensitive and a comprehensive indicator of the past of a group or population. This is amply demonstrated by the work that has been done, as well as by modern evidence both from the developing and from the industrialized world. As Martorell, Klein, and Delgado[20] put it:

> the results of the present study suggest that simple and well-known measures such as weight and supine length (height) should be utilised in evaluating public health programs. These are not only among the most sensitive of measures but also among the most reliable.

Since this is so, we can rely on the fact that (provided we can estimate changes in height in the past with reasonable accuracy) height data do accurately reflect the nutritional status of populations in the past and, in

[18] Eveleth and Tanner, op. cit. in n. 10, p. 261.

[19] Steckel, op. cit. in n. 9; C. Power, K. Fogelman, and A.J. Fox, 'Health and Social Mobility during the Early Years of Life', *Quarterly Journal of Social Affairs*, 2 (1986), pp. 397–414.

[20] R. Martorell, R.E. Klein, and H. Delgado, 'Improved Nutrition and its Effects on Anthropometric Indicators of Nutritional Status', *Nutrition Reports*, 21 (2) (1980), pp. 219–30.

particular, the nutritional status of cohorts of populations during their early childhood.

More speculative, but even more fascinating, is the likelihood that height is important as an indicator of the future of such populations, in the sense of their experience during adult life. In some ways, height can be seen as a measure of human capital, acquired during childhood and adolescence and used in adult life.[21] It represents accumulated experience, the balance between inputs and outputs up to the time of measurement or the cessation of growth. In addition, however, it represents future potential. This was clear to military recruiters, who explicitly sought tall recruits on the grounds that they would be healthier and better able to withstand military life. It was also clear to slave owners, who were prepared to pay more for taller slaves and who selected relatively small slaves for élite tasks.[22] It seems, therefore, that relative height confers both a physical and a psychological advantage, a supposition that is confirmed in studies of social mobility.[23]

However, the epidemiological studies which have shown a consistent inverse relationship between height and mortality from cardiovascular and respiratory diseases are of particular significance.[24] It has long been observed, of course, that deprivation and disease in childhood can affect life-chances and there have been numerous studies of the effects of childhood infection on subsequent mortality and morbidity.[25] In addition, Barker and Osmond[26] have recently observed ecological correlations between mortality rates by geographical regions in a given modern cohort and mortality rates in the same region at the time that the cohort was born. But whereas such studies operate within the closed circle of mortality and poorly observed morbidity, without considering the wider character of the society as a whole, the studies which relate height to mortality make a direct connection between nutritional status and health experience much later in life.

Finally, studies of nutritional status emphasize the need for, as well as the complexity of, considering separately the welfare of different social and

[21] Floud, op. cit. in n. 8.

[22] R.W. Fogel, *Without Consent or Contract* (New York, 1989).

[23] R. Illsley, 'Social Class Selection and Class Differences in Relation to Stillbirths and Infant Deaths', *British Medical Journal* (1955) (ii), p. 1520; Power, Fogelman, and Fox, op. cit. in n. 19; Knight and Eldridge, op. cit. in n. 12.

[24] Waaler, op. cit. in n. 14; Marmot, Shipley, and Ross, op. cit. in n. 14.

[25] F. Falkner (ed.), *Prevention in Childhood of Health Problems in Adult Life* (WHO, Geneva, 1980); W.T. Hughes, 'The Sequelae of Infectious Diseases of Childhood'. In Falkner (ed.), op. cit. in this note; A. Forsdahl, 'Are Poor Living Conditions in Childhood and Adolescence an Important Risk Factor for Arteriosclerotic Heart Disease?', *British Journal of Preventive and Social Medicine*, 31 (1977), pp. 91–95.

[26] D.J.P. Barker, and C. Osmond, 'Infant Mortality, Childhood Nutrition and Ischaemic Heart Disease in England and Wales', *The Lancet* (1986) (i), pp. 1077–81; 'Childhood Respiratory Infection and Adult Chronic Bronchitis in England and Wales', *British Medical Journal* (1986) (ii), pp. 1271–75.

income groups within a society. In considering the impact of famine in pre-industrial England, Fogel has recently[27] shown the importance of discussing the nutrient intake of different classes in explaining the impact of dearth and famine on mortality and, by implication, on morbidity and productivity. These studies require further refinement, but demonstrate what can be done.

4. Height and the European Mortality Decline

What then can indicators of nutritional status contribute to the investigation of the European mortality decline and in particular to the role of medicine within that decline? It is necessary, first, to distinguish sharply between the role of nutritional status and the role of nutrition as it was seen by a number of earlier writers, most notably McKeown. As every demographer knows, he argued by exclusion in *The Modern Rise of Population*[28] that improved nutrition was the primary cause of the mortality decline in England and, by implication, in Europe as a whole. It is clear that McKeown thought of nutrition in the sense of food intake—indeed, he devoted part of his book to a discussion of improvements in agricultural technology—and that he saw nutrition as clearly distinct from medical intervention either in the sense of public-health measures or of drug or other therapy.

Nutritional status is much more than nutrition, and certainly comprises public-health measures and, indeed, therapies which reduce the incidence or mitigate the effects of the diseases of childhood and adolescence. In this sense, the demonstration that heights increased in Europe alongside the mortality decline does not provide any direct support for McKeown's thesis; nutrition may have improved, but so may public health or other forms of medical intervention, and height data do not currently, as I argued above, make it possible for us easily to distinguish between these possible causes. The evidence of improved nutritional status is not, in other words, evidence of improved nutrition.

At the same time, the height evidence focuses attention on the role of improved nutritional status of a given group in the past, by contrast with improved medical knowledge, public-health measures, or other influences on mortality in the present life of that group. This is the importance of the role of nutritional status as an indicator of the future, as it was described in the last section. It directs our attention to cohort rather than period effects in explaining the decline of mortality.

[27] R. W. Fogel, 'Biomedical Approaches to the Estimation and Interpretation of Secular Trends in Equity, Morbidity, Mortality and Labor Productivity in Europe 1750–1980', (Mimeo, University of Chicago, Center for Population Studies, 1987).

[28] T. McKeown, *The Modern Rise in Population* (London, 1976).

It is particularly interesting, therefore, to observe the time pattern of declining mortality in Britain in relation to the evidence of heights. It is a well-known feature of British mortality decline that improvements were first seen during the late 1860s or early 1870s for children under 15, that females aged 15–24 benefited at the same time, and males of the same age during the next decade and that improvements then continued, age group by age group and decade by decade; infant mortality, finally, fell early during the twentieth century.[29] Kermack, McKendrick, and McKinley[30] observed long ago that this pattern was one in which mortality rates fell in each successive cohort and suggested that such a pattern could best be explained by improvements in the health of children.

This pattern matches very well with the evidence of heights, which began to rise with the birth cohorts of the 1860s and rose consistently, if slowly, thereafter until the end of the century and beyond. Taken together with the clear correlations which have been established in modern studies between height and subsequent mortality, this appears to establish a strong case for the view that the mortality decline was linked to improved nutritional status.

Since, as was suggested above, modern evidence from the developing world suggests that it is nutritional status after the period of weaning which is particularly important in determining height and thus long-term health chances, this suggested link between height and the mortality decline does not founder on the fact that neonatal and post-neonatal mortality were slow to fall. Many of the causes of this mortality seem to be largely unaffected by the environment of the very young child. In addition, if such mortality is, as some modern studies would suggest, linked to the health of the mother, one would expect a delay of at least a generation before the improved nutritional status of female children would be translated into an improvement in the life-chances of their children.

To say that the mortality decline may plausibly be linked to improved nutritional status does not, of course, settle the issue of which inputs into nutritional status changed so as to produce a net improvement. There is not space, in this brief chapter, to do more than suggest that the most likely candidate is that rising real incomes overcame, during the third and fourth quarters of the century, the urban diseases which had become so prevalent during the first and second quarters of that century. Nor is it yet possible to estimate with any certitude the likely elasticity of mortality with respect to height, and thus to estimate the extent to which the mortality decline can be attributed to improved nutritional status, although Fogel has made some suggestive attempts to do so.[31]

[29] M. Greenwood, 'English Death Rates, Past, Present and Future' , *Journal of the Royal Statistical Society*, 99 (1936), pp. 674–707.

[30] W.O. Kermack, A.G. McKendrick, and P.L. McKinley, 'Death Rates in Great Britain and Sweden: Some General Regularities and Their Significance'. *The Lancet* (1934) (i), pp. 698–703.

[31] Fogel, op. cit. in n. 5.

5. Directions for Future Research

This brief survey has indicated a number of areas where further research is required. First, the military records of Europe must be exploited to yield additional information on the socio-economic and spatial covariates of height differentials; it is unsatisfactory that so much information on this subject is currently drawn from the countries with volunteer armies, where the problems of statistical estimation of the parameters of truncated distributions are inextricably mixed with the complexities of social stratification.

Secondly, despite the substantial efforts of Komlos and Ward in their studies of Austria-Hungary and of Steckel in his work on American slaves,[32] much more effort needs to be devoted to the discovery and exploitation of sources of data on young children. It is unsatisfactory that, when the literature of the subject in the developing world suggests that the younger ages are particularly influential in determining the pattern of growth, we still know so little about growth during the early years or even about birthweight.

Thirdly, much more effort must be devoted to the investigation of the long-term sequelae of nutritional status in childhood. This will require further investigation of the evidence on Norway used by Waaler, together with the exploitation over the next few decades of longitudinal samples and a search for more relevant historical evidence which can be fitted into the suggestive, but still inconclusive, patterns which are now developing. The possibilities are exciting, not least because of the very rapid improvements in nutritional status since the Second World War which are evident in the data on the heights of Europeans and which are almost certainly taking place in many parts of the developing world. There is every reason to believe that, as the mean heights of populations move towards the optimum levels for life expectancy identified by Waaler and found, over one century ago, in the Union Army data, 'we ain't seen nothing yet'!

[32] Komlos, (1986), op. cit. in n. 7; W.P. Ward, 'Weight at Birth in Vienna, Austria, 1865–1930', *Annals of Human Biology*, 14(6) (1988), pp. 495–596; Steckel, op. cit. in n. 16.

9 Housing and the Decline of Mortality

JOHN BURNETT *Brunel University*

Between the middle of the eighteenth century and 1914 many Western European countries experienced, at differing times and rates, population growth, industrialization, and urbanization, which resulted in fundamental changes in the ways people lived, worked, and were housed. Nowhere were these changes more dramatic than in England, 'the first industrial nation'. Here, an estimated population of little more than 6 million in 1750 grew to 8,893,000 at the first Census in 1801, doubled to 17,928,000 in 1851, and doubled again to 36,070,000 by 1911;[1] meanwhile, the distribution between urban and rural population was completely reversed, the proportion of town-dwellers rising from 20 per cent in 1801 to 80 per cent in 1911. By then, England and Wales was the most highly urbanized society in Western Europe, and contained 15 per cent of its total population. The fastest rates of growth were recorded in some of the new industrial towns of the North and Midlands, which considerably outpaced the growth of London from 1,088,000 in 1801 to 4,541,000 in 1911. Thus, Manchester grew by no less than 40.4 per cent between 1811 and 1821, and by a further 47.2 per cent during the next decade: Liverpool increased by 43.6 per cent between 1821 and 1831, while Bradford grew eightfold in 50 years, from 13,000 in 1801 to 104,000 by 1851.

By the later decades of the century, however, the rate of growth of most English industrial towns was slackening. The characteristic feature now was the rapid growth of residential suburban areas around existing towns, following improved communications and an increasing separation of home from work. The migration of the better-off classes out of crowded city centres, which had begun in London during the late eighteenth century, and had been observed by Engels in Manchester in the 1840s[2] was now typical of all large towns, and this resulted in physical segregation of the populations by differing qualities of environment and housing which clearly reflected social status.

This rapid growth of numbers and of towns from the later eighteenth century offered major opportunities for builders to provide accommodation

[1] B. R. Mitchell and P. Deane, *Abstract of British Historical Statistics* (Cambridge, 1962), pp. 5–6.

[2] F. Engels, *The Condition of the Working Class in England* (1845), trans. and ed. W. O. Henderson and W. H. Chaloner, (Stanford, Calif., 1968), pp. 54–55.

for people at different income levels. The rate of house-building fluctuated in complex ways in relation to the general state of the economy, interest rates, the cost of labour and materials, and local demand, and varied in England and Wales between an increase of 20.6 per cent in 1821–31 (the fastest in the century), and 10.1 per cent in 1841–51 (the slowest).[3] The number of houses increased from 1,576,000 in 1801 to 7,550,000 in 1911, and given its small-scale, unrevolutionized nature, the building industry responded surprisingly closely to overall demand, the average number of persons per house falling from 5.67 in 1801 to 5.46 in 1851 and 5.05 in 1911.[4] Such averages fail to reflect the overwhelming opinion of contemporaries that much working-class housing was grossly overcrowded, and becoming increasingly so, but since they took no account of regional, class, income, or other variables, it is impossible to verify this belief. Industrialization widened income differences within and between classes, enabling the skilled and better-paid workers to move up in the housing hierarchy, and increasing the numbers and wealth of the middle classes who occupied large houses with many rooms. 'In this event', Professor Flinn has commented, 'the constancy of the national density over the whole period must, as a result, have involved increased crowding of those in the lower income groups'.[5]

In fact, throughout the nineteenth century in north-western Europe as a whole, urban death rates were consistently higher than those in rural areas. Furthermore, infant mortality was strongly and positively correlated with the proportion of population living in cities of more than 20,000 inhabitants, suggesting that 'the urban effect' was a major determinant of life chances. During the 1880s infant mortality rates in the three countries with the largest proportions of such city-dwellers—England and Wales, Belgium, and the Netherlands—were high at 142, 158, and 175 per 1,000 respectively, while in Norway and Sweden with fewer than 14 per cent of city-dwellers, were found the lowest rates of 96 and 107 per 1,000 respectively: crude death rates also followed the same pattern, though in a less pronounced way.[6] In discussing the likely effects of housing on mortality decline it is, therefore, essential to have regard to its location. In the search for prime causes, accommodation was not an independent variable whose effect can be measured separately from the environment in which it occurred or from a range of socio-economic factors which affected its occupants.

[3] J. Burnett, *A Social History of Housing 1815–1985* (London, 1986), p. 16.

[4] H. Barnes, *Housing: The Facts and the Future* (London, 1923), p. 340.

[5] M. W. Flinn, introd. to E. Chadwick, *Report on the Sanitary Condition of the Labouring Population of Great Britain* (1842; Edinburgh, 1965), p. 5.

[6] S. J. Kunitz, 'Speculations on the European Mortality Decline', *Economic History Review*,[2] 36(3) (1983), p. 359.

1. The Quality of Accommodation

Although it was the squalor of urban slums which aroused most contemporary alarm, in the case of Britain it was the rural labourer who was the worst housed of any large, regularly employed class. This was due to a variety of causes, but fundamentally because the labourer's small wage did not enable him to pay a rent large enough to encourage speculative builders to erect healthy, sanitary cottages. Even in the decade 1841–51, when half the population of England and Wales was still rural, only 81,000 cottages were built in the countryside compared with 234,000 houses in towns.[7] Throughout the eighteenth and nineteenth centuries there remained an absolute shortage of accommodation for the farm labourer, estimated even in 1913 after a rapid 'flight from the land', at 120,000.[8] Cottages were not only deficient in number, but much too small for the families they now contained: they were dark, damp, dilapidated, and ill-ventilated, lacking in almost every requirement of civilised life. Speaking at a conference in 1860 on the subject of 'Overcrowded Villages', Revd. John Montgomery noted that while overcrowding in towns had received some attention from reformers, the grave problems in the countryside had remained unnoticed. Yet here, there was 'a mass of accumulated misery and corruption. . . . If human beings are crowded together, moral corruption takes place as certainly as fermentation or putrefaction in a heap of organic matter.'[9]

For observers like this, the moral effects of 'cottage herding' were paramount, but others stressed its sanitary and medical consequences. In a Parliamentary Report in 1843 it was found that dilapidation and decay were present almost everywhere in the countryside—wattle and daub walls so thin as to be worn into holes, rotting thatch roofs, floors of broken brick or even earth, wet throughout the winter, a total absence of drainage and sanitation. Although there was a scattering of new 'model' cottages built by philanthropic employers for estate workers, most labourers' cottages had been built a century or two before, and typically consisted of a single room which served all the purposes of living, cooking, eating, and washing: out of this a narrow staircase or ladder led to one or two tiny loft bedrooms, unheated and open to the rafters. At Stourpain in Dorset a family of eleven inhabited a two-roomed cottage, the single bedroom 10 square feet containing three beds, one occupied by four sons aged 10–17 years, one by twin daughters aged 20 and another girl, the third by the parents and two younger children: there was only one tiny window, 15 square inches. The investigator was told that almost every bedroom in the village was similarly crowded, and that

[7] R. Weber, 'A New Index of Residential Construction and Long Cycles in House-Building in Great Britain 1838–1950', *Scottish Journal of Political Economy*, 2 (1955), pp. 120–21.

[8] *Report of the Land Enquiry Committee*, i. *Rural* (1913), p. 131.

[9] J. Montgomery, 'On Overcrowded Villages', *Transactions of the National Association for the Promotion of Social Science 1860* (1861), pp. 787–89.

at Studley no fewer than 29 people occupied one small cottage. A surgeon in Blandford reported that he had recently treated three typhus patients, a woman and her two children, who were all lying in the same bed in an out-house which contained a well and a large tub of pig-food: there was a bare earth floor and no ceiling.[10]

Individual cases did not convince contemporaries who cherished a romantic view of the countryside, but the results of a national enquiry in 1864 clearly showed that the problems were general and increasing. The survey covered 821 rural parishes, in which the population had increased from 305,567 in 1851 to 322,064 in 1861 while the number of cottages had actually diminished from 69,225 to 66,109: of these, 40.8 per cent had only one bedroom, 54.5 per cent two, and a mere 4.7 per cent three – the ideal of the housing reformers. The average air-space per person was 156 cubic feet, whereas the law required 500 cubic feet in workhouses and other Poor Law institutions.[11]

It is likely that similar conditions prevailed in peasant communities throughout most of Western Europe during the eighteenth and much of the nineteenth centuries. Cottages were constructed of whatever local materials were available – frequently a timber frame supporting walls of mud, wattle and daub, sometimes mixed with cow-dung. A single, all-purpose room, not always with a loft bedroom, accommodated the family, and often directly adjoined a cowshed or pigsty. The one advantage of such a domestic environment was that, given the nature of agricultural work, relatively little time was spent in it. Rural cottages might be densely occupied but were not usually densely congregated: most had gardens or allotments and all had nearby fields where most working hours of men, many children, and some women were spent. Compared with that of the industrial town, the external environment of the rural labourer's cottage was benign.

Unlike the uniformly low standards of rural housing for the working class, urban housing presented a clear hierarchy of quality, with extremes both worse and better than those of the countryside. At the lowest and cheapest level was the cellar-dwelling, described by contemporaries as dark, damp, and airless, the abode of the lowest-paid workers, the feckless, improvident, and intemperate. Consisting of one or, at most, two rooms, with light and air only from a grating or skylight at ground level, these underground dwellings came into widespread use in north-west England during the rapid Irish immigration between the 1830s and the 1850s. By then, there were an estimated 40,000 cellar-dwellers in Liverpool, representing about 20 per cent of the population, and between 15,000 and 20,000 in the central borough

[10] *Report of Special Assistant Poor Law Commissioners on the Employment of Women and Children in Agriculture* [510] xii (1843), p. 89.

[11] *Seventh Report of the Medical Officer of the Privy Council*, app. 6, 'Inquiry into the State of the Dwellings of Rural Labourers, by Dr H. J. Hunter' [3484] xxvi (1865).

of Manchester, probably between 10 and 15 per cent of the total.[12] Cellar-dwellings were, however, largely restricted to cities in which there was sudden pressure by the poor on existing accommodation: other industrial towns such as Leeds, Birmingham, and Nottingham contained either few, or none at all.

Only slightly higher in the scale were the lodging-houses found in all large towns and originally intended for the temporary accommodation of migrant workers. They were usually former middle-class houses of considerable size, but now split up into single rooms, each containing the maximum number of beds the floor-space would allow. A contemporary, Peter Gaskell, described such places in Manchester where there were five, six, or seven mattresses crammed into each room, covered with filthy clothes. 'Young men and young women; men, wives and their children—all living in a noisome atmosphere, swarming with vermin, and often intoxicated'.[13] Although intended only for temporary lodging, they often became more or less permanent homes for the near-destitute and semi-criminal classes, and were almost indistinguishable from a normal tenemented house, except for their gross overcrowding and promiscuity. Their number must be conjectural, but Mayhew in 1861 estimated that they accommodated some 80,000 people.[14]

For many workers in English towns, and especially in London, the next step up in the housing hierarchy was to occupy rooms in a tenemented house—that is, an existing house subdivided into separately-let floors or single rooms. The origins of the slums, or what contemporaries called 'rookeries', were found here, in the poorest parts of London like St Giles and Jacob's Island, in Little Ireland and Gibraltar in Manchester, or in Boot-and-Shoe Yard in Leeds. This was residual housing, often built originally for better-off tenants who had now fled to the more salubrious suburbs. An observer in 1850 described houses in London in which the average number of persons per room was 12, and in one instance 17,[15] while in a Manchester slum in 1832 one privy served 380 inhabitants.[16] By the later nineteenth century there had been some improvement in most towns, but the scarcity of accommodation in London perpetuated the tenement as a normal form of accommodation for the working classes: here in 1901 6.7 per cent of the whole population lived in one room, 15.5 per

[12] Burnett, op. cit. in n. 3, p. 61.

[13] P. Gaskell, *The Manufacturing Population of England* (1838; repr. Leicester, 1972), pp. 141–42.

[14] H. Mayhew, *London Labour and the London Poor, London Street Folk* (London, 1861), pp. 269–81, 454.

[15] T. Beames, *The Rookeries of London* (London, 1850; repr. 1970).

[16] J.P. Kay, *The Moral and Physical Condition of the Working Classes Employed in the Cotton Manufacture in Manchester* (1832; repr. Didsbury, Lancs., 1969), p. 36.

cent in two, and 16.6 per cent in three, a total of 38.8 per cent compared with 18 per cent as the average for English towns.[17]

New housing specifically designed for working-class occupation by speculative builders was overwhelmingly of a terraced type,[18] detached or semi-detached houses being too expensive of land and materials for the mass market. The simplest terrace house, widely adopted in midland and northern industrial towns, was the 'back-to-back', a house only one room deep, sharing a common back wall and side walls with its neighbours. Such houses were usually built in long, double rows on a gridiron pattern, the front houses abutting directly onto the road while the rear houses faced onto a narrow court and another double row. The smallest versions were simply 'one up and one down'—that is, a living-room and a bedroom, each approximately 12 square feet: larger types had a second storey and a basement, providing four rooms in all, though in this case the cellar was often separately let. Unlike the types of accommodation previously described, the 'back-to-back' provided for family privacy at a minimal level, and despite the criticisms of sanitary reformers was not unpopular with residents: in Leeds there were 49,000 'back-to-backs' in 1886, and building was not prohibited until 1909.

South of Birmingham, however, such houses were rare, and in London and Bristol almost unknown. Here, the typical form of new building throughout the eighteenth and nineteenth centuries was the 'through' terrace—rows of houses, usually two rooms deep, each with a yard or small garden at the rear: here there was light at both ends of the house, through circulation of air and private territory which could contain a privy or, later, a water-closet. Such houses spanned the social spectrum from plebeian to aristocratic, depending on the width of the plot, the number of storeys, ranging from two to five or six, and the amount of ornamental elaboration. Well-paid artisans could hope to occupy one of the smallest types with two living-rooms (kitchen and parlour), possibly a small scullery at the rear, and two or three bedrooms on the upper floor. Beyond this, houses on three or more floors would be rented by middle-class families with servants, or split up for multi-occupation. The terraced house fell increasingly out of favour with the wealthier classes from around the mid-nineteenth century, partly because it lacked scope for individualization, partly because a suburban lifestyle in a detached house with a large garden became more attractive.

Except in London and the poorest parts of other cities, where families squeezed into one or two rooms of larger houses, the individual cottage was the characteristic form of English urban housing. This was not so in

[17] *Cost of Living of the Working-Classes: Report of an Enquiry by the Board of Trade into Working-Class Rents, Housing and Retail Prices, 1905* [1861] (1908), pp. 592–93.

[18] S. Muthesius, *The English Terraced House* (New Haven, Conn., and London, 1982), p. 1.

neighbouring Scotland. In Edinburgh, Glasgow, and other cities, purpose-built tenements of three or four storeys were the normal type, a common staircase giving access to flats of two or three rooms. Room sizes were usually larger than in England, and additional sleeping accommodation was provided by bed recesses in the living-room. In Edinburgh the typical tenement contained four flats to each floor, sixteen to the block: washing and toilet facilities were shared on each floor. The Scottish tenement system therefore resulted in higher densities and greater overcrowding than in any English city: in Glasgow in 1911 (population 784,496) 85.2 per cent of dwellings had three or fewer rooms, and 55.7 per cent of the population lived in 'overcrowded' conditions, defined as more than two adults per room.[19]

Scottish housing was much more akin to that in most Western European towns than the English form: indeed, in the European context the English cottage was almost the exception, and the tenement the rule. Closest to the English model of cottage accommodation was Belgium, where working-class houses were not normally divided, and 'back-to-backs' were widely built in Brussels, Ghent, and Antwerp throughout the nineteenth century. In industrial towns like Ghent—'the Manchester of the Continent'—urban housing conditions deteriorated during the first half of the century under the impact of rapid population growth: here, between 1830 and 1855 population increased by 41 per cent, dwellings by only 28 per cent.[20] As elsewhere, the result was a sharp rise in rents, which absorbed an increasing proportion of working-class budgets: Schollier has estimated that cotton-workers in Ghent occupying the lowest-rented 15 per cent of houses, spent 11.2 per cent of their earnings on rent in 1835, 25.4 per cent in 1875, and 30.1 per cent in 1910. As in England, housing conditions in Belgian towns were probably at their worst during the 1830s and 1840s, before sanitation began to be brought to the old town centres, and better building standards were required in the new wards: the major improvements in the urban environment, however, date from the 1890s, by which time the average number of persons in Ghent 'back-to-backs' had fallen to 3.6.[21] Here, and in other Belgian cities, much depended on the energy and ability of local administrators. When Dr Thomas Legge surveyed sanitary arrangements in six European countries in the early 1890s, he particularly praised those in Brussels where a Bureau d'Hygiène with wide powers had been established by the burgomaster in 1874. Legge believed that future improvements in public health might follow the Brussels model, rather than the British.[22]

[19] M. J. Daunton, *House and Home in the Victorian City: Working-Class Housing 1850–1914* (London, 1983), pp. 54–55.

[20] P. Schollier, 'The Cost and Quality of Housing in Belgium in the Nineteenth Century', paper presented at International Colloquium on the Standard of Living in Western Europe, Sept. 1983 (Amsterdam and Leiden, 1983), p. 1.

[21] Ibid., pp. 5, 9.

[22] T. M. Legge, *Public Health in European Capitals* (London, 1896), p. 128, cited by R. Woods, Ch. 13 in this vol.

If Belgium and parts of northern France were closest to the English housing pattern, German towns paralleled the Scottish. Here the tenement was the dominant form, with the one exception of Bremen, where single-family houses were the norm. France and the Swiss Romande lay somewhere between these two extremes, cottages predominated in around a third of French towns, tenements in about half. Urban growth was considerably slower here than in England or Germany, only one-quarter of the French population being town-dwellers in 1851.[23] Paris had adopted a building code as early as 1783 which covered the width of main roads, paving, and drainage (the *alignements*), but did not extend to unhealthy side-streets, courts, or new suburbs like Belleville, and the cholera outbreak in 1832 caused much the same panic as in England. Densely packed tenement blocks were rapidly built in Paris and other French towns during the modernization schemes of the Second Empire, although Haussmann's work concentrated mainly on improved street communications, and a permissive law of 1852 which allowed towns to draw up public-health and housing regulations was not widely adopted until the 1880s and 1890s: by 1900 they were enforced in 200 towns. But in Paris the sewerage system was not completed until the first decade of the twentieth century; doubtless a cholera outbreak in 1892 had something to do with this.

One possible explanation of the prevalence of tenement building in European towns is the late survival of fortifications which restricted outward expansion and necessitated building upwards. This would seem to have been the case in the Swiss Romande, where in Geneva before the fortifications were demolished in 1851 housing normally consisted of tenements with three to five storeys which contained two- or three-roomed flats with shared toilets and washhouses. Concern about the state of public health in mid-century led to improved tenement designs which owed something to the influence of Henry Roberts in London. Reformers like Barde condemned the overcrowding, lack of ventilation, sunlight, and privacy in such buildings. There was much debate about the relative merits of tenements and cottages, 'associated' and self-contained units. The trend here, as in England, was towards more individualized space, away from collective or shared space which had formerly been used for washing, cooking, and sanitary purposes. Genevan flats of the later nineteenth century were usually self-contained rather than 'associated', and increasingly controlled by codes of conduct laid down by the canton and landlords: in particular, regulations of 1893 controlled the use of the remaining collective space in tenement blocks, and resulted in a more privatized, if coercive, residential environment.[24]

Precisely how housing conditions evolved in a nineteenth-century town

[23] A. Sutcliffe, *Towards the Planned City: Germany, Britain, the United States and France 1780–1914* (Oxford, 1981), p. 131.

[24] R.J. Lawrence *Le Seuil franchi: Logement populaire et vie quotidienne, en Suisse Romande 1860–1960* (Geneva, 1986), pp. 285–91.

can best be understood at the micro- rather than the macro-level, and has been well demonstrated in a recent study of Odense, Denmark by Professor Hans Johansen. Population in Odense, the largest provincial town until 1879, increased rapidly after the middle of the century with the onset of industrialization, when building activity spread beyond the confines of the medieval town. In Hans Jensens Stroede, a side-street in the old town (where Hans Andersen was born in 1805), there were 36 houses, all single-storey, the majority consisted of only one room and a kitchen: water was supplied, sometimes irregularly, from outside pumps, while sewage flowed down the street in an open ditch. In 1845 these houses were occupied by 178 persons, an average density of five persons per house, but during the second half of the century numbers began to fall with migration outwards: moreover, most houses now had a second storey added and outhouses for kitchens or sculleries built: Johansen estimated that living space increased by about 20 per cent per person between 1870 and 1914. Sanitary improvements in the old town began in 1853 when supplies of filtered running water were laid on, and continued in the 1880s when pig-keeping in back yards was controlled, and cesspits were replaced. New building in the developing areas of the town was generally of a much improved standard of design and space, conforming to a Housing Act of 1858: by the end of the century the typical new working-class dwelling consisted of three rooms and a kitchen, and the density of occupation was only about half that in the old town.[25] The evolution of housing in Odense therefore followed the same directions that were noted elsewhere—towards more, larger rooms, more privatized amenities, and stricter building and sanitary regulations.

2. Housing Problems

This brief survey of the quality of accommodation available to the mass of the population has already suggested the existence of widespread housing problems both in town and country. Contemporaries identified the hazards to health as arising mainly from overcrowding, unhygienic methods of construction, lack of ventilation, inadequate and impure water supplies, and imperfect or non-existent sewerage. To this formidable list may be added some less obvious problems which also had implications for health—the levels of rent which tenants had to pay for their accommodation, the arrangements for cooking and storage of food, and wider social problems which, at least in part, resulted from poor housing.

The earliest housing anxieties were, in fact, about none of these, but about fire hazards caused by the crowding of timber houses in the narrow lanes

[25] H. C. Johansen and P. Boje, 'Working Class Housing in Odense 1750–1914', *Scandinavian Economic History Review*, 34(2) (1986), pp. 132–52.

and courts of London and other cities. The Great Fire of London in 1666 resulted in attempts to control new building by Acts in 1667 and 1707, extended by the London Building Act of 1774. This introduced a concept of status by dividing houses into 'rates' or classes by size and value: there was a structural code for each 'rate' which specified foundations, thickness of walls, size and position of windows, and heights of ceilings, as well as the width of streets onto which different 'rates' faced. By this time, brick was the normal building material in London and other towns, unless local supplies of stone were available, but in the countryside it did not become general until well into the nineteenth century when railways made it possible to distribute bricks and roofing slates easily and cheaply.

In his pioneering *Report on the Sanitary Condition of the Labouring Population of Great Britain* in 1842, Edwin Chadwick was concerned to point out the relationship between disease, poverty, bad housing, and other environmental factors. He revealed a frightening picture of the squalor and decay of rural housing—of cottages built directly onto marshy ground without foundations or flooring, of open sewers immediately in the front of houses, full of decaying animal and vegetable refuse, and roofs of thatch, rotten and saturated with wet. Tiny, broken windows were stuffed with rags in vain attempts to keep out the cold and the smell from adjacent dung-heaps, while walls and floors were constantly damp throughout the winter: in 1838 there had been 5,893 deaths from endemic, epidemic, and contagious diseases in the rural counties of Cornwall and Devon alone.[26] But contemporaries believed that the greatest dangers, both sanitary and moral, resulted from the overcrowded sleeping arrangements in cottages, where a single bedroom, 10 feet square, often accommodated five, six, or seven people. Dr Edward Smith thought that 'A man may carry his rheumatism, acquired from the sweating walls and "heaving" floor of his ruinous dwelling to a good old age: the peasant, gaining immunity from his open-air existence, may escape the noxious results of stagnant drains and even of impure water; but it is his sleeping accommodation which produces the most insidious (and often fatal) results upon his health. Overcrowding has probably killed more than all other evil conditions whatever.'[27]

By the beginning of the nineteenth century house-building in most English towns was in brick, with roofing of slate or tile. Although brick had been regarded as a superior material in earlier times, that used for cheaper, working-class housing was often of poor quality, not thoroughly baked, and porous. Moreover, many such houses, especially the 'back-to-backs', were built only of single brick (4½ inches) instead of the proper double. Writing of such houses in Manchester in 1842, Chadwick observed:

[26] Chadwick, op. cit. in n. 5, pp. 80–81.
[27] E. Smith, *The Peasant's Home 1760–1875* (London, 1876), p. 10.

They have certainly avoided the objectionable mode of forming underground dwellings, but have run into the opposite extreme, having neither cellar nor foundation. . . . The whole of the materials are slight and unfit for the purpose. . . . They are built back-to-back, without ventilation or drainage, and, like a honeycomb, every particle of space is occupied. Double rows of these houses form courts, with perhaps a pump at one end and a privy at the other, common to the occupants of about twenty houses.[28]

The extract encapsulates the problems of much urban housing during the mid-nineteenth century. In tenemented houses overcrowding and the necessary sharing of amenities were the principal targets of reformers: in 'back-to-back' cottages serious overcrowding might or might not exist depending on the size of the family and numbers of other occupants, but the main objection was the lack of through-ventilation, both within the house and externally in the narrow, enclosed courts where foul air was trapped. Courts and alleys, unlike principal streets and shopping thoroughfares, were rarely cleaned by local authorities, receiving all kind of rubbish and, not infrequently, human excrement from choked, overflowing privies which served a hundred or more inhabitants. In such conditions of prevailing filth, where sewers, if they existed at all, ran open through the courts, it probably mattered little whether one accepted the contagionist or miasmatic theory of disease, since there was abundant material, human and non-human, for its generation and transmission. Statisticians had no difficulty in demonstrating how widely mortality rates varied in town and country, between different towns and between 'healthy' and 'unhealthy' districts of the same town depending on environmental factors. In 1841, when the average expectation of life at birth in England and Wales was 41 years, in rural Surrey it was 45, in London 37, in Liverpool 26, and in Manchester only 24.[29] More revealing still, within any one town the expectations of life varied directly with social class and economic status, and the implications which these carried for standards of housing and hygiene: thus, in Leeds in 1841 expectation of life in the gentry and professional classes was 44 years, for tradesmen 27, and for labourers only 19.[30]

'Overcrowding' was defined by statute in Britain in 1891 as more than two adults per room, children under 10 years counting as half and those under 1 year not at all: the size of rooms was not taken into account, though sculleries and bathrooms (where they existed) were not included. On this generous definition, in 1901 8.2 per cent of the population of England and Wales lived in 'overcrowded' conditions, but the national average concealed wide variations. In that year the range was between 0.6 per cent in Bournemouth, 1.0 per cent in Leicester, 16.0 per cent in London (Finsbury

[28] Chadwick, op. cit. in n. 5, pp. 343–44.
[29] W. Farr, *Vital Statistics*, ed. N.A. Humphreys (London, 1885), p. 467.
[30] Chadwick, op. cit. in n. 5, p. 224.

35.2), 30.5 per cent in Newcastle, and 35.5 per cent in Gateshead. In the last two towns, it is true, flats on Scottish lines, with rather larger, but fewer, rooms than in the English cottage, were a common type, but in Glasgow, with its preponderance of tenements, the average overcrowding in 1911 reached 55.7 per cent.

In his *Report* Chadwick also commented on 'the domestic habits affecting the health of the labouring classes'. The difficulty of keeping homes clean, especially when in multi-occupation, was an obvious factor, and contemporary accounts make constant reference to vermin, fleas, flies, lice, and bed-bugs which residents found almost impossible to exterminate. The storage, preparation, and cooking of food was another difficulty, particularly in tenemented houses where an open fireplace was often the only provision: by mid-century new working-class cottages usually contained a fitted iron range with an oven and a water-boiler, but for many town dwellers the real improvement came only after the 1890s when it became possible to rent gas-cookers on a meter system. Inadequate storage facilities, as well as lack of capital, meant that food was often bought in tiny quantities for each meal, for which the housewife paid dearly.[31]

Irregular needs could always be economised to some extent in hard times, but rent was a fixed demand which had to be given priority. The clear evidence from Britain and other European countries is that rent was in inverse proportion to income—that although the middle classes usually devoted around 10 per cent of income to it, the fraction increased rapidly as income fell. In York in 1900, average rents took 14.9 per cent of working-class earnings, but the poorest wage-earners with less than 18*s*. a week had to spend 29 per cent on rent while the best-paid (over 60*s*. a week) spent only 9 per cent.[32] An American enquiry carried out in 1890–91 indicated that the English worker spent a rather higher proportion of income on rent (11.8 per cent) than the French (10.4 per cent), Belgian (9.7 per cent), Swiss (9 per cent), or German (8.7 per cent), though lower than in the United States (15.1 per cent).[33] Rents also varied over time in the same area, depending on local demographic pressure and the ability of the building industry to respond to demand; the proportion that rents bore to wages also depended on the success of workers in the labour market. Thus, in Odense at the beginning of the nineteenth century, rent took around 10 per cent of the worker's wage, but as pressure on accommodation increased during the 1840s, between 15 and 20 per cent: by 1900 wage levels had risen and the proportion had returned to nearer 10 per cent.[34] Economic considerations

[31] J. Burnett, *Plenty and Want: A Social History of Diet in England from 1815 to the Present Day*. (London, 1983), ch. 8.

[32] B.S. Rowntree, *Poverty: A Study of Town Life* (London, 1902), p. 165.

[33] British and Foreign Trade and Industrial Conditions, *Memoranda: Statistical Tables and Charts Prepared in the Board of Trade* [1761] (1903), p. 220.

[34] Johansen and Boje, op. cit. in n. 25 pp. 150–52.

were paramount in housing, and, in the absence of subsidized provision, rent and wages were always the ultimate, limiting factors governing the extent and quality of accommodation.

3. Housing, Disease and Mortality

A leading Environmental Health Officer and Housing Hygiene Consultant to WHO has recently written

> Housing and health studies have usually failed to separate or take into account the multi-factoral non-housing variables which affect health e.g. poverty, ignorance, poor nutrition and lack of medical care. It is even less clear whether these various factors are equally important or not, and how they should be evaluated in a research programme.[35]

This difficulty, of isolating the effects of bad housing on health from other predisposing factors which often accompany it, is compounded as we move back in time. That life chances were related to degrees of urbanization was clearly established by Chadwick in 1842, and the 'urban effect' has since received more sophisticated analysis. In England and Wales in 1811 the expectation of life at birth for inhabitants of the largest towns was 30 years, for those in smaller towns 32 years, and in rural areas 41: in 1861 the figures were 35, 40, and 45, while by 1911 they had narrowed to 51, 53, and 55 years.[36] The periods of substantial improvement occurred after the middle of the century, when sanitary reforms began to take effect, and after 1900 when infant mortality was reduced.

In general, there was also a clear relationship between mortality and density of population, first established by William Farr in 1843, although he recognized that the unhealthy tendency of density could be 'counteracted by artificial agencies' such as adequate ventilation, water supplies, and sewage disposal. Thus, in the 'model' Peabody tenements in London in 1889, where a high density of 751 persons to the acre was reached, the death rate was 16.49 compared with 17.4 for the whole of London, where the average density was 58 to the acre.[37] High densities could be made tolerable, even healthy, by careful planning and investment, but 'improved dwellings' of this kind were still exceptional in Britain at the end of the period, and charged rents beyond the reach of the poorer working classes.

Sir Arthur Newsholme, the former Principal Medical Officer of the Local

[35] R. Ranson, 'Relating Housing Standards to Health Hazards', *Journal of the Royal Society of Health* 107(6) (1987), p. 231.

[36] R. Woods, 'The Effects of Population Redistribution on the Level of Mortality in Nineteenth Century England and Wales', *Journal of Economic History* 45(3) (1985), p. 650.

[37] A. Newsholme, *The Elements of Vital Statistics in their Bearing on Social and Public Health Problems* (London, 1923), p. 285.

Government Board, wrote in 1923: 'The relation between housing and health illustrates the intricacy of the connection between any two connected social events. Is the excessive death-rate and sickness-rate in small tenements due to the drifting of the physically and mentally inferior section of the people into these dwellings by a process of selection, or are the dwellers themselves responsible for the result?'[38] Earlier writers had asked the same question without the neo-Darwinian explanation—did the pig make the sty or the sty the pig? Medical Officers of Health generally avoided the awkward question, preferring merely to demonstrate the statistical relationship between density and mortality in cities like Glasgow where in 1911 the standardized death rate in one-room dwellings was 20.1, in two-room 16.8, in three-room 12.6, and in four or more 10.3.[39]

Examination of some of the major fatal diseases of the eighteenth and nineteenth centuries strongly suggests a relationship with housing and associated problems. Infectious diseases were the major causes of death in Western Europe for most of the nineteenth century. In England and Wales in 1850 they were responsible for some 60 per cent of all deaths, air-borne diseases being about twice as significant as water- and food-borne,[40] though in French cities, where pure water supplies developed more slowly, the latter became more important. Smallpox, one of the most widespread diseases of the eighteenth century, recurred at frequent intervals in the major industrial towns; less frequently and less seriously in smaller towns and villages. In densely populated Glasgow it is estimated to have caused 19 per cent of all deaths during the last quarter of the eighteenth century, children under 5 years often made up half the total, and in London there were eleven peak years during the century, each with over 3,000 deaths.[41] Highly infectious, it was caused by direct or indirect contact with a preceding case, and therefore easily transmitted in overcrowded living conditions. Typhus, transmitted by the body louse, was equally serious during the eighteenth century, and particularly associated with poverty and unhygienic, crowded housing: in 1741 it caused 7,500 deaths in London, one-quarter of the total, and one-fifth of those in Edinburgh, but it was also very common in the cellars and 'back-to-backs' of Manchester, Liverpool, Leeds, and other northern industrial towns. It continued in both its endemic and epidemic forms until the mid-nineteenth century, with serious outbreaks in 1817–19, 1826–27, 1831–32, 1837–38, and 1846–48, the last associated with the flood of Irish immigrants during the Potato Famine.

[38] Ibid., pp. 305–06.

[39] A.K. Chalmers, 'The House as a Contributory Factor in the Death Rate', *Proceedings of the Royal Society of Medicine* (1913), cited in Newsholme, op. cit. in n. 37, pp. 305–306.

[40] S.J. Kunitz, 'Mortality since Malthus', in D. Coleman and R. Schofield (eds.), *The State of Population Theory*, (Oxford, 1986), p. 283.

[41] G.M. Howe, *Man, Environment and Disease in Britain: A Medical Geography* (New York, 1972), p. 143.

Typhoid, another frequent cause of death, was a water-borne disease spread by contamination with sewage, or by contaminated food, and was not suppressed until pure water supplies and sewage disposal systems were developed during the later nineteenth century. But the new, and most dreaded, disease was cholera, which first appeared in Britain in 1831. This first outbreak of 1831–34 caused 21,882 deaths in England and Wales, 9,592 in Scotland and 25,378 in Ireland: the second, even more serious, epidemic in 1848–49 resulted in 52,293 deaths in England and Wales. A water-borne disease, the conditions favourable to its spread were water rich in organic matter and salts, overcrowding, and dark, sunless dwellings: the outbreak of 1848–49 was particularly severe in overcrowded Glasgow (3,800 deaths) and the mushrooming mining towns of South Wales like Merthyr Tydfil (1,400 deaths) in which sanitation had been neglected.

Phthisis (pulmonary tuberculosis) was also at its height during the first half of the nineteenth century, accounting for an estimated 17.6 per cent of all deaths in 1838.[42] Although not class-specific, it was particularly associated with overcrowding and lack of ventilation in houses and work-places, and was prevalent among those in domestic occupations, such as handloom-weaving and framework-knitting. Both its forms—bovine tuberculosis caused by infected cow's milk, and human, caused by inhaling bacilli from infected sputum—declined after the mid-century peak of 360 deaths per 100,000 and had fallen to 150 per 100,000 by 1914.

Most of the improvement in mortality rates after about 1850 was due to the reduction of the death rate among children and young adults—not significantly among infants under 1 year nor the elderly. Children were particularly at risk from the water-borne and food-borne diseases, and from zymotic diseases where overcrowding was a predisposing cause. As late as 1901–10, 35 per cent of all deaths of males occurred among boys less than 5 years old, their principal causes being, in order: whooping cough, measles, diarrhoeal diseases, diphtheria, scarlet fever, pneumonia, and bronchitis.[43] The distribution of death rates from zymotic diseases in 1901 was positively correlated with population density and domestic overcrowding, being highest in London, industrial Lancashire, Tyneside, and the West Riding of Yorkshire, where tenemented houses or 'back-to-backs' were the commonest dwelling types. In 1911 children under 10 years of age formed 10.7 per cent of the population of all dwellings in England and Wales, but 38.2 per cent of the population of all 'overcrowded' dwellings;[44] in these, the conditions for transmission of infectious and contagious diseases were most favourable.

[42] Ibid., p. 179.
[43] Newsholme op. cit. in n. 37, p. 371.
[44] Ibid., p. 304.

4. Housing Reform

Improvements in the quality of mass housing came about from a variety of causes—the rising standards of living of many working-class families during the later nineteenth century, the concerns of philanthropists for the poor, and the growth of intervention by the state and local authorities in housing policy. It is only possible here to outline the course of change.

The state of English rural housing had been an object of concern for a minority of landowners since the late eighteenth century. Designs for 'model' cottages, which usually consisted of a living-room, scullery, and two bedrooms, were adopted by some large estate owners, partly to ensure a contented labour supply, and partly as picturesque adornments to their properties. By the mid-nineteenth century three bedrooms had become the ideal, enabling a moral separation of parents, male, and female children. Although this movement for cottage reform, and in a few cases for the building of entire 'model villages' is interesting architecturally,[45] it is unlikely that it was sufficiently widespread to have had any significant effects on general health or mortality.

In British towns, housing reform began as a by-product of the 'sanitary idea' which the cholera outbreak of 1831 had inspired. Arguments for effective legislation met powerful opposition, however, and the first Public Health Act of 1848 was a very inadequate measure which gave limited powers to local authorities to control drainage, water supply, and the removal of refuse, but left housing itself untouched.[46] In the view of most Victorians, 'the Englishman's castle' was inviolable.

Potentially more important changes came from two sources. From 1844, when Lord Ashley was instrumental in establishing the Society for Improving the Condition of the Labouring Classes, numerous philanthropic housing trusts were founded, especially in London, to build sanitary accommodation in 'model' tenements and lodging-houses: some began with donations from philanthropists, or raised their capital from investors willing to limit their annual dividend to 5 per cent. By 1885, there were 28 such housing trusts, accommodating 147,000 people or 4 per cent of London's population. 'Five Per Cent Philanthropy', as it was termed, was scarcely significant as a contribution to national housing need, though it did have exemplary effect in demonstrating that improved standards of sanitation and convenience were appropriate for working-class accommodation and could make crowded tenement life healthy.[47]

The other source of improvement came from the actions of some progressive local authorities which, from the 1840s onwards, began to control

[45] G. Darley, *Villages of Vision* (London, 1975).

[46] S.E. Finer, *The Life and Times of Sir Edwin Chadwick* (1952–70).

[47] J.N. Tarn, *Five Per Cent Philanthropy: An Account of Housing in Urban Areas 1840–1914* (Cambridge, 1974).

the standards of new housing and urban development. A principal target was the 'back-to-back' and the court system which accompanied it: Manchester prohibited the building of 'back-to-backs' by by-laws in 1844, Nottingham in 1845, Liverpool in 1864, and Birmingham in 1876. Liverpool, with its special problems of mass immigration, was the first city to appoint a Medical Officer of Health in 1846, and also the first to embark on council building in 1869. Intervention by central government was usually limited to granting permissive powers to local authorities which they could adopt or not as they chose, a freedom which led to great variations in housing policies in different British towns. Manchester prohibited cellar-dwellings in 1853, and in 1867 drew up regulations governing room sizes, window areas, and the provision of private yards to all new houses. Many town councils adopted sets of model by-laws under the terms of the Public Health Act 1875. Local authorities could now control the width of new streets, the construction of new houses, the spaces around them, and the sanitary provisions relating to them: regulations extended to ceiling heights, window sizes, and ventilation within the house, and externally to details of paving, drainage, and sewerage.[48] These led, in the period from 1880–1914, to what has become known as 'by-law housing' in many English towns—architecturally monotonous terraces of two-storey 'through' houses consisting of two living-rooms, a scullery 'out-shot', and three bedrooms: each had a small yard containing its own privy, soon to be converted to a water-closet. Such houses, uninspired but sanitary, represented a major improvement in the standard of working-class accommodation. Similar tightening of building controls was introduced into many European cities during the 1880s and 1890s. As tenements of five to seven storeys became increasingly common, and occupational densities correspondingly higher, it was even more important to plan adequate ventilation, light, and removal of refuse, and to control the use of collective internal and external space. Stricter design requirements for multi-storey blocks were introduced in London, Geneva, Odense, and many other cities at this time in attempts to mitigate the potential dangers of crowded environments.

But although new housing came under increasing public control during the last quarter of the century, there remained the inheritance of old, insanitary property, much of it decaying into slums, which yielded high profits to landlords but high death rates to occupants. In Britain, an Act of 1868 permitted, but did not require, local authorities to declare individual houses unfit for human habitation, to enforce their improvement or, alternatively, demolition, while in 1875 a further statute gave powers to councils to deal with areas of insanitary property by slum clearance. In fact, more slums were removed as a result of commercial developments and the

[48] S. M. Gaskell, *Building Control: National Legislation and the Introduction of Local Bye-Laws in Victorian England* (London, 1983), p. 48.

building of railway termini than by public action, most councils preferring to repair and modernise unfit property. From the 1880s onwards, many enclosed courts were opened up, 'back-to-backs' were converted into 'through' houses, water-closets replaced cesspools and earth middens, and piped water was laid on to individual houses. 'The Great Clean Up', it has been said 'did inch forward'[49] but many English towns did not acquire proper water supplies and sewerage systems until the 1890s, and then only, as in the case of Cambridge, when rising rates of typhoid and scarlet fever prompted action. It was not difficult for energetic Medical Officers of Health to demonstrate the good effects of such action—how in Merthyr Tydfil draining, watering, and sewering between 1855 and 1885 halved the infant death rate, reduced typhoid mortality from 2.1 to 0.3 per 1,000 and added 10 years to the average expectation of life, or how in West Bromwich the substitution of piped water for polluted wells was accompanied by a fall in deaths from scarlet fever from 63 a year to 5.[50]

The course of housing and sanitary reform in other European cities followed a similar pattern to that in England, modified in some cases by the different timing of urban growth. In Belgium, early urbanization and deterioration of working-class housing resulted in official inquiries in Brussels in 1838 and in Ghent in 1845 which mirrored Chadwick's condemnations of 'overcrowded, unhygienic, tumbledown hovels'. As in England, sanitary reforms began around 1850, especially in new quarters of towns, but there was little improvement in the old wards until the 1890s, by which time piped water and sewerage were being introduced and the average number of persons per house was falling.[51] In Swiss Romande there was similarly a proliferation of official reports on housing and sanitation from mid-century, which led to 'the inspection of dwellings by health officials, the founding of benevolent societies concerned with housing issues. . . . [and] the organization of architectural competitions to resolve the shortage'.[52] Housing reform in France suffered, as it did in England, from the permissive nature of much of the legislation. The building controls of 1852 were only widely adopted during the 1880s and 1890s, at the same time as water-borne sewerage systems were laid: 'social hygiene' became an important public issue in France during the 1890s, with widespread concern about unhealthy housing, tuberculosis, and alcoholism. An Act of 1902 finally required all sizeable towns to draw up public-health regulations, including the inspection and demolition of insanitary dwellings,[53] the

[49] F.B. Smith *The People's Health 1830–1910* (London, 1979), p. 226.

[50] Ibid., p. 227.

[51] Schollier, op. cit. in n. 20. pp. 6–9.

[52] R.J. Lawrence, 'Public Space—Collective Space—Private Space: The Morphogenesis of Popular House Types in Swiss Romande', Unpublished paper, p. 16.

[53] Sutcliffe, op. cit. in n. 23, pp. 137 ff.

later adoption of such measures perhaps reflecting the smaller extent of urbanization in France.

5. Conclusion

It is beyond dispute that housing was one of the important environmental factors which influenced disease and mortality. When housing conditions were at their worst in the early industrial towns, so also were mortality rates: when conditions improved during the later nineteenth century, mortality improved significantly. But the fact that rural death rates were consistently lower than urban, despite the generally inferior quality of rural housing, suggests that the house itself was not the principal determining factor. Although bad housing could clearly facilitate the transfer of communicable diseases, interfere with physiological needs, and cause injury to health and safety, so also could other factors, and it would be unwise to attempt to assign a quantifiable 'weight' to the specific influence of the house. In this chapter I have argued that it is not possible to isolate the house as a physical structure from associated amenities such as water supplies and sewerage, from the external environment in which it was located, or from the wider social and economic environment of its occupants; poor housing almost always went with overcrowding, poor sanitation, poor diet, and a generally poor standard of living as part of the cycle of deprivation. Improved housing could even result in an increase in mortality when higher rents meant there was less to spend on food.[54] Finally, the relatively late period at which standards of accommodation, in terms of structure, space, density, and hygiene, generally improved lends little support to the contention that housing was one of the environmental improvements which accounted for the fall in mortality from as early as the eighteenth century onwards.[55]

[54] G.C.M. M'Gonigle and J. Kirby, *Poverty and Public Health* (London, 1936), pp. 108–129.

[55] T. McKeown and R.G. Brown, 'Medical Evidence related to English Population Changes in the Eighteenth Century', *Population Studies*, 9(2) (1955), repr. in M. Drake (ed.), *Population in Industrialisation* (London, 1969).

10 Conditions of Work and the Decline of Mortality

MICHAEL R. HAINES *Wayne State University, Detroit*

It now seems evident that conditions in the workplace, whether factory, farm, workshop, mine, commercial establishment, or elsewhere, influence health and, by extension, mortality. We are aware of numerous conditions related to workplace hazards, such as 'brown lung' disease among textile workers, asbestosis, 'black lung' disease among coal miners, other lung conditions among coal and hard-rock miners and workers in dusty environments, lead and other metal and chemical poisoning, and a variety of cancers. And, of course, there is the ever-present danger of debilitating or fatal accidents, as well as the many physical conditions resulting from particular aspects of repetitive arduous tasks. Indeed, we now have an entire speciality, which evolved early in the twentieth century, known as industrial medicine.[1] But it is not always easy to identify such phenomena historically.

The first systematic treatise on occupational disease, *De morbis artificum diatriba* by Bernardino Ramazzini, appeared as early as 1713. The advent of the Industrial Revolution in Britain focused attention more clearly on these issues. By the nineteenth century, concern for factory safety and health motivated several British government inquiries, including the Sadler Committee (1832), the Ashley Mines Committee (1842), and finally Edwin Chadwick's well-known *Report on the Sanitary Condition of the Labouring Population of Great Britain* (1842) and the *Health of Towns* (1844). A number of pieces of factory and industrial legislation resulted, but most of the early laws simply regulated hours or conditions for women and child workers in mines and factories. After about 1850, however, specific issues of ventilation, machinery safety, dust, noxious chemicals, and other problems began to be considered in Great Britain. Industrial safety and hygiene also began to feature in legislation in France after 1874, in Germany after 1869, and in the United States at the end of the nineteenth century.[2]

Contemporaries were aware of the apparent ill-effects of employment in industry and mining on health. Chadwick noted, for instance, that crowding

[1] See e.g. P. A. B. Raffle, W. R. Lee, R. I. McCallum, and R. Murray, *Hunter's Diseases of Occupations* (Boston, Mass., 1987).

[2] G. M. Kober and E. M. Hayhurst, *Industrial Health* (Phil., 1924), pp. xi–xxxvi.

in tailors' workshops was associated with an excess incidence of tuberculosis, and that the conditions of handloom weavers were leading to rapid physical deterioration: '[T]he whole race of them is rapidly descending to the size of Lilliputians . . . You could not raise a grenadier company among them at all'.[3] Similar comments were made about the deleterious effects of employment in the mines. Subsequent work by John Simon and Dr Edward Greenhow began to establish the statistical connection between excess mortality in particular districts and the concentration of certain hazardous employments.[4] This early interest led Britain to be a pioneer in the collection and publication of statistics on mortality by age, sex, location, occupation, and (sometimes) cause.

One of the chief pieces of historical evidence for the effect of conditions of work on mortality has thus been occupation-specific death rates. Because the information was often so copious and diffuse, these were later often grouped into social-class categories or socio-economic strata. A well-known example is the grouping into five social classes originally developed by the Registrar-General of England and Wales for the analysis of the Census of 1911, which was subsequently considerably modified and is still used.[5]

One problem with the study of differential mortality by occupation, occupational group, or social class is the interpretation of the results. Occupations, or their combinations into social classes, do not in themselves cause higher mortality, but these categories do represent 'bundles' of biological, behavioural, and environmental circumstances and variables which have a causal role. Unfortunately, many of these variables are interrelated; and occupation, or social class, is often taken as an index of these:

> [T]hese various factors affecting mortality are interdependent – occupation is related to education; income is related to occupation; and both income and education may influence diet, housing conditions and living habits. Since it is not feasible to attempt to assess the influence on mortality of these factors individually, writers have often

[3] E. Chadwick, *Report on the Sanitary Condition of the Labouring Population of Great Britain* (London, 1842), p. 252.

[4] Sir John Simon became Medical Officer to the Privy Council and in 1856 secured the first lectureship in Public Health at St Thomas's Hospital for his colleague Dr Edward Greenhow. They produced *Papers Relating to the Sanitary State of the People of England* in 1858, and an annual series of reports thereafter, which provided much more specific evidence.

[5] This was created by T. H. C. Stevenson to organize his analysis of vital and census data around 1911 for the Registrar-General. It has been seriously challenged as being *ad hoc* and arbitrary. For critical discussion of the social stratification schemes for England and Wales, see S. Szreter, 'The Genesis of the Registrar General's Social Classification of Occupations', *British Journal of Sociology*, 35(4) (1984), pp. 522–46; W. A. Armstrong, 'The Use of Information about Occupation', in E. A. Wrigley (ed.), *Nineteenth Century Society: Essays in the Use of Quantitative Methods for the Study of Social Data* (Cambridge, 1972), pp. 191–310; R. Leete and J. Fox, 'Registrar General's Social Classes: Origins and Uses', *Population Trends*, 6 (1977); J. A. Banks, 'The Social Structure of Nineteenth Century England as seen through the Censuses', in R. Lawton (ed.), *The Census and Social Structure: An Interpretative Guide to Nineteenth Century Censuses for England and Wales* (London, 1978), pp. 179–223.

taken one factor as an index of all others. The factor most frequently studied is occupation, or social class based on occupation.[6]

Hence the conditions of work would only be one among many influences on historical differentials in occupational mortality.

There are other types of problem with these data, notably the difficulty experienced in correctly matching numerators and denominators when calculating rates.[7] Since occupation is not an inherent characteristic of individuals, some individuals change occupations or retire before they finally die of a condition contracted previously in other lines of work. Hence, occupation at time of death may incorrectly identify the activity related to death. This is not to mention the problem of properly calculating person-years at risk. In other words, it is often difficult to identify the period of exposure to risk of particular occupational hazards. None the less, occupational death rates are available for the past and can be used effectively. But there is also reason to use data on small geographical areas with high concentrations of particular activities.

In addition to occupation itself, however, one of the most pervasive historical influences on differential mortality at all ages has been urbanization. While residence in urban areas was not precisely a condition of work, relocation in crowded urban neighbourhoods, often but indifferently supplied with basic water supplies, sanitation, paving, ventilation, etc. was often necessary as structural economic change proceeded. There is abundant evidence that urbanization had a distinct effect on mortality. It is believed that mortality was very high in larger urban areas in medieval and early modern Western Europe and that the populations of towns were not always replacing themselves.[8] Nineteenth-century evidence suggests that urban mortality was well above rural.[9] For instance in 1881–90 the expectation of life at birth in Sweden was 43.4 in urban and 51.6 in rural areas and in 1871–80 the infant mortality rate was 193 in urban and 119 in rural regions. Similarly, in Norway standardized death rates were considerably higher in urban areas in 1889–92 (23.0 and 19.2 per 1,000 for men and women) than in rural places (17.2 and 15.8 per 1,000 for men and women), while infant mortality rates reflected the same differential (125.7 for urban and 83.0 in rural areas in 1896–1900).

This situation was made worse by rapid urban growth induced by industrial development. In England and Wales in 1841, the expectation of

[6] UN, *The Determinants and Consequences of Population Trends: New Summary of Findings on Interactions of Demographic, Economic, and Social Factors* (New York, 1979), p. 137.

[7] J. Vallin, 'Facteurs socio-économiques de la mortalité dans les pays développés', in UN/WHO, *Proceedings of the Meeting on Socioeconomic Determinants and Consequences of Mortality* (New York, 1979), pp. 266–302.

[8] E.A. Wrigley, *Population and History* (London, 1969), pp. 95–98; J. De Vries, *European Urbanization 1500–1800* (Cambridge, Mass., 1984), ch. 9.

[9] UN, op. cit. in n. 6, pp. 132–43.

life at birth was 40.2 for men, but only 35 in London, 25 in Liverpool, and 24 in Manchester. This contrasts with a value of 44 years for the then largely rural, agrarian county of Surrey. By 1881–90 men's expectation of life at birth in Manchester was still 29, while in selected healthy districts it stood at 51, and in the country as a whole at about 44 years. In Scotland in 1871–80, the expectation of life for men was 41.0 years in the country as a whole and 30.9 in Glasgow.[10] In one recent work on living standards in Britain during the industrial revolution infant mortality was used as an index of 'urban disamenities' and showed that city size, density, and an employment mix that favoured mining and manufacturing were all positively and significantly related to infant mortality in both 1838–44 and 1905.[11]

When the Death Registration Area (of ten states and the District of Columbia) was finally formed in the United States in 1900, the expectation of life at birth for the white population was 49.6 years, but in urban areas it was 45.9 in contrast to 54.7 for rural locations.[12] In seven upstate New York counties, urban child mortality exceeded rural between 1850 and 1865, and mortality in Massachusetts towns in 1859–61 increased regularly with town size.[13] Results from the censuses of 1890 and 1900 also confirm the less favourable character of cities in the United States, particularly larger ones.[14]

Researchers on urban French mortality in the nineteenth century found considerably higher mortality in the three largest French cities (Paris, Lyons, Marseilles) than the average for the remainder of the country. The differentials tended to disappear (partly in a cohort fashion) as public-health and especially sanitary improvements were introduced.[15] Indeed, from the late nineteenth century onwards, urban and rural mortality tended to converge, with more rapid declines in urban areas, especially in the largest cities with the greatest resources. This was certainly true of the United States

[10] D. V. Glass, 'Some Indicators of Differences between Urban and Rural Mortality in England and Wales and Scotland', *Population Studies*, 17(3) (1964), pp. 263–67; A. F. Weber, *The Growth of Cities in the Nineteenth Century: A Study in Statistics* (New York, 1899), p. 347.

[11] J. G. Williamson, 'Was the Industrial Revolution Worth It? Disamenities and Death in Nineteenth Century British Towns', *Explorations in Economic History*, 19(3) (1982), pp. 221–45.

[12] J. W. Glover, *United States Life Tables 1890, 1901, 1910 and 1901–10* (Washington, DC, 1921).

[13] M. R. Haines, 'Mortality in Nineteenth Century America: Estimates from New York and Pennsylvania Census Data 1865 and 1900', *Demography*, 14(3) (1977), pp. 311–31; M. A. Vinovskis, 'Mortality Rates and Trends in Massachusetts before 1860', *Journal of Economic History*, 32(1) (1972), pp. 184–213.

[14] G. Condran and E. Crimmins, 'Mortality Differentials between Rural and Urban Areas of States in the Northeastern United States 1890–1900', *Journal of Historical Geography*, 6(2) (1980), pp. 179–202.

[15] S. H. Preston and E. van de Walle, 'Urban French Mortality in the Nineteenth Century', *Population Studies*, 32(2) (1978), pp. 275–97.

and Britain.[16] Similar results were reported for Sweden by Davis[17] and for Prussia by Weber,[18] who also noted:

> The death rate is the lowest in the rural parts and steadily increases with the size of the city . . . There is no inherent reason why men should die faster in large communities than in small hamlets . . . In some degree, doubtless, the mortality of city adults must exceed that of rural adults, on account of the dangerous nature of city occupations . . . But leaving aside accidental causes, it may be affirmed that the excessive urban mortality is due to lack of pure air, water and sunlight, together with the uncleanly habits of life induced thereby. Part cause, part effect, poverty often accompanies uncleanliness: poverty, overcrowding, high rate of mortality, are usually found together in city tenements.[19]

The evidence for contemporary developed nations strongly indicates that these historical differences between rural and urban areas have virtually disappeared or have even been reversed. This appears to be the consequence of the increased effectiveness of public health, sanitation, and medical science in reducing overall mortality in a variety of disease environments.[20] Indeed, the convergence or urban and rural mortality was so rapid during the late nineteenth and early twentieth centuries that Kingsley Davis has reported historical rates of urban mortality decline which exceeded the recent experience of developing nations.[21] Some of this decline was undoubtedly related to improved conditions of work, although this was probably swamped by general improvements in public health and sanitation.[22]

The effect of conditions of work and industrialization *per se* on mortality is often much more difficult to discern. The expectation is that specific occupational hazards would lead to higher mortality among the working population. It is difficult to separate this from the effects of urban environments. In an early study, for Copenhagen and other towns in Denmark for 1865–74, it was found that death rates for men aged 20 and over

[16] M. R. Haines and S. H. Preston, 'Cities, Ethnicity, and Child Mortality in the United States in 1900', paper presented at the Annual Meeting of the Social Science History Association, Toronto, Oct. 1984; D. Friedlander, J. Schellekens, E. Ben-Moshe, and A. Keyser, 'Socio-economic Characteristics and Life Expectancies in Nineteenth-Century England: A District Analysis', *Population Studies*, 39(1) (1985), pp. 137–51.

[17] K. Davis, 'Cities and Mortality', in IUSSP, *International Population Conference, Liège, 1973*, iii (Liège, 1973), pp. 259–82.

[18] Weber, op. cit. in n. 10, pp. 343–67.

[19] Ibid. pp. 344, 348.

[20] UN, op. cit. in n. 6, pp. 132–33.

[21] Davis, op. cit. in n. 17.

[22] Excellent summaries of some of this evidence can be found in UN, op. cit. in n. 6, pp. 137–40; A. Antonovsky, 'Social Class, Life Expectancy and Overall Mortality', *Milbank Memorial Fund Quarterly*, 45(2), pt. 1 (1967), pp. 31–73; and for infant and child mortality see A. Antonovsky and J. Bernstein, 'Social Class and Infant Mortality', *Social Science and Medicine* 11(8/9) (1977), pp. 453–77.

increased monotonically from the higher class (capitalists, professionals, wholesale dealers, higher officers) to the middle class (master mechanics, petty officers, teachers, clerks, small shopkeepers) to the poorest class (workmen, servants, almshouse inmates). Mortality among the poorest was 89 per cent higher than that of the richest class in Copenhagen and 69 per cent higher in other towns. And, further, men's mortality differentials were greater than those for women from the same socioeconomic status groups.[23] In a study of working men in France in 1907–08, based on the Census of 1906, Huber found that mortality among employers (managers and officials) was consistently lower than among wage and salary earners, while death rates of salaried workers (clerks) were generally lower than among wage earners (craftsmen and kindred workers), except at ages 25–34.[24] Mortality of male private household workers was surprisingly low, possibly reflecting the affluence of households able to employ butlers, footmen, coachmen, etc. Wide variations between death rates for specific occupations were reported (e.g., mortality of plumbers was roughly double that of textile workers at all ages).

In England and Wales data on mortality for specific occupations began to be collected in the mid-nineteenth century.[25] In the twentieth century these were condensed into social classes. In Table 10.1 we show men's death rates for over 100 specific occupational titles and groups for 1860/71, 1880/82, and 1890/92. Notable was the high mortality among publicans, innkeepers, and servants in inns and hotels. These individuals often suffered from the ill-effects of excessive alcohol consumption. (See Table 10.2 below.) Low mortality was characteristic of many professions (clergymen, teachers, barristers, and solicitors) as well as of persons working in agriculture and healthier rural and outdoor settings (farmers, graziers, farm labourers, gardeners, nurserymen, fishermen). Many who were engaged in commerce (shopkeepers, merchants) did better than average, provided that they were not impoverished street sellers (hawkers, costermongers). Surprisingly, many coal miners did not do so badly, the effect varied by region.[26] Mortality was above average, however, in employments with

[23] Reported in S.D. Collins, *Economic Status and Health: A Review and Study of the Relevant Morbidity and Mortality Data*, US Public Health Service. *Public Health Bulletin*, 165 (Washington, DC, 1927), pp. 34–38.

[24] M. Huber, 'Mortalité suivant la profession, d'après les décès enregistrés en France en 1907 et 1908', *Bulletin de la statistique générale de France*, 1(4) (1912), pp. 402–39.

[25] England and Wales, Registrar-General, *Supplement to the Forty-Fifth Annual Report (1882): Mortality 1871–1880* (London, 1885) and *Supplement to the Fifty-Fifth Annual Report* (London, 1897).

[26] The lower than expected mortality of coal miners during the late 19th and early 20th cents. from lung diseases, despite the incidence of 'black lung' disease (coalworkers' pneumoconiosis) even prompted some experts to speculate that coal dust protected against tuberculosis. Coal mining even came to be regarded as a relatively healthy occupation. This changed during the 20th cent., as cutting-machinery and more work in hard rock increased the amount of dust in the mines. It became relatively more serious and widespread as technology changed and more difficult seams were worked. See Raffle *et al.*, op. cit. in n. 1, pp. 663–69.

Table 10.1 Death rates by occupation for males aged 25–65 in England and Wales 1860/1871, 1880/1882, and 1890/1892

Occupation	Mean annual death rates per 1,000 living						
	1860/61–1871		1880/82		1880/82	1890/92	
	Age 25–45	45–65	Age 25–45	45–65	Index 25–65	Age 45–54	Index
All males	11.27	23.98	10.16	25.27	1,000	21,37	1,000
Occupied males			9.71	24.63	967		
Unoccupied males			32.43	36.20	2,182		
Males in selected healthy districts[a]			8.47	19.74	804		
1 Clergy, priest, minister	5.96	17.31	4.64	15.93	556	10.52	492
2 Barrister, solicitor	9.87	22.97	7.54	23.13	842	17.72	829
3 Physician, surgeon, GP	13.81	24.55	11.57	28.03	1,122	21.04	985
4 Schoolmaster, teacher	9.82	23.56	6.41	19.84	719	14.31	670
5 Artist, engraver, sculptor, architect	11.73	22.91	8.39	25.07	921		
6 Musician, music master	18.94	34.76	13.78	32.39	1,314	26.01	1,217
7 Farmer, grazier	7.66	17.32	6.09	16.53	631	10.16	475
8 Labourer, in agricultural counties[b]		7.13	5.52	17.68	701		
Farm labourer						13.56	635
9 Gardener, nurseryman	6.74	17.54	5.52	16.19	599		
10 Fisherman	11.26	15.84	8.32	19.74	797	18.61	871
11 Cab driver, omnibus serviceman	15.94	35.38	15.39	36.83	1,482		
12 Bargeman, lighterman, waterman	14.99	30.78	14.25	31.13	1,305		
13 Carter, carrier, haulier			12.52	33.00	1,275	28.01	1,311
14 Groom, domestic coachman			8.53	23.28	887		
15 Commercial traveller	12.28	29.00	9.04	25.03	948		
16 Brewer	19.26	36.86	13.90	34.25	1,361		
17 Innkeeper, publican, spirit, wine, beer dealer	18.01	34.14	18.02	33.68	1,521	44.48	2,081
18 Inn, hotel servant	21.91	42.19	22.63	53.30	2,205		
19 Maltster	7.04	22.26	7.28	23.11	830		
20 Law clerk	18.75	37.05	10.77	30.79	1,151		
21 Commercial clerk, insurance service	14.28	28.88	10.48	24.29	996		
22 Bookseller, stationer	10.84	21.36	8.53	20.57	825		
23 Chemist, pharmacist	13.92	23.56	10.58	25.16	1,015		
24 Tobacconist	13.19	21.76	11.14	23.46	1,000		
25 Grocer	9.49	17.15	8.00	10.16	771	14.34	671
26 Draper, Manchester warehouseman	14.34	26.33	9.70	20.96	883		
27 Ironmonger	10.38	22.95	8.42	23.87	895		
28 Coal merchant	8.83	22.59	6.90	20.62	758		
29 General shopkeeper			9.12	21.23	865		

Table 10.1 (*Continued*)

Occupation	Mean annual death rates per 1,000 living						
	1860/61–1871		1880/82		1880/82	1890/92	
	Age 25–45	45–65	Age 25–45	45–65	Index 25–65	Age 45–54	Index
30 Cheesemonger, milkman, butter-man			9.48	26.90	1,009		
31 Greengrocer, fruiterer	11.41	24.51	10.04	26.57	1,025		
32 Fishmonger, poulterer	15.62	29.21	10.53	23.45	974	20.13	942
33 Shopkeeper (nos. 22–32)			9.04	21.90	877		
34 Butcher	13.19	28.37	12.16	29.08	1,170	22.65	1,060
35 Baker, confectioner	10.72	26.39	8.70	26.12	958		
36 Corn miller		26.65	8.40	26.62	957		
37 Hatter	12.81	31.76	10.78	26.95	1,064		
38 Hairdresser	15.11	30.10	13.64	33.25	1,327		
39 Tailor	12.92	24.79	10.73	26.47	1,051	21.98	1,029
40 Shoemaker	10.39	22.30	9.31	23.36	921		
41 Tanner, fellmonger	10.43	26.57	7.97	25.37	911		
42 Currier	11.32	25.09	8.56	24.07	906		
43 Saddler, harnessmaker	12.29	25.21	9.19	26.49	987		
44 Tallow chandler, soap-boilder	11.75	27.24	7.74	26.10	920		
45 Tallow, soap, glue, manure manufacture			7.31	27.57	933		
46 Printer	13.02	29.38	11.12	26.60	1,071		
47 Bookbinder	12.76	31.56	11.73	29.72	1,167		
48 Watch and clock maker	10.78	24.90	9.26	22.64	963		
49 Watch, clock, philosophical instrument and jeweller			9.22	23.99	932		
50 Paper manufacture	10.33	20.19	6.48	19.62	717	18.84	882
51 Glass manufacture	13.19	29.32	11.21	31.71	1,190	32.74	1,504
52 Earthenware manufacture	12.59	41.75	13.70	51.39	1,742	42.97	2,011
53 Cotton, linen, manufacture (Lanc.)[c]	10.65	27.90	9.99	29.44	1,088	25.11	1,175
54 Silk manufacture	9.89	20.08	7.81	22.79	845		
55 Wool, worsted manufacture (West riding)[c]	9.35	23.26	9.71	27.50	1,032	20.58	963
56 Carpet, rug-manufacture	9.92	25.57	9.48	24.10	945		
57 Lace manufacture			6.78	20.71	755		
58 Hosiery manufacture (Leics., Notts.)			6.69	19.22	717	1215	569
59 Dyer, bleacher, printer, etc. of textile fabrics	11.19	25.99	9.46	27.08	1,012		
60 Rope-, twine-, cord-maker	9.19	29.35	7.95	22.25	839		
61 Builder, mason, bricklayer	11.43	27.16	9.25	25.59	969	22.04	1,031
62 Slater, tiler	10.66	30.76	8.97	24.93	942		
63 Plasterer, whitewasher	9.50	27.90	7.79	25.07	896		

Occupation	Mean annual death rates per 1,000 living						
	1860/61–1871		1880/82		1880/82	1890/92	
	Age 25–45	45–65	Age 25–45	45–65	Index 25–65	Age 45–54	Index
64 Plumber, painter, glazier	12.48	34.66	11.07	32.49	1,202		
65 Upholsterer, cabinet-maker, French polisher	11.09	24.09	9.55	24.77	963		
66 Carpenter, joiner	9.44	21.36	7.77	21.74	820		
67 Sawyer	8.67	21.27	7.46	23.74	852		
68 Wood turner, box-maker, cooper	11.80	26.13	10.56	28.55	1,091		
69 Coach builder	10.43	29.57	9.13	24.72	944		
70 Wheelwright	8.40	21.17	6.83	19.21	723		
71 Shipbuilder, shipwright	10.68	26.26	6.95	21.29	775		
72 Locksmith, bellhanger, gas-fitter	11.04	27.90	9.15	25.66	967		
73 Gunsmith	10.62	25.32	10.62	25.78	1,031		
74 Cutler, scissors-maker			12.30	34.94	1,309	35.60	1,666
75 File-maker	16.27	42.30	15.29	45.14	1,667	40.06	1,875
76 Cutler, scissors, file, needle, saw, toolmaker[d]	11.86	32.74	11.71	34.42	1.273		
77 Engine, machine-maker, fitter, millwright			7.97	23.27	803		
78 Boiler-maker			9.27	26.65	994		
79 Nos. 77–78	10.61	23.81	8.23	23.89	888		
80 Blacksmith	10.07	23.88	9.29	25.67	973	20.74	971
81 Other iron and steel workers			8.36	22.84	869		
82 Tin worker	10.36	23.67	8.00	24.17	885	20.08	940
83 Cooper, lead, zinc, brass, etc. worker	10.74	26.17	9.15	26.79	992		
Lead worker						36.72	1,760
Brass worker						26.05	1,219
84 Metal worker (nos. 72–83) Coal Mining[e]			8.30	25.03	938		
85 Miner (Durham, North.)	11.30	22.01	7.79	24.04	873	16.35	765
86 Miner (Lancs.)			7.91	26.30	929		
87 Miner (West Riding)			6.59	21.80	772		
88 Miner (Derby., Notts.)			6.54	20.23	734		
89 Miner (Staffs.)	11.33	30.45	7.81	26.50	929		
90 Miner (S. Wales, Monmouth)	14.72	20.66	9.05	30.87	1,081	24.27	1,136
91 Coal Miner (nos. 85–90)			7.64	25.11	891	19.42	909
92 Miner (North Riding and other iron-stone districts)			8.05	21.85	834		
93 Miner (Cornwall)	11.84	41.73	14.77	53.69	1,839	33.20	1,554
94 Stone, slate quarrier	10.88	28.67	9.95	31.04	1,122		
95 Railway, road, clay, sand, etc. labourer			11.01	24.80	1,025		
96 Coalheaver			10.22	23.77	968		

Table 10.1 (*Continued*)

Occupation	Mean annual death rates per 1,000 living						
	1860/61–1871		1880/82		1880/82	1890/92	
	Age 25–45	45–65	Age 25–45	45–65	Index 25–65	Age 45–54	Index
97 Chimney sweep	17.53	42.87	13.73	41.54	1,519	31.43	1,471
98 Messenger, porter, watchman (not government)			17.07	37.37	1,565		
99 Costermonger, hawker, street seller	18.35	40.04	20.62	50.85	2,020	31.94	1,495
100 General labourer (London)	18.35	40.04	20.62	50.85	2,020	31.94	1,495
101 Dock, wharf labourer						40.71	1,905
102 Railway porter						16.98	795
103 Railway engine driver						16.09	753

[a] Selected healthy districts include registration districts with a mean annual death rate (for both sexes) below 17.00 per 1,000 for 1871/80.
[b] Includes Herts., Oxon., Beds., Cambs., Suffolk, Wilts., Dorset., Hereford, and Lincs.
[c] For England and Wales for 1860/61–71.
[d] 1871 only for the period 1860/61–71.
[e] For the period 1860/61–71, based on a return to an inquiry into the condition of miners in Great Britain made in connection with the Census of 1861. Covers 1860/62 for coal miners and miners in Cornwall.

Source: 1860–82: England and Wales, Registrar-General, *Supplement to the Forty-Fifth Annual Report 1882* (London, 1885), table J; 1890–92: England and Wales, Registrar-General, *Supplement to the Fifth-Fifth Annual Report 1892* (London, 1897), pp. CXIX ff.

heavy exposure to certain other kinds of dust and noxious substances such as tin mining (Cornwall), pottery and earthenware manufacture, among file-makers, cutlery- and scissors-makers, other non-ferrous metal miners and workers (brass, zinc, copper, lead), and chimney sweeps. In 1890–92, if the death rate from respiratory diseases for male agricultural workers is taken as 100, the index for coal miners was 133, for workers in cotton textiles 244, for copper miners and workers 307 and 317 respectively, for file makers 373, for tin miners 400, for cutlery- and scissors-makers 407, and for pottery and earthenware workers 453 — four and a half times the rate for agricultural workers. The death rate from gout for file makers was more than double the national average for gout, phthisis (respiratory tuberculosis), other respiratory diseases, and nervous and urinary tract diseases. The mortality of lead workers from nervous diseases was about three times the national average, from digestive diseases, two and a half times, and from urinary tract conditions, four times.[27] The effects of exposure to heavy metals

[27] England and Wales, Registrar-General (1897), op. cit. in n. 25, reported in A.S. Wohl, *Endangered Lives: Public Health in Victorian Britain* (Cambridge, Mass., 1983), pp. 279–82.

was already suspected and is now well established.[28] The unfavourable mortality experience of poor outdoor workers, such as general labourers in London, costermongers, porters, and dock and wharf labourers (Table 10.1), was due, in part, to low incomes and bad living conditions (resulting in poor nutrition and housing) and to the fact that sanitation and public-health improvements generally reached these groups very late.

Obviously, it is important to inquire further into cause of death, since this provides clues about causation. In Table 10.2 we show some data for England and Wales for 1880/82 for the occupations with the highest mortality from selected causes. The serious effects of certain dusty environments on respiratory tuberculosis and other lung diseases are apparent from the table, especially among hard-rock miners and quarrymen, earthenware and pottery workers, file-makers, cutlers, and textile workers. Innkeepers suffered in the extreme from alcoholism, liver disease, gout, nervous and urinary tract disorders, and suicide. Diseases of the nervous, circulatory, and urinary systems, substantial cause categories, all suggest effects of environmental contamination on such groups as file-makers, painters, plumbers and glaziers, earthenware workers, and cutlers. Mortality in other occupations, such as cabmen and omnibus servicemen and costermongers, points to the effects of poverty. Although these historical cause-of-death schemes changed over time, and some of the gross categories (e.g. diseases of the nervous system or circulatory system) were sometimes used as 'catch all' residuals for poor or unclear diagnoses, such information is useful and needs further exploration.

During the twentieth century, the emphasis in England and Wales was focused more closely on social class, and variations of the five social-class groupings pioneered for the Census of 1911 were used.[29] In Table 10.3 we show some of these results for the period 1909–12 to 1949–53.[30] Mortality generally rose from the highest social class (I) (including professional and higher administrative positions) through II (other administrative, professional, managerial, and shopkeepers), III (clerical workers, shop assistants, personal service, foremen, skilled manual workers), and IV (semi-skilled manual workers), down to the lowest socio-economic status group V (unskilled manual workers, especially labourers). By 1950, however, mortality was lowest in social class II, but it continued to be highest in social class V. The lower-ranking of class I possibly reflected stress and other factors associated with higher supervisory positions. Recently Pamuk[31] has noted that mortality differentials between social classes among occupied and retired adult men in England and Wales declined from the 1920s to about

[28] Raffle *et al.*, op. cit. in n. 1, ch. 6.
[29] For a history of these social groupings, see Szreter, op. cit. in n. 5.
[30] This table was reproduced from Antonovsky, op. cit. in n. 22, table 17.
[31] E. Pamuk, 'Social Class Inequality in Mortality from 1921 to 1972 in England and Wales', *Population Studies*, 39(1) (1985), pp. 17–31.

Table 10.2 Industries with the highest mortality from selected causes, in England and Wales 1880/1882[a]

Diseases of the: Respiratory system		Nervous system		Circulatory system	
Total	402	Total	119	Total	120
Cornish miner	1,148	File-maker[b]	262	Costermonger	227
Earthenware manufacturer	1,118	Costermonger	207	File-maker	180
File-maker	783	Innkeeper	200	Brewer	165
Cutler	760	Cutler[b]	190	Cab-driver, omnibus serviceman	160
Printer	627	Plumber, painter, glazier	167	Earthenware manufacturer	160
Quarryman	582			Fisherman	153
Cotton manufacturer	543	Brewer	144	Woollen manufacturer	142
Tailor	471	Tailor	144	Innkeeper	140
Wool manufacturer	462	Cotton manufacturer[b]	142	Plumber, painter, glazier	
Mason, builder, bricklayer	453	Earthernware manufacturer[b]	140		
		Butcher	139	Butcher	132
Draper	430	Commercial traveller	139	Baker	131
Baker, confectioner	398	Baker	136	Tailor	127
Carpenter, joiner	337	Cab-driver, omnibus serviceman	134	Blacksmith	121
Coal miner	328	Woollen manufacturer	127	Miner (South Wales)	120
Grocer	283	Shoemaker	122		
Agriculturalist	237				
Fisherman	198				

Urinary system		Liver disease		Suicide	
Total		Total	39	Total	14
File-maker	123	Innkeeper	240	Costermonger, etc.	31
Painter, plumber, glazier	100	Brewer	96	Commercial traveller	26
		Butcher	96	Innkeeper, etc.	26
Innkeeper	83	Commercial traveller	61	Baker	23

Costermonger	69	Cab-driver, omnibus serviceman	54	Butcher	22
Cab-driver, omnibus serviceman	65	Grocer	52	Hosiery manufacturer	21
Brewer	55	Earthenware manufacturer	49	Painter	17
Butcher	55	Painter, plumber, glazier	48	Farmer	17
Builder	49			Carpenter	17
Earthenware manufacturer	49	Tailor	48	Shoemaker	17
Grocer	48	Costermonger	47	Grocer	16
Tailor	45	Baker	46	Cab-driver omnibus serviceman	16
Commercial traveller	44	Cotton manufacturer	43	Tailor	15
Shoemaker	44	Farmer	41	Woollen manufacturer	14
Blacksmith	44	File-maker	41	Builder, mason, etc.	14
Hosiery manufacturer	42	Cornish miner	40		
Alcoholism		Gout			
Total	10	Total	3		
Innkeeper	55	Innkeeper	13		
Cab-driver, omnibus serviceman	33	Cab-driver, omnibus serviceman	11		
Brewer	25	Painter, plumber glazier	10		
Butcher	23				
Commercial traveller	23	Brewer	9		
Costermonger	19	Commercial traveller	6		
Baker	15	Butcher	5		
Painter, plumber, glazier	12	Tailor	4		
		Costermonger	3		
Tailor	11	Builder, mason, etc.	3		
Grocer	10				

[a] The numbers are the deaths that would occur in a population of 64,641 persons, aged 25–64, of whom 41,920 were aged 25–44 and 22,721 were aged 45–64. The death rates in Table 10.1 were multiplied by this standard population to obtain the deaths in this table.
[b] Includes deaths from suicide.

Source: England and Wales, Registrar-General, *Supplement to the Forty-Fifth Annual Report 1882* (London, 1885), tables N. O. P.

Table 10.3 Standardized death rates per 1,000 and standardized mortality ratios in England and Wales 1910–1953 by social class

Period/Rate[a]	Class					Population Group
	I	II	III	IV	V	
1910/12						
Death rate per 1,000	12.0	–	13.6	–	18.7	Occupied and retired males, aged 15+ excluding miners, textile workers, agricultural labourers
Ratio (1 = 100)	100	–	114	–	156	
SMR	88	94	96	93	142	Males aged 25–64, excluding miners textile workers, agricultural labourers
SMR	88	94	96	107	128	As above, modified by Stevenson
1921/23						
Death rate per 1,000	7.4	8.6	8.7	9.2	11.5	Males
Ratio (I = 100)	100	116	117	124	155	
SMR	82	94	95	101	125	Males aged 20–64
1930/32						
SMR	90	94	97	102	111	Males aged 20–64
SMR	81	89	99	103	113	Married women aged 20–64
1949/53						
SMR	98	86	101	94	118	Males aged 20–64
SMR	96	88	101	104	110	Married women aged 20–64
SMR	100	90	101	104	118	Occupied males 20–64, adjusted to control for occupational changes since 1930/32
Death rate per 1,000	6.6	–	6.4	–	9.5	Males 20–64, excluding agricultural workers
Ratio (I = 100)	100	–	97	–	144	

[a] SMR is the standardized mortality ratio.

Source: A. Antonovsky, 'Social Class, Life Expectancy, and Overall Mortality,' *Milbank Memorial Fund Quarterly*, 45(2) part 1 (1967), table 17.

1950, but then began to increase again (in relative terms). These more recent increases in inequalities of mortality probably had more to do with income, general levels of well-being, and access to medical care than with specific conditions of work. While such social-class categories may be useful as indices of overall socio-economic progress, they do not lend themselves to the study of conditions of work. Detailed information on occupational mortality (and morbidity) is required for this purpose.

A good deal of work has been done on the relation between mortality and occupation in the United States since the end of the nineteenth century. The censuses of 1890, 1900, and 1910 furnished extensive data on adult men's mortality by industry. Paul Uselding has analysed this information for states with adequate death registration and found generally (though not consistently) higher mortality among workers in mining, manufacturing,

Table 10.4 Age-standardized death rates by occupation/industry: males in the United States, Death Registration Area, 1890, 1900 and 1908/1910

Occupation/Industry	Age-Standardized Death Rates per 1000			Index		
	1890	1900	1908/10	1980	1900	1908/10
Professional	14.15	14.60	12.56	101	97	99
Clerical and official	11.10	14.35	10.93	79	95	86
Mercantile and trade	12.78	13.27	8.34	91	88	66
Entertainment, personal service, police, military	15.74	13.75	11.31	113	91	89
Labouring and servant	24.54	25.12	18.45	176	167	145
Manufacturing and mechanical	14.62	14.23	14.22	105	94	112
Agriculture	7.72	11.75	11.22	55	78	88
Forestry and fishing	7.80	9.67	7.82	56	64	61
Mining	9.94	15.78	13.06	71	105	103
Transport and communication	16.13	14.92	13.59	115	99	107
Overall Death Rate	13.98	15.06	12.73	100	100	100

Source: P. Uselding. 'In Dispraise of Muckrakers: United States Occupational Mortality 1890–1910'. *Research in Economic History*, 1 (1976), p. 347.

and mechanical industries, and transport and communications.[32] Some of his results are given in Table 10.4. The very high mortality among the labouring and servant population indicates, however, that a substantial part was played by urban residence and poverty, as is also suggested by the low rates for agriculture and for forestry and fishing.

There has been some narrowing of differences between industrial workers and other groups in the population of the United States during the twentieth century. For example, in 1911–12 the mean expectation of life at age 20 was only 36.9 years for white male industrial workers, whereas it was 42.7 years for all white men in the Death Registration Area in 1909/11. This was not due to urban residence alone, since the expectation of life at age 20 was 40.5 years for urban white men. In 1930 mortality rates for unskilled workers were still twice as high as for professionals. By 1949 the expectation of life at age 20 for industrial workers had risen to 48.4 years, only one year lower than that for all white men (49.5 years for 1919/51).[33] In an extensive study of vital registration for 1950, Moriyama and Guralnick found continuing

[32] P. Uselding, 'In Dispraise of Muckrakers: United States Occupational Mortality 1890–1910', *Research in Economic History*, 1 (1976), pp. 334–71.

[33] Metropolitan Life Insurance Company, 'Longevity of Industrial Workers', *Statistical Bulletin*, 31(11) (1950), pp. 4–7; J.S. Whitney (ed.), *Death Rates by Occupations Based on Data of the US Census Bureau* (New York, 1934); Glover, op. cit. in n. 12; US Bureau of the Census, *Historical Statistics of the United States: Colonial Times to 1970*, i (Washington, DC, 1975).

large relative mortality variations between occupational groups.[34] For example, among white men aged 20–64 the mortality rate was 10.6 per 1,000 for labourers, but only 6.4 for professionals and 7.6 for the equivalent of English social classes II–IV. Differences were smallest at the older ages (55–64) and largest at younger ages. In a matched-records study for the United States in 1960, Kitagawa and Hauser found persistent mortality differentials for white men aged 25–64 between white-collar workers (with a mortality ratio of 0.94) and blue-collar workers (mortality ratio 1.06), and especially relative to service workers and non-farm labourers (with a mortality ratio of 1.16). But agricultural labourers still did relatively well (a mortality ratio of 0.82).[35]

In an extensive summary of mortality differentials by socio-economic status, Antonovsky concluded that, although mortality differentials between the lowest and highest social class/occupational groups may have been as high as two to one during the nineteenth and early twentieth centuries, they may have fallen to as low as 1.3–1.4 to one by the 1940s.[36] The differences tended to be lowest at older ages and highest at younger and middle ages. The differences had not disappeared by the date (1967) of his work.

It is apparent from the available historical statistics that men's occupational mortality was much better covered than women's. Indeed, we seem to know rather more about the relationship of infant and child mortality to the occupation and social class of the father. It is fairly clear that the mortality of children was inversely related to the social class or income of the father.[37] The risk of dying was higher for children of mothers who worked outside the home than for children of non-working mothers at the end of the nineteenth century, but the causal mechanisms are not entirely clear.[38] Most of the studies of the mortality of women by socio-economic status have been based on their hushands' status or occupation.[39] In

[34] I.M. Moriyama, and L. Guralnick, 'Occupational and Social Class Differences in Mortality', in Milbank Memorial Fund, *Trends and Differentials in Mortality* (New York, 1956), pp. 61–73; L. Guralnick, 'Mortality by Occupation and Industry among Men 20 to 64 Years of Age: United States 1950', in US Public Health Service: National Vital Statistics Division, *Vital Statistics: Special Reports*, 53(2) (Washington, DC, 1962).

[35] E.M. Kitagawa and P.M. Hauser, *Differential Mortality in the United States* (Cambridge, Mass., 1973), pp. 34–46.

[36] Antonovsky, op. cit. in n. 22.

[37] UN, op. cit. in n. 6., pp. 138–39; Antonovsky and Bernstein, op. cit. in n. 22; M.R. Haines, 'Inequality and Childhood Mortality: A Comparison of England and Wales, 1911 and the United States, 1900', *Journal of Economic History*, 45(4) (1985), pp. 885–912; P.A. Waterston 'Infant Mortality by Father's Occupation from the 1911 Census of England and Wales', *Demography*, 25(2) (1988), pp. 289–306.

[38] S.H. Preston, M.R. Haines, and E. Pamuk, 'Effects of Industrialization and Urbanization on Mortality in Developed Countries', in IUSSP, *International Population Conference, Manila 1981*, ii (Liège, 1981), table 1; R.M. Woodbury, *Infant Mortality and its Causes* (Baltimore, 1926), ch. 3.

[39] Antonovsky, op. cit. in n. 22.

general, the patterns for these women were similar to those for their husbands, i.e. an inverse association between mortality and social class. We do, however, need more extensive information on the mortality of working women themselves, whether working outside the home, in handicraft industry, domestic service, or as unpaid family labour.

The confounding effect of urbanization and industrialization continues to complicate the study of mortality and conditions of work. In a study of industrial areas of northwest Europe in the late nineteenth century, Wrigley found that mortality in coal-mining and industrial districts in France and Germany seldom differed much from that of the surrounding rural areas. High mortality was characteristic of the large cities, some of which happened also to be partly industrial (e.g. Paris, Berlin, Marseilles).[40] Again, in England and Wales, random samples of 125 registration districts in 1851, 1861, and 1871 showed that the zero-order correlations between infant mortality rates and adult men's death rates on one hand, and the proportion of men employed in mining and metallurgy on the other, were insignificant, but that the correlations with the proportion of the districts that were urban were positive, significant, and large.[41] In a recent study of expectation of life in the registration districts of England and Wales during the nineteenth and early twentieth centuries stronger relations were found (in a regression analysis) between population density and mortality than for industrial structure (as measured by proportions of the labour force in professional, commercial, industrial, textile, mining, and domestic employments).[42] This was true for 1851–60 and especially for 1871–80, but economic structure seems to have been more important by 1901–10. Mortality gradients by density were reduced, as mortality, particularly from infectious diseases, declined.

An instructive example is furnished by the study of two mining and industrial districts in England and Wales between 1851 and 1870: Durham and Easington in northern England, and Merthyr Tydfil in South Wales. Durham and Easington was not very urban and mortality rates were close to or below the national average. Adult men's mortality was below the national average. Mortality from respiratory disease (an expected hazard) was not above the national level for adult men, but mortality from accidents was well above. Mortality from this cause was high even for male children, an indication of general environmental hazards as well as of specific occupational risks. In Merthyr Tydfil, on the other hand, mortality was consistently above the national rate at all ages and for both sexes (except for women aged 55 and older). This was mainly due to the unhealthy urban

[40] E.A. Wrigley, *Industrial Growth and Population Change: A Regional Study of the Coalfield Area of Northwest Europe in the Later Nineteenth Century* (Cambridge, 1961), ch. 4.

[41] M.R. Haines, *Fertility and Occupation: Population Patterns in Industrialization* (New York, 1979), p. 35.

[42] Friedlander *et al.*, op. cit. in n. 16.

environment. Mortality from accidents among men was quite high in Merthyr as well, but the overall high death rate was found for almost all causes of death, notably gastro-intestinal infections, an indicator of poor sanitation.[43] The investigation of mortality differences between men and women within districts of different types can be especially instructive, since general environmental hazards from poor urban sanitation and housing would be expected to affect both sexes equally, while conditions of work would influence death rates among the working population, in which mortality differences by sex were important. The conclusion must be that the urban environment had a much greater impact than the specific occupational situation, although this diminished over time as urban/rural mortality differentials converged in consequence of public-health and sanitary improvements. In a study of trends in occupational mortality in England and Wales conducted in 1938, Stocks concluded that 'it is evident that the contribution made by the actual work done to the men's social [i.e. occupational] mortality gradient from all causes must be very small compared with the contributions made by the accompanying environmental, economic or selective factors'.[44]

Despite this, the study of the effects of occupation, employment, and conditions of work on mortality is of great historical interest, partly because of the essential importance of structural change to historical socio-economic development, and partly because of basic concern with improving the quality of human life. There are a number of possible approaches and directions, all of which may be pursued in a complementary fashion. The one emphasized here is the study of mortality differentials in the cross-section and over time by age, sex, occupation (or industry), and cause. Related to this is the analysis of small, more economically homogeneous geographical areas. There is still a great deal of published and archival material remaining to be exploited here. Studies of individual occupational titles and of alternative industrial, occupational, or social class groupings over time will clarify the role of occupation and working conditions on mortality decline.

Another possibility is the study of historical morbidity data. This has been actively pursued in recent years by, for example, Riley and Alter.[45] While morbidity and mortality did not necessarily move closely together

[43] Haines, op. cit. in n. 41, pp. 199–202.

[44] P. Stocks, 'The Effect of Occupation and its Accompanying Environment on Mortality', *Journal of the Royal Statistical Society*, 101(4) (1938), p. 690.

[45] J.C. Riley, 'Disease without Death: New Sources for a History of Sickness', *Journal of Interdisciplinary History*, 17(3) (1987), pp. 537–63; J.C. Riley and G. Alter, 'Mortality and Morbidity: Measuring Ill-Health across Time', paper presented at the Ninth International Congress on Economic History, Berne, 24–29 Aug. 1986; J.C. Riley and G. Alter, 'The Epidemiologic Transition and the Morbidity Trend: Sickness Risk by Age and Form', paper presented at the Annual Meeting of the Social Science History Association, New Orleans, 29 Oct.–1 Nov. 1987.

historically, analysis of morbidity data from sickness and insurance funds and from friendly and benevolent societies can also yield clues as to the contribution of improved conditions of work to increases in human longevity. Insurance company records and data from government social insurance schemes may be able to furnish more detailed evidence on the incidence, severity, and causes of occupation-related accidents and other debilitating conditions. Workmen's compensation data can also provide useful sources of both morbidity and mortality information. Hospital records can be a most fruitful source of micro-level data, especially since occupation-related conditions may be revealed after admission for other causes. Statistics on human stature and other anthropometric data constitute yet another possible source.[46] While heights of adults and various measures of height-for-weight (e.g. Quetelet's index) may be rather imprecise measures of the effect of recent socio-economic conditions (such as occupation) on well-being, it may be possible to examine some impact of work on the health and welfare of adolescent and young adult workers. And, finally, there is the literature from the history of medicine, which has been only briefly mentioned here. There is the large field of industrial medicine and hygiene which also has a detailed and rich history.[47] There we find information on the dates of scientific discoveries and the extent of their application to reduce work-related mortality and morbidity. While ultimate emphasis should be on such outcomes as mortality and morbidity, institutional history can be of value in explaining trends, differentials, and the timing of specific changes in these outcomes.

[46] J.M. Tanner, *A History of the Study of Human Growth* (Cambridge, 1981); id., 'The Potential of Auxological Data for Monitoring Economic and Social Well-Being', *Social Science History*, 6(4) (1982), pp. 571–81; R.W. Fogel, S.L. Engerman, and J. Trussell, 'Exploring the Use of Data on Height: The Analysis of Long-Term Trends in Nutrition, Labor Welfare and Labor Productivity', *Social Science History*, 6(4) (1982), pp. 401–21; R.W. Fogel, 'Nutrition and the Decline in Mortality since 1700: Some Preliminary Findings', (National Bureau of Economic Research, Working Paper, 1402, 1984).

[47] See e.g. Raffle *et al.*, op. cit. in n. 1; A.J. Fleming, C.A. D'Alonzo, and J.A. Zapp, *Modern Occupational Medicine* (2nd edn., Phil., 1960); Kober and Hayhurst, op. cit. in n. 2; ILO, *Occupation and Health: Encyclopaedia of Hygiene, Psychology and Social Welfare* (2 vols., Geneva, 1934); H.S. Selleck and A.H. Whittaker, *Occupational Health in America* (Detroit, 1962).

11 The Care of Children: the Influence of Medical Innovation and Medical Institutions on Infant Mortality 1750–1914

MARIE-FRANCE MOREL *École Normale Supérieure de Fontenay-Saint-Cloud*

The many historical demographic studies that have been undertaken during the last 20 years have shown, in spite of the disparity of available data, that infant and child mortality fell significantly everywhere, and that the fall gathered pace after the First World War. This decline is well documented, even though in some cases it was irregular, and the initial levels, the rate of fall, and the conditions associated with the decline have differed in different countries.

As is true of overall mortality, the mortality of infants and small children may be interpreted in different ways. Its decline could be seen as a consequence of the improvements of the general standard of living of the population (improved nutrition, higher standards of personal hygiene, better water supply, higher quality of foodstuffs, better housing), or it could be attributed more specifically to increases in medical knowledge and a wider diffusion of this knowledge among mothers. Since 1970 the medical explanation has been strongly criticized, particularly by Ivan Ilich and Thomas McKeown, whose arguments are well known.

I do not accept the a priori assumption that medicine has only played a minor part in improving the survival rates of infants. It is not correct to consider only the direct effects of progress, account must also be taken of the indirect effects and of changing attitudes to life and death. As Jacques Léonard has written: 'we must appreciate the true role played by physicians in the past. Some historians who have looked at the slow and relatively insignificant changes in mortality appear to believe that the effectiveness of medical measures was low before 1890 and that all demographic improvements can be related to social and economic changes'.[1]

I would like to thank Nicole Pellegrin, Chantal Beauchamp, and Christopher Duhamelle for their help in collecting the data for this chapter. Michael Haines, Ludmilla Jordanova, Catherine Rollet, and Christopher Wilson helped with their constructive and critical comments when this chapter was originally presented as a paper at the IUSPP Seminar on Medicine and the Decline of Mortality, Annecy, France, June 1988.

[1] J. Léonard, *La France médicale au XIXe siècle* (Paris, 1978), p. 11.

However, medical intervention was traditionally least frequent in early infancy. In this field it was largely women who were active, and practical advice was passed from mother to daughter between different generations with very little change. However, the period of transition in which we are interested, was the very period when medical men began to intervene in this area of childbirth, early infancy, and the care of sick children which had hitherto been reserved to women. It is, therefore, necessary to understand why medicine took an increased interest in children and became more effective, and how it came about that physicians acquired the central place in child-rearing that they occupy today. Moreover, and this is much more difficult, it will be necessary to go beyond medical discussions to evaluate how mothers and wet-nurses reacted to medical advice and to consider the effects of such advice on them. The important question is when and how attitudes towards the life and death of small children changed.

Throughout this period, infant mortality rates were high, of the order of 100 to 350 per 1,000 births. What did these infants die of? During the neonatal period (the first four weeks of life), the main causes of death were congenital malformations, prematurity, difficult labour, and poor health of the mother. Slightly older children who died (post-neonatal deaths) tended to die of diseases of the digestive system (particularly children given out to be wet-nursed, or those who were not breast-fed), or of respiratory diseases largely caused by cold winters against which there was little protection, or of epidemic diseases, such as smallpox, measles, diphtheria, dysentery, etc.

The risk of dying continued to be high during the second and third years of children's lives, particularly during the critical period of weaning. Our discussions must, therefore, extend beyond infant mortality to the mortality of children between their first and fifth birthdays.

Could the reduction in mortality between 1750 and 1914 have been due to improvements in treatment given by physicians? In this chapter, we shall try to assess the extent to which they could have exercised such an influence. We shall take a particular interest in those periods in which infant mortality fell most steeply. In France, where there is a long tradition of research in historical demography, it has been shown that a reduction in infant mortality first occurred between the second half of the eighteenth and the early part of the nineteenth centuries, and that this was followed by a period of relative stagnation which lasted throughout most of the remainder of the nineteenth century. A significant fall was then resumed between 1880 and 1890, and again after 1914.[2] Whereas the first phase of the decline appears to have been specific to France, the second occurred in all developed countries, and after 1890 coincided with the revolution in medicine which followed the work of Louis Pasteur. (Fig. 11.1.)

[2] J. Dupâquier, *et al.*, *Histoire de la population française*, ii. *De la renaissance à 1789* (Paris, 1987–88); M. Poulain and D. Tabutin, 'La Mortalité aux jeunes âges en Europe et en Amérique du Nord du XIXe siècle à nos jours', in P.M. Boulanger and D. Tabutin (eds.), *La Mortalité des enfants dans l'histoire*.

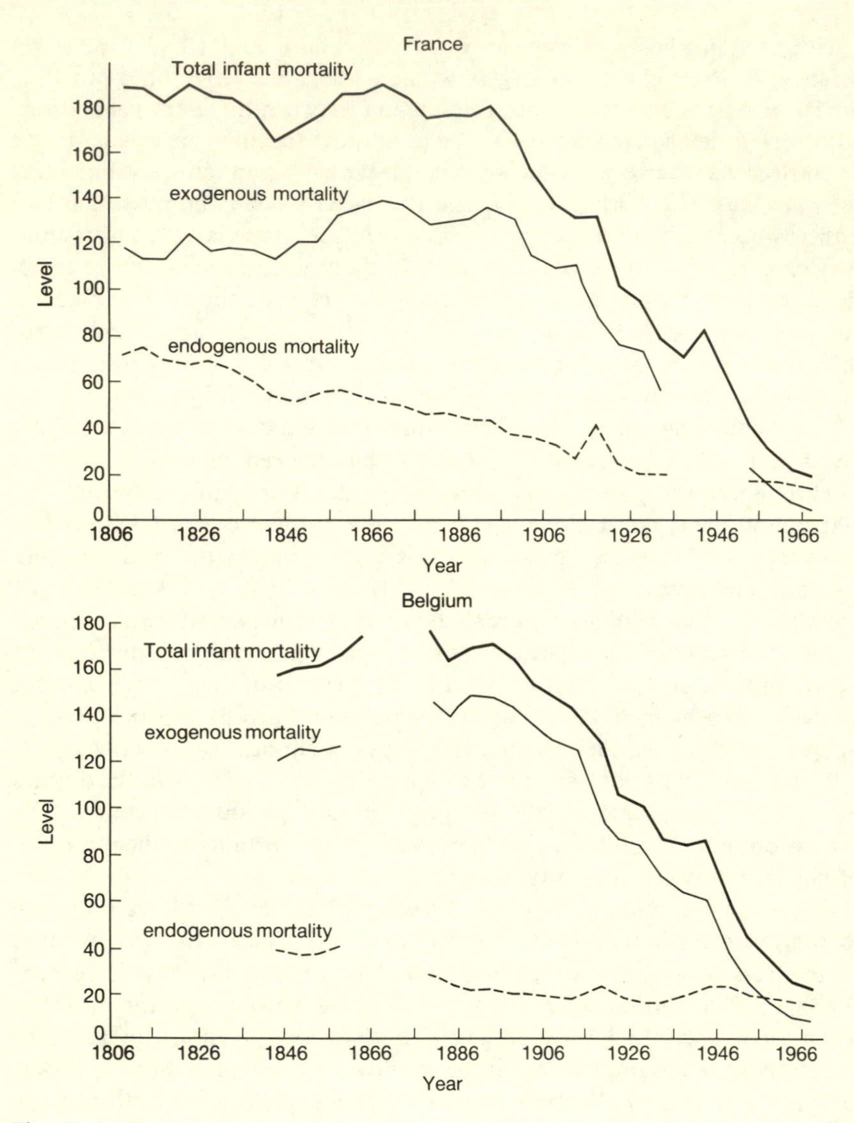

Fig. 11.1 Development of endogenous, exogenous, and total infant mortality: France and Belgium

Source: M. Poulain and D. Tabutin, 'La Mortalité aux jeunes âges en Europe et en Amérique du Nord du XIXe siècle à nos jours', La Mortalité des enfants dans l'histoire (Liège, 1980), p. 131.

1. The First Stage of Medicalization

The slight but significant reduction in infant mortality in France between 1790 and 1829 has not been adequately explained by demographers; it seems to have been unrelated to advances in medical knowledge.[3] However, in my view it would be wrong to judge the effectiveness of medicine in the eighteenth century in the light of twentieth-century knowledge. It is true that during that period there was no medical breakthrough which changed the chances of infant survival radically, but medical men took a new and increasingly passionate interest in saving children's lives. This was manifest by a new willingness to change both the environment and the behaviour that were responsible for a majority of diseases. In the élite groups of society, whose members had the opportunity both to understand the new ideas and to act upon them, the entire climate of opinion changed and a new dynamic appeared, even though it took some time for it to become effective.

Throughout Europe, infancy was on the agenda during the period of the Enlightenment: in art, philosophy, morals, medicine, and political economy. The gracious nature of childhood was stressed, as was the need to preserve its innocence, and attention was drawn to the need for investment in children's education and to the desirability of a large number of births to preserve the power of the State. In many countries, censuses began to be taken in order to assess the quantity of available human resources[4] and medical advice was sought to preserve the public health, and particularly the health of young children, whose special vulnerability was recognized. A whole new literature of more or less scientific treatises appeared, dealing with the best method of conducting confinements and of caring for children. This literature was not confined to France, and the best books (by W. Cadogan, J. Franck, J. Raulin, Tissot, J.C. Desessartz, and, above all, Rousseau's famous *Émile* which was published in 1762) were translated into several languages and inspired the work of other authors.[5]

What were the common themes in this European campaign to save children's lives? There was condemnation of midwives who conducted deliveries in the villages; their ignorance resulted in the loss of a large number of mothers in childbirth, and of babies. Their lethal procedures were always

[3] Y. Blayo, 'La Mortalité en France de 1740 à 1829', *Démographie historique* (*Population*, 30, special issue, (1975)).

[4] Jacqueline Hecht, 'L'Évaluation de la mortalité aux jeunes âges dans la littérature économique et démographique de l'Ancien Régime', in Boulanger and Tabutin (eds.), op. cit. in n. 2.

[5] Cf. M.F. Morel, 'Théories et pratiques de l'allaitement en France au XVIIIe siècle', *Annales de démographie historique* (1976); 'Mère, enfant, médecin: La Médicalisation de la petite enfance en France (XVIIIe–XIXe siècles)', in A. Imhof (ed.), *Mensch und Gesundheit in der Geschichte* (Husum, 1980); R. Spree, 'Sozialisationsnormen in ärztlichen Ratgebern zur Säuglings und Kleinkinderpflege: Von der Aufklärung zur naturwissenschaftlichen Pediatrie', in J. Martin and A. Nitschke, *Zur Sozialgeschichte der Kindheit* (Freiburg and Munich, 1986).

the same: they were in a hurry to get labour over with, and used violent methods in cases of malpresentation, so that the babies sustained damage at birth or were stillborn.[6] A second important feature of the literature was the importance attached to breast-feeding. The plea to mothers to breast-feed their children had formed part of the moral code from ancient times, but during the eighteenth century it was supported for the first time by medical rather than by purely moral arguments, and these arguments were presented systematically. During the period of the Englightenment, physicians acquired knowledge about the chemical composition of mother's milk and began to attach greater importance to clinical observations that showed its superiority over other forms of nourishment; they discovered that mother's milk, and particularly colostrum, was the most suitable feed for the newborn child, and protected it against disease. The first numerical estimates were published: children fed on their mothers' milk were less liable to die than those nourished on 'mercenary' milk or, even worse, on cows' milk. Moreover, mothers who used their bosoms for the purpose that nature had provided also protected their own health by doing so; indeed, those women who attempted to evade this sacred duty by having their milk dried up were likely to contract all manners of diseases, the sole cause of which was the 'resorption of the milk', which would lead them to an early grave.[7]

Other themes that were common in the discussion of early infancy were condemnation of the practice of swaddling babies, a practice which impeded their proper growth, and which was held responsible for rickets and other deformations. Equally, the administration of pap during the early weeks of life was criticized, as it was completely indigestible and merely resulted in stuffing the baby and ultimately in intestinal obstruction and death.

Advice on hygiene also began to be given in the medical literature: babies were to be bathed daily in lukewarm water in order to counteract damaging humours that were concentrated in their skins.

The final conclusion of the medical literature was a condemnation of wet-nurses who indulged in this practice for profit. Their deplorable practices, condemned as being made up of 'errors and prejudice', were regarded as the main reason responsible for depopulation. It was above all in France that this vicious practice needed to be discouraged if infant mortality were to be reduced. (It was widespread in all French towns during the eighteenth century.)

How can we measure the effect of these campaigns directed to mothers and children by physicians and administrators? French historians have maintained that it did not result in major changes of behaviour. In my view this conclusion needs modification. It is true that at a time when most

[6] J. Gelis, *L'Arbre et la fruit: La Naissance dans l'Occident moderne* (Paris, 1984); id., *La Sage-femme ou le médecin: Une nouvelle conception de la vie* (Paris, 1988).

[7] V. A. Fildes, *Breasts, Bottles and Babies: A History of Infant Feeding* (Edinburgh, 1986). ead., *Wet Nursing: A History from Antiquity to the Present* (Oxford, 1988).

women were illiterate, few could read even the simplest manuals (e.g. the so-called 'catechisms' published by some authorities for the use of midwives), and only the most enlightened mothers were able to read the medical literature and above all Rousseau's writings. However, some of them were so impressed that they accepted the advice given them. Such a one was Mme Roland who, acting against the advice of her friends, decided to breast-feed her little daughter Eudora who was born in 1781; nor was she by any means the only one to do so.[8] In the countryside, midwives who had been educated in the new courses which were arranged throughout the kingdom (10,000 attended such courses between 1780 and 1790) were able to conduct confinements more safely and counsel mothers during the first months of their children's lives. In the large towns, where the habit of giving children out to be wet-nursed had been most lethal, officials tried to exercise some measure of control over wet-nurses in the country (surgeon inspectors had been appointed to tour the environs of Paris since 1760). Institutions with openly populationist objectives were founded with the advice of physicians. During the last decade of the *ancien régime*, philanthropists in Lyons and Paris provided allowances for working women among the deserving poor which enabled them to breast-feed their own children instead of sending them out to be wet-nursed.[9] In Rouen, the General Infirmary, which used to help poor families by paying the wet-nurses' fees for a year, adopted a completely new policy in 1764 which left the children with their natural mothers who were paid an allowance for breast-feeding them.[10] It is difficult to estimate accurately the demographic gains achieved by these measures; the limited statistics that are available appear to show that the mortality amongst breast-fed children was lower than amongst others, even in the poorest classes.

Wet-nursing was much less common in other European countries, and no comparative studies exist which make it possible to assess and understand the reasons for this French practice. In Germany, only a few wealthy families used wet-nurses, and the practice had little effect on the level of infant mortality. On the other hand, artificial feeding was widespread; throughout southern Germany children were rarely breast-fed and this had considerable demographic consequences.[11] Imhof has studied two particularly striking

[8] F.M. Morel, 'Madame Roland, sa fille et les médecins: Prime éducation et médicalisation à l'époque des Lumières', *La Médicalisation en France du XVIIIe au début du XXe siècle* (*Annales de Bretagne et des Pays de l'Ouest* special issue 86(3) (1979)).

[9] Morel, op. cit. in n. 5, pp. 407–408.

[10] J.P. Bardet, 'Enfants abandonnés et enfants assistés à Rouen dans la seconde moitié du XVIIIe siècle', in *Hommage à Marcel Reinhard: Sur la population française au XVIIIe et XIXe siècles* Société de Démographie historique, (Paris, 1973), p. 24.

[11] C. Duhamelle, 'La Petite Enfance sous le regard médical dans l'Allemagne des Lumières (fin XVIIIe–début XIXe siècles)', master's thesis (Univ. of Paris I 1987); J.N. Biraben, 'Les Aspects médico-écologiques de la mortalité différentielle des enfants au XVIIIe et XIXe siècles', in IUSSP *Proceedings of the International Population Conference* ii (Manila, 1981).

examples:[12] the villages of Gabelsbach in Bavaria where infant mortality was extremely high at 339 per 1,000 births, and Hesel in the Hanover region where it was very low at 130. These differences can be explained by differences in the method of infant-feeding: in Gabelsbach infants were hardly ever breast-fed, nor given cows' milk, but were nourished on porridge, soup, and bread; in Hesel, on the other hand, almost all children were breast-fed by their mothers. Until the beginning of the present century, infant mortality in Germany shows a definite contrast between the regions in which children were breast-fed and those in which they were fed artificially. Breast-feeding increases as one passes from south-east to north-west Germany, and there is an associated fall in infant mortality from levels exceeding 300 per 1,000 in the south-west and Bavaria to 200–250 in middle Germany and to less than 150 in the north-west and on the North Sea coast. Physicians resident at the German courts during the period of *Aufklärung* recognized this state of affairs and were instrumental in interesting the authorities in the maintenance of public health and in alerting their sovereigns and officials to the disastrous effects of infant-feeding methods. Studies in medical geography were published and, following the example of their French colleagues, German physicians advocated action to prevent disease and promote public health.[13]

In addition to these books on hygiene and giving advice to parents, physicians during the eighteenth century also took an interest in sick children. Leading practitioners with clinical experience of children's diseases had isolated certain conditions and had suggested new methods of treatment. The most famous of them were found in England: Harris who was physician to the royal family, Underwood who was attached to the Lying-in Hospital, and above all Armstrong, who in 1769 founded the first hospital for poor children in London and acted as its director until its closure in 1781. We should also mention the Swede Rosen von Rosenstein, and among the French physicians Astruc, Desessartz, Raulin, Ballexserd, Brouzet, and Baudelocque. The Royal Society of Medicine was founded in Paris in 1776 and contained many physicians who were interested in public health. It frequently organized competitions which were concerned with children's diseases, and supervised pilot studies made on foundlings in the Paris region. It became possible to diagnose some children's diseases with certainty: e.g. smallpox, croup, whooping cough, measles, scarlet fever, and a disease particularly lethal among foundlings—'hardening of subcutaneous fat' or *scleroma neonatorum*—, thrush, rickets, and syphilis. On the other hand, diphtheria, rubella, and typhoid tended to be classed together under the

[12] A.H. Imhof, 'Unterschiedliche Säuglingssterblichkeit in Deutschland. 18–20 Jahrhundert', *Zeitschrift für Bevölkerungswissenschaft und Demographie*, 3 (1981).

[13] Cf. Duhamelle, op. cit. in n. 11; J.P. Goubert (ed.), *La Médicalisation de la société française 1770–1830* (Waterloo, Ont., 1982).

somewhat nebulous rubric of 'fevers' or 'anginas', and physicians depended upon their symptoms for their identification. However, these improvements in medical knowledge were not accompanied by major changes in treatment. In the Hippocratic tradition, the physician could only drive out or neutralize 'noxious humours' by the old method of bleeding (either by lancet or by leeches), purgation (cream of tartar or rhubarb), emetics (ipecacuanha or antimony), and quinine mixtures for fevers.[14] All these medicines had a violent effect and were not particularly effective. How could rickets be cured by emetics or enemas, or whooping cough by bleeding? The parents were not deceived: they dreaded the application of these official treatments to their little ones, and in wealthy families the physician was called in much less frequently to treat children than to treat adults; instead, women continued to pass on their knowledge of traditional treatments from one to another by word of mouth; the little invalids were kept as warm as possible by blankets or drinks (often with a vinous basis), they were surrounded by red colours which, by analogy with fever or blood, were believed to restore vitality,[15] and amulets and magic spells were used for protection, as were prayers and pilgrimages to saints who were thought to be concerned with certain specific diseases.[16]

Some diseases escaped this rough treatment by official medicine: one such was smallpox against which inoculation provided protection, though the reason why it did so was not then understood. However, the practice of inoculation was not widespread in eighteenth-century France, apart from a few well-known cases. Another disease was *scleroma neonatorum* for which the physicians at the Foundling Hospital (including Auvity) had established empirically that the child patients needed to be kept warm by all possible means (by being covered with hot sand, by massage, or by hot baths) i.e. essentially by substitutes for modern incubators, which were not used until the beginning of the present century.[17] The application of these methods at the Foundling Hospital was successful in saving the lives of some of these babies.

Is it possible to evaluate the effects of these new attitudes and of the desire to save children's lives? Some historians have taken a very pessimistic view, e.g. F. Lebrun writing about Anjou:

> There remains the art of healing. A fossilized method of teaching, an ineffective armamentarium of therapies, hospitals with inadequate or useless equipment, a majority of unqualified practitioners, particularly in the countryside, all this left the

[14] M.-F. Morel, 'Médecins et enfants malades dans la France du XVIIIe siècle', *L'Enfant malade et son corps* (*Lieu de l'enfance*, 9–10 (1987)).

[15] Y.M. Berce, *Le Chaudron et la lancette: Croyances populaires et médecine préventive 1798–1830* (Paris, 1984), p. 197.

[16] F. Loux, *Le Jeune enfant et son corps dans la médecine traditionnelle* (Paris, 1978), pp. 238–40.

[17] Dupâquier *et al.*, op. cit. in n. 2, p. 273.

field wide open for all sorts of healers. The picture is certainly not a brilliant one. Only a few enlightened spirits saw the possibility of not continuing the passivity of previous generations in the face of death, and to take new initiatives. They dreamt of filling the countryside with trained midwives, they foresaw a complete revision of the medical curriculum which would be linked more strongly to clinical practice, they accepted inoculation as a means of preventing disease, they planned a rational campaign against epidemics and misery. But although they obtained support from the central authorities, they were struggling against the mistrust and apathy of local populations—whether the municipality of Angers or rural communities, and above all against the absence of any progress in the healing art: inoculation was not the same as vaccination, ipecacuanha as penicillin, Pierre Hunauld was no Pasteur. . . . it is necessary not to confuse the principles that were expressed with everyday reality, the efforts that were made with what was actually achieved. . . . Even if we were to give due recognition to the small improvements that occurred during the eighteenth century, the cumulative effects of which laid the foundations for decisive later progress it would seem that any attempt to speak of. . . . a revolution in mortality in Anjou during the second half of the eighteenth century (and this would also apply to Normandy, Brittany and Maine i.e a large part of western France in which the population was constant or even declining during a period when in the rest of France mortality was beginning to fall) would be to anticipate the course of history for at least 50 years.[18]

It seems probable that the slight fall in infant mortality registered in France was due to non-medical causes. Amongst these we must include contraception; families had fewer children, but these were more precious and were treated better. The medicalization of childbirth and care in early infancy had begun and continued to make progress.

2. Relative Stagnation of Medicalization to 1870

We have already shown that infant mortality rates did not decline during most of the nineteenth century. But if we divide infant mortality into its 'endogenous' and 'exogenous' components as it is possible to do in France and Belgium (Fig. 11.1), it is seen that whereas exogenous mortality either remained constant, or even increased slightly in some years, endogenous mortality appears to have declined relatively regularly and continuously. What were the reasons for this difference? Clearly, conditions of childbirth improved as the number of better-trained and more efficient midwives increased, but there were additional non-medical reasons: improved nutritional standards among the mothers resulted in a lower incidence of premature births and in increasing the natural resistance of the newborn.

The relative constancy of endogenous mortality rates was partly due to

[18] F. Lebrun, *Les Hommes et la mort en Anjou au XVIIe et XVIIIe siècles* (Paris and The Hague, 1972), conclusion.

lack of progress in medicine. Throughout most of the nineteenth century there was relatively little advance in methods of child care, compared with the eighteenth century. Handbooks for mothers were more numerous and were probably more widely read in middle-class households, where the ideal of the mother as a carer was dominant.[19] However, there were some innovations: hygiene was stricter, regular schedules were recommended for the infant to prepare him or her for adult life, swaddling was discouraged, and the gradual introduction of artificial foods was recommended in order to avoid the problems associated with abrupt weaning at the end of the second year of life.[20] In French middle-class families this new regime coincided with the emergence of the family physician and also led to changes in the practice of wet-nursing. Whereas during the eighteenth century wealthier parents were prepared to accept separation from their infants and were glad to send them to the country for a year or two to be wet-nursed, they now preferred to employ a 'resident' wet-nurse and engaged a young mother from the country who would send her own child back to the country, to come and live with the family in the town. The wet-nurse, who was often the highest-paid member of the domestic staff, spent her entire time in feeding the baby, taking it for walks, and generally caring for it, and her work was closely supervised by the mother and the family physician.[21] Child-care was to some extent becoming professionalized and carried out under medical supervision. For the privileged infants who benefited from this form of nursing (some 4,000 in Paris in 1850), it is clear that the infant mortality rate was lower than among their precursors during the previous century.

Progress among the less wealthy classes was less pronounced. However, the total number of physicians increased, even though there continued to be a considerable difference between town and country in this respect. In 1844 there was one physician for every 662 inhabitants in the *département* of the Seine, compared with one for every 5,274 in Morbihan in Brittany. There was some reduction in medical manpower during the second half of the nineteenth century a result of the disappearance of health officers, but in any case some three-quarters of the population at the time never received any medical advice or assistance throughout their lives.

Although physicians were more numerous in towns, the infant death rate there was higher than in the country, particularly in areas like Belgium, where the industrial revolution resulted in a deterioration of living conditions for the workers.[22] During the nineteenth century the infant mortality rate actually increased in some towns: during the 1890s, for

[19] C. Fouquet and Y. Knibiehler, *Histoire des mères du Moyen-Age à nos jours* (Paris, 1980), p. 180.

[20] P. Ariès, G. Duby, *et al.*, *Histoire de la vie privée*, iv. *De la Révolution à la grande guerre* (Paris, 1987), pp. 596–99.

[21] F. Fay-Sallois, *Les Nourrices à Paris au XIXe siècle* (Paris, 1980).

[22] Poulain and Tabutin, op. cit. in n. 2.

instance in West Flanders (Bruges, Ypres, Courtrai, Ostend),[23] and also in Gimont, a small town of 3,000 inhabitants in the Gers region of the south-west of France, where infant mortality amounted to 126 per 1,000 live births in 1850–59, 195 in 1870–79, and 233 in 1890–99.[24] As it was primarily exogenous mortality that increased, it seems reasonable to assume that reduced frequency of breast-feeding (resulting from more women being employed outside their homes) may have been one cause, together with a general decline in sanitary conditions, in spite of the larger number of physicians in the towns who were both better trained and more interested in public health.

In Germany, and particularly in the southern part of the country, infant mortality rates hardly declined at all. However, in some German states, e.g. in Bavaria, there was a quantum leap in medicalization. Between 1820 and 1860 public expenditure on health doubled, the number of medical personnel including midwives and country physicians increased, and their training improved. Since 1816, newly trained midwives were required as part of their duties to promote breast-feeding and to campaign against the traditional forms of artificial feeding.[25] A larger medical establishment will lead to a reduction in infant mortality in the long run, and this is what happened, albeit very slowly, in Bavaria. It was only after 1870 that the very high rates of infant mortality in that country began to fall by 10 per cent. Paradoxically, a similar fall of 10 per cent was only achieved in the north German states after 1910, although the initial levels of infant mortality in these states were much lower.[26] In other parts of the country, an increase in the numbers of medical personnel did not result in lower infant mortality, e.g. in Swabia in 1843, or the Palatinate in 1863. The countryside in Prussia towards the end of the nineteenth century shows results which seem paradoxical at first sight; smaller numbers of trained midwives than in the towns, yet a lower infant mortality rate.[27] If an increase in the numbers of medical personnel only had a small effect on the mortality of young children, the principal reason for the high mortality rates of children would seem to have lain in deficiencies of nutrition. In spite of all the efforts of the health professionals, traditional feeding practices remained unchanged until the beginning of the twentieth century, because mothers could not or would not breast-feed their children, either because of economic constraints or because of a psychological resistance to the practice.[28]

[23] G. Masuy-Stroobant, 'La Surmortalité infantile des Flandres au cours de la deuxième moitié du XIXe siècle: Mode d'alimentation ou mode de développement?', *Annales de démographie historique* (1973), p. 235.

[24] A. Fine-Souriac, 'Mortalité infantile et allaitement dans le sud-ouest de la France au XIXe siècle', *La Mortalité du passé* (*Annales de démographie historique* (1978)), p. 96.

[25] R.W. Lee, 'Medicalisation and Mortality Trends in South Germany in the Early Nineteenth Century', In Imhof (ed.) op. cit. in n. 5, pp. 80–88.

[26] J. Knodel, *The Decline of Fertility in Germany 1871–1939* (Princeton, NJ, 1974).

[27] Lee, op. cit. in n. 25, p. 89.

[28] Imhof, op. cit. in n. 12.

This situation changed only slowly during the nineteenth century as the quality of infant foods and the milk supply began to improve. Attitudes and behaviour to small children in Germany did not change before the middle of the nineteenth century and the change only affected the wealthier groups.

> In Germany, on the other hand, we find no evidence of a new orientation towards infants until the mid-nineteenth century, and even then only in the cities among middle-class patients. . . . possibly Germany never experienced a breast-feeding revolution; mothers there simply going over to safe 'artificial' foods as they became available towards the end of the nineteenth century.[29]

We should add that the most famous German paediatricians of the nineteenth century (Virchow, Schlossman, Heubner, Czerny) were particularly interested in the struggle against nutritionally induced gastro-intestinal disorders. Their researches resulted in the study of the composition and calorific value of foodstuffs, of digestion, of the amount and quality of nutrition, of metabolism, and of weight gain. All these researches at the beginning of the present century led to an increase in the survival rate of artificially fed infants.

Even before the Pasteurian revolution in medicine, the influence of medical men on the survival of children was not insignificant. Its effects were indirect, mainly through improvements in hygiene.

> Lack of understanding of aetiology and limited treatments resulted in the physician becoming active in the promotion of hygiene which made it possible for him, in spite of being unable to control the health situation effectively, to occupy the position of expert in the social aspects of disease, which influenced both the advice he gave and his prescriptions.[30]

Physicians tried to inspire, stimulate, and be active in different forms of hygienic, cultural, agricultural, and administrative activities which were part of the social process. They were to be found working in health authorities and elected assemblies, in learned societies, and within families. Little by little, their patient endeavours transformed people's lives and postponed the hour of decline and death.[31]

In response to these hygienic campaigns, a demand for medical care gradually emerged among the population, even in country areas in which physicians had previously hardly been seen. Even the poor demanded medical care, though their demands were rarely expressed in clear and explicit fashion, but rather can be seen in a number of examples.[32] For example, at Souesmes in central France, we hear complaints that people were

[29] E. Shorter, *The Making of the Modern Family* (New York, 1975), p. 203.

[30] C. Beauchamp, *Délivrez-nous du mal! Epidémies, endémies, médecine et hygiène dans l'Indie, l'Ondre-et-Loire et le Loir-et-Cher* (Maulévner, 1990), p. 350.

[31] Léonard, op. cit. in n. 1, p. 16.

[32] O. Faure, 'La Médecine gratuite au XIXe siècle: De la charité à l'assistance', Santé, médicine et politique de santé' (*Histoire, Économie et Société*, 4, special issue, (1984)), pp. 593–608.

unable to see their doctors frequently enough, particularly when their children were seriously ill: 'some nine out of ten are cured of dysentery; fewer than half, on the other hand, survive diphtheria'.[33]

The mass vaccination campaigns not only offered protection against smallpox, but also resulted in a recognition of the value of scientific medicine among sections of the population that had hitherto been ignorant. The conflicts engendered when urban medicine was first brought to the countryside have been frequently described. Thus, the Savoy physician Daquin recounted the difficulties that he met in attempting to vaccinate the mountain populations: 'As regards the countryfolk, I am not surprised that the majority do not wish to be vaccinated; their heads are full of misguided opinions on a large variety of subjects, and they cling to these views with incredible tenacity'.[34]

However, later attitudes to the vaccinators became more favourable: some mothers explicitly asked for their children to be treated, and were prepared to do anything to save them from a death which they no longer regarded as inevitable. Often urged on by their husbands, they jostled to approach the vaccinator when there were epidemics, they cried and beseeched him by brandishing their infants, because they were frightened that the supplies of vaccine would be exhausted or that the vaccinator would refuse to treat an infant who was already suffering from the disease; others, who had observed the vaccinator's actions tried to vaccinate their children themselves by using sewing needles.[35] In many distant areas vaccination campaigns familiarized the population with scientific medicine and resulted in medical personnel (physicians, health officers, and midwives) gaining their confidence.

After the beginning of the nineteenth century medical progress was not confined to vaccination: clinical practice improved and methods of diagnosing and identifying illnesses became more certain. However, there were hardly any changes in the means available to the physician to treat these conditions, and the effectiveness of medicine remained limited. Consider, for instance, diphtheria: one of the most cruel afflictions of infancy in the past.[36] In 1868, 85 per cent of those who died from diphtheria in France were infants; in 1875 in Veroli to the south of Rome they made up 84 per cent of the patients and 81 per cent of the deaths. In 1826, the famous Tours physician Bretonneau succeeded in identifying the disease and in separating it from the vague category of 'malign, gangrenous or scarlatinous afflictions' which were used previously. He demonstrated clearly that diphtheria was a specific disease manifested by a characteristic lesion, the pseudo-membranes of the larynx which could obstruct the trachea or

[33] Beauchamp, op. cit. in n. 30.
[34] Bercé, op. cit. in n. 15.
[35] Ibid., p. 104.
[36] Beauchamp, op. cit. in n. 30.

bronchus, that its progress exhibited an orderly succession of symptoms, and that it was spread by contagion. However, treatment raised problems; there were two different schools of thought. Bretonneau concentrated on the local specific manifestations of the disease, that is to say on the membranes, and tried to treat them by local cauterization. He and his disciple Trousseau experimented with many different remedies which ranged from the harmful (hydrochloric acid or mercury) to the less violent (calomel, silver nitrate, or insufflation with powdered alum, according to the old prescription by Arete of Capodoccia which he had rediscovered empirically). The other school of thought was headed by Broussais, a dogmatic partisan of physiologism, who regarded every inflammation as a symptom of a more general disorder which needed to be attacked by treating the organism as a whole. Diphtheria, therefore, would have to be treated by external anti-phlogistic medicines (bleeding or leeches), and by internal means, such as antinomy of tartar, emetics, or skin irritants. Cauterization was not included among the remedies; Brousseau's followers regarded the treatment of an inflammation by the heat of cauterization as a heresy.

In spite of these quarrels about theory, the majority of physicians unashamedly practised a mixture of these two treatments: bleeding, purgatives, and emetics were used to reassure the patient who was used to these traditional procedures which were designed to draw out the 'humours'; local cauterization by powdered alum or silver nitrate flattered the physician who wished to apply a scientific remedy with precision and effectiveness. Those in central France who knew Bretonneau or Trousseau took pride in using their specific treatments and in belonging to the 'Tours school of medicine' which was in the vanguard of modern developments. Finally, in some desperate cases after 1818, the leading physicians tried tracheotomy. The first success only dates back to 1825, and even the most skilled practitioner could not achieve a success rate higher than 25 per cent, in spite of the technical improvements that had been introduced during the 1840s (Trousseau's double canula). Moreover, it was necessary for the parents to agree to have the operation performed on their child as a last chance, and many refused, as is attested by Dr Yvonneau, a physician who treated epidemic diseases and who wrote in 1855: 'We would be told that they knew well that there was nothing that could be done, and we would rather allow our child to die peacefully than to see it suffer'. A cruel sentence for a physician who was trying to do his best to save his patient at all costs.

After several decades during which diagnosis became more accurate and treatment improved, we can witness a certain disenchantment during the 1850s and 1860s. Dr Haime, the public physician appointed to deal with epidemics for the *arrondissement* of Tours expressed his impotence in face of the absence of advances in treatment: 'truly effective measures have not yet been found'. We would add that at the time the majority of physicians were not convinced that diphtheria was a contagious disease and returned to the classical, somewhat vague, generalizations of the epidemical influence of poor sanitary conditions, or of the constitution of the atmosphere. All these considerations had already been advanced in the programme of the Royal Society of Medicine a century earlier. Given these attitudes, it is not surprising that Pasteur's views and bacteriological discoveries took some time before being reflected in the treatment prescribed by physicians. During the epidemic in Sonzay in the *département* of Indre-et-Loire in 1884, some medical men continued to advocate basic measures of hygiene: to treat rivers, public wash-houses, and stagnant pools, to remove manure heaps and put cemeteries in order, to dry out humid dwellings, rather than to concentrate on the influence of bacteria and the places where they spread.[37] It was only after 1890 that the adoption of strict procedures of asepsis and antisepsis completely revolutionized the forms of medical intervention.

3. Pasteur's Revolution and Its First Applications 1890–1914

All historical demographers are agreed that infant mortality only began to fall significantly during the 1890s. This is the date when Pasteur's new techniques of hygiene first spread throughout the population, and when the discovery of the first new vaccines seemed to justify the belief that, on this occasion, medical progress had provided effective weapons in the struggle against disease. We shall show how these discoveries were applied to transform child care practices both by the medical profession and by women who looked after infants and small children. The latter effect is much more difficult to document.

The medical view was that the care and upbringing of children could no longer be left exclusively in the hands of women, and that the State would have to intervene, because the survival of children was of fundamental importance for the polity. In an age of resurgent nationalism, particularly in France and Germany, the old populationist ideals were once again taken up by the medical profession.

In Germany after 1890 progress in bacteriology resulted in the paediatricians, who had previously limited their interest to the physiology and pathology of childhood, becoming interested in hygiene and in methods of diffusing knowledge about the subject. They worried about the high rates of infant mortality in their country (the rate in Germany was 220 per 1,000, a little better than in Russia, where it was 270, or in Austria where it was 240, but well above the figure of 160 in France or 150 in England). They became almost militant in their endeavours to promote infant hygiene, and stressed the economic, political, and military costs of high infant mortality. A national campaign, supported by the empress, was organized. In 1906 the

[37] Ibid., p. 349.

famous paediatrician Seiffert affirmed in an article which appeared in the catalogue of an exhibition devoted to infant care, that it was:

> the national duty of parents, and of mothers in particular, to protect the health of their children. . . . a nation that fights against infant mortality half-heartedly or even gives up the fight surrenders itself. . . . It is the duty of a nation that believes in its future not only to look after those who are bearing arms, but also to care for those generations who are destined to take up arms in the future to fight for the security of their mother country.[38]

The motives of the French physicians were very similar. Because fertility had begun to fall earlier in France than in Germany, and in the context of the preparation for *revanche*, the need to safeguard the lives of infants appeared to be even more urgent. It followed that mothers would have to change their methods of rearing infants in order to ensure their survival, and this implied that they, and others charged with the duty of bringing up children, would have to be provided with strict and coherent rules relating to the new methods of medicalized education, some of which contradicted those that had been hallowed by tradition. These new methods which had different intellectual origins were moulded into a coherent whole by the new Pasteurian medicine which carried all before it. Some dated back to the first attempts at medicalization during the period of the Enlightenment: a light diet consisting entirely of milk adapted to the infant's weak digestive system during the first months of its life, prohibition of feeding with pap, daily baths that were no longer designed to eliminate 'bad humours' but rather to kill microbes. Others issued from the bourgeois morality of the nineteenth century and were internalized by the medical profession even though medical justification for them was limited: regular breast-feeding at fixed times and early indoctrination in cleanliness. Yet others were the results of technical progress achieved during the second industrial revolution: the introduction of glass feeding-bottles and rubber teats which could be thoroughly washed and disinfected, and which replaced bottles with long feeding-tubes or siphons which were a breeding ground for microbes.[39] Lastly and most importantly, there were rules which stemmed from Pasteur's discoveries about asepsis and antisepsis and which made it possible to feed infants on cows' milk which had previously been a dangerous food, and to use boiled milk and boiled water to make up baby mixtures. There were also rules relating to the sterilization of feeding-bottles and teats and about the need to wash hands before beginning to breast-feed.[40]

In contrast to their eighteenth-century predecessors, physicians of the

[38] Quoted by S. Lilienthal, 'Paediatrics and Nationalism in Imperial Germany', *Bulletin of the Society for the Social History of Medicine*, 39 (1986), pp. 66–67.

[39] Fay-Sallois, op. cit. in n. 21, pp. 166–69.

[40] L. Boltanski, *Prime éducation et morale de classe* (Paris and The Hague, 1969; 2nd edn., 1977), pp. 41–42.

Pasteur period understood the reasons why their rules worked, and they tried to persuade all mothers to follow their advice: unless they did so, mothers were told, they would be responsible for their children's deaths. This was a complete change of attitude; it was no longer necessary to accept the death of a small child fatalistically; parents (and especially mothers) asked themselves whether they had done all in their power to minimize the likelihood of death. Guilt feelings came to be associated with parenthood and acted as a driving force for further medicalization. Most historians are agreed that these new methods were of decisive importance in increasing the survival chances of infants:

> and the great decline in infant mortality which occurred everywhere in Western society between the end of the nineteenth century and the 1920s and 1930s faithfully mirrors improvements in sterile food, the Pasteurisation of milk, green soap in the nursery, and other forms of the fight against pathogens.[41]

However, medical progress on its own was not sufficient, changes in attitudes and behaviour were also needed. Those who cared for young children had to be convinced of the need for these new medicalized practices. In France, the government attempted to popularize the new rules of hygiene, particularly in those groups of the population in which infant mortality was highest, the new proletariat in the towns, where families often lived in conditions of squalor and promiscuity. A number of different methods were used in an attempt to reach these groups: child-care was taught in domestic-science lessons to girls in primary schools, free medical advice was provided for nursing mothers, and distributions of sterilized milk were organized in working-class districts from 1892. Leaders of the medical profession (Pinard, Marfan, Budin, Variot) participated in conferences in which the new techniques were presented to the public. A League against Infant Mortality was founded in 1902 and published leaflets and articles in the popular press in which advice was given for the prevention and cure of children's illnesses.[42]

It is tempting to relate these exceptional publicity efforts to the decline in infant mortality. It should be noted, however, that the decline began well before the new methods of child-rearing had become widespread, and that even after Pasteur's discoveries, mortality among bottle-fed children continued to be higher than among those who had been breast-fed.[43] If one wishes to look for evidence on changing methods of child-rearing within families, the causal link appears weaker; medical advice did not always result

[41] Shorter, op. cit. in n. 29, p. 200.

[42] J.Léonard, *Archives du corps: La Santé au XIXe siècle* (Rennes, 1986), p. 197.

[43] C. Rollet, 'Allaitement, mise en nourrice, et mortalité infantile en France à la fin du XIXe siècle', *Population*, 33 (1978); id., L'Allaitement artificiel de nourrissons avant Pasteur', *Mères et nourissons* (*Annales de démographie historique*, special issue, (1983)); id., *La Politique à l'égard de la petite enfance sous la Troisième République 1865–1939* (Paris, 1990).

in changes in behaviour, particularly when mothers saw it as a rule imposed by outsiders which contradicted many of their traditional beliefs and practices. In particular, many mothers did not accept that the new rules were a coherent whole and often practised what might be called 'cultural do-it-yourself' methods, accepting some of the new rules whilst ignoring others.

Thus, mothers might boil the water and milk when making up the baby's feed, but would not sterilize the feeding-bottles, or would content themselves with merely scalding them.[44] In so doing, they followed old beliefs which suggested that it was the contents, rather than the containers, that were dangerous to the baby's health. As Guillon, a medical practitioner, remarked towards the end of the nineteenth century: 'It is extremely difficult to change behaviour. . . . once the feeding-bottle with a simple teat has been adopted, many mothers believe that they have done all that is required for hygiene; they do not realize that after use the teat needs to be taken off, washed, and kept in clean water until it is next used'.[45] As late as 1895, the practitioners in the General Council of Nièvre complained of the persistence of old practices, particularly that of

> mixing milk with infected beverages, such as tisanes, barley water, marshmallow and other mixtures, all of which had been prepared in sufficient quantities to last for a whole day or even longer. The liquids turn sour and become veritable cultures and infect the infant's digestive tract which has been put at risk by using a dirty feeding bottle, or even a clean bottle in which the milk has been allowed to go off. The Robert feeding bottle is still being used in spite of the fact that bottles without tubes have been distributed; nursing mothers continue to use it because it permits them to continue working without having to look after the infant.[46]

In 1905 the same council noted that progress had been slow:

> The use of boiled milk and boiled water is widespread, but there has hardly been any progress in the use of sterilized milk, the labour involved in sterilizing bottles puts nursing mothers off. . . . The use of sterilized milk is the exception and nursing mothers do not follow medical advice in this respect.

In the less-favoured rural districts, schooling did not become universal until about 1880, and it would be necessary to wait until the 1930s for 'popular prejudices' relating to child rearing to disappear.

However, after Roussel's law which provided for the protection of children who were sent out to be nursed was enacted in 1874, all children

[44] Boltanski, op. cit. in n. 40, p. 109; F. Loux, *Pratiques traditionnelles et pratiques modernes d'hygiène et de prévention de la maladie chez les mères et leurs enfants* (Paris, 1975), p. 169.

[45] E. Guillon, *Essai sur la mortalité infantile dans le département de la Vienne*, (Orléans, 1897), cited by N. Pellegrin and M. C. Planchard, *Entrer dans la vie en Poitou du XVIe siècle à nos jours* Catalogue de l'exposition, Poitiers, Dec. 1987–Mar. 1988, (1987) p. 88.

[46] G. Thuillier, *Pour une histoire du quotidien au XIXe siècle en Nivernais* (Paris and The Hague, 1977), p. 93.

should have benefited from progress in hygiene and medical science. Paradoxically, it was the children from the least privileged classes who benefited most from protection and supervision; in 1882 Théophile Roussel, the deputy who gave his name to the law congratulated himself on its success in relation to poor children. 'The only children who are well cared for in the poorer *départements* are those of girl-mothers who receive monthly help from the authorities, and who are specially supervised by an Inspector from the Prefecture, of whom they stand in awe and whose advice they listen to.'

After 1880, when Roussel's law had become effective, children given out to be nursed (some 80,000 a year, or a little less that 10 per cent of all births) were supervised by medical inspectors. The records of their visits provide a valuable source which makes it possible to trace how children were cared for in the country; in 1883 the inspectors still complained that milk was often mixed with various other liquids—wine, cider, or chicory,[47] in 1892 sterilized milk began to be distributed in Paris and its suburbs, and later sterilizers were also distributed.[48] Nurses increasingly replaced breast-feeding by bottle-feeding, except in the southern French *départements*, where cows' milk was used less frequently. As the new rules of hygiene came to be adopted and the bacteriological quality of the food sold, and particularly that of milk, improved, especially after the law of 1 August 1905 had become operative, the excess mortality of bottle-fed infants declined. In this connection, we must mention the part played by medical practitioners who pressed the health authorities to enforce the controls and to improve the quality of the milk on sale and of the process used for sterilization. Milk sold in the cities was now more easily available, better controlled, and of higher quality than in the countryside.[49]

In England the decline in the birth rate and the stagnation of infant mortality led in about 1900 to the emergence of an active infant- and child-welfare movement, and this was also true of Germany and France. Medical practitioners and health officials put pressure on the central and local authorities to adopt new measures (infant milk depots, health visitors to visit the newborn, school medical and school meal services). These measures which had been begun before 1914, became more widespread during the war, because the country was in need of soldiers! The decisive fall in infant mortality rates at the time can be attributed to these energetic measures.[50]

Child health, too, began to emerge as a medical speciality of its own in the hospitals. In France, the first Hospital for Sick Children was founded

[47] Rollet, op. cit. in n. 43, p. 87.

[48] G. D. Sussman, *Selling Mother's Milk: The Wet Nursing Business in France 1715–1914* (Urbana, Ill., 1982), p. 165; cf. also Rollet op. cit. in n. 43.

[49] M. A. Beaver, 'Population, infant mortality and milk', *Population Studies*, 27(2) (1973); Rollet, op. cit. in n. 43.

[50] D. Dwork, *What is Good for Babies and Other Young Children: A History of the Infant and Child Welfare Movement in England 1898–1918* (London, 1987).

in 1802. In England Charles West founded the first modern hospital for sick children at 49 Great Ormond Street in 1852; by 1900 all the teaching hospitals in England contained some beds for sick children, and the founder of modern paediatrics, G.F. Still, was consultant physician to the Great Ormond Street Hospital. However, paediatrics as a speciality took some time to develop; the first chair in the subject was not founded until 1924 in Glasgow.[51] In Germany, paediatrics as a discipline developed a little earlier in connection with the building of modern hospitals which contained laboratories where diagnosis and treatment achieved some astounding successes, e.g. in the treatment of diphtheria. The discovery of the diphtheria bacillus by Klebs and Loeffler in 1883–84 was followed by the production of a serum in Berlin by Behring, and simultaneously in Paris at the Institut Pasteur by Roux, the effectiveness of which was immediately tested in specialist children's hospitals. It became clear that, provided the serum was administered early enough in the disease, it would save children's lives. The pioneers of this serum therapy were appointed to chairs in paediatrics, and pursued their work on two fronts simultaneously: curing patients by popularizing the new treatment and establishing depots throughout the country where the serum was kept, and preventing diphtheria and other infectious diseases by reinforcing children's natural immunity through improvements in diet and hygiene. The leaders of the profession in the hospitals and laboratories were pioneers of the child health movement in the field of preventive medicine which started at the same time.[52]

However, parents' attitudes were still slow to change; they refused to have a child treated in hospital, or even to call in a physician even when the child became seriously ill, either for reasons of economy, or because of a long tradition of fatalism. However, the problem of cost became less important, as free medical attention came to be provided in northern Europe, and particularly in France, towards the end of the nineteenth century. The law of 15 July 1893 acknowledged the right of all citizens to medical treatment either at home or in hospital in case of illness, and two million Frenchmen benefited from this law.[53] However, there remained a gap between theory and practice; in 1905 the General Council of Nièvre stated that 'free medical attention is not generally available for sick infants'.

Moreover, it took some time for parents to recognize the achievements of modern medicine. Many local practitioners commented on parents' reservations to the serum treatment of diphtheria that had been pioneered by Roux, and on their continuing beliefs in traditional nostrums such as

[51] See A.D.M. Jackson's account of his paper presented at the Conference of the Society for the Social History of Medicine, 'Child Health, Healing and Mortality' (Oct. 1987), *Social History of Medicine*, 1 (1988), p. 115.

[52] See P. Weindling's account of his paper presented at the conference mentioned in n. 51 above, in *Social History of Medicine*, 1 (1988) p. 120.

[53] Faure, op. cit.in n. 32, p. 603.

lemon juice. In 1898 Dr Broussard of Poitiers gave an account of one of these cases to the Medical Society of Poitiers:

[the parents] whose child I had proposed to inject with Roux's serum on the following morning refused, saying that the injection would kill the child; also the child had a good appetite, was not ill and would soon recover with the administration of lemon juice. . . . the little patient who did not receive treatment died a few days later, whereas his brother who had received the injection was rapidly cured.

Another practitioner added: 'Thanks to the serum, I no longer rely on lemon juice, apart from the fact that its administration satisfies the parents'.[54] Similarly, in a completely different area, Flanders, there was no reduction in the number of deaths from diphtheria between 1878 and 1900, even though sufficient quantities of the serum were available. A possible explanation for this was the poor education received by girls who were sent to work in the textile industry at an early age (compulsory schooling was not introduced in Belgium until 1914). Mothers were not aware of Pasteur's and Roux's discoveries, or of modern methods of child-rearing, and towards the end of the century, medical commissions complained of the poor quality of the diet given to children, who were weaned much too early (feeding-bottles with long tubes, beer, mashed potatoes, decoctions of poppy, mashed bread, gruel, etc.). This poor quality of nutrition made young children particularly vulnerable to infectious diseases.[55]

In the United States, the federal government did not limit its actions to propaganda in favour of the medicalization of births and infancy, as was the case in other Western countries, but adopted a massive policy of active intervention to deal with infant mortality, targeted on families who were at greatest risk. From 1909, the Children's Bureau organized an exemplary collection of data. Each family which had lost a child through death was visited during the following year by an investigator who asked questions about income, number of rooms, ethnicity, occupation of husband and wife, and number of children. Questions concerned with the deceased baby related to the length of the period of breast-feeding and of mixed feeding, age at weaning, and cause of death. Some of the information for eight towns was published. This exceptionally complete data source made it possible to study differences between the behaviour of different ethnic and social groups, and of the impact of medicalization upon behaviour.[56]

There was also no doubt about progress in the treatment of children's diseases, which became much less lethal. In Fig. 11.2 we compare death rates from the principal contagious diseases in different European countries between 1861–65 and 1911–15. These show that mortality from smallpox

[54] *Bulletin de la Société des Sciences Médicales de Poitiers*, 1 (1899), pp. 177, 181, cited by Pellegrin and Planchard, op. cit. in n. 45.

[55] Masuy-Stroobant, op. cit. in n. 23, p. 242.

[56] R.M. Woodbury, *Infant Mortality and its Causes* (Washington, DC, 1926).

Development of mortality from measles, scarlet fever, whooping cough, diphtheria, and smallpox 1861/65–1911/15 in Belgium, Denmark (urban population), and Sweden.

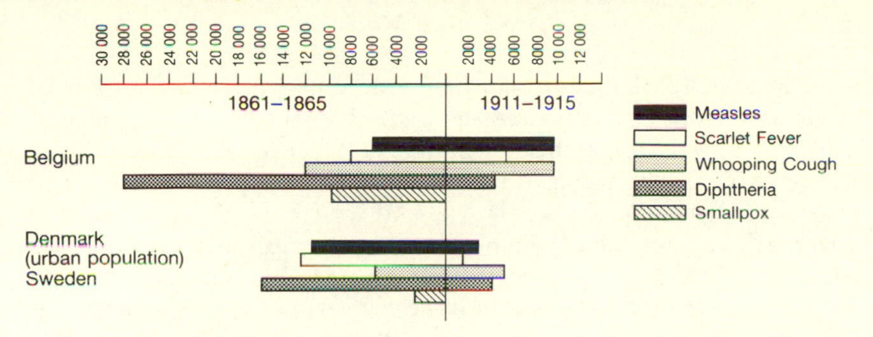

Development of mortality from measles, scarlet fever, whooping cough, diphtheria, and smallpox 1861/65–1911/15 in England, Wales, and Scotland.

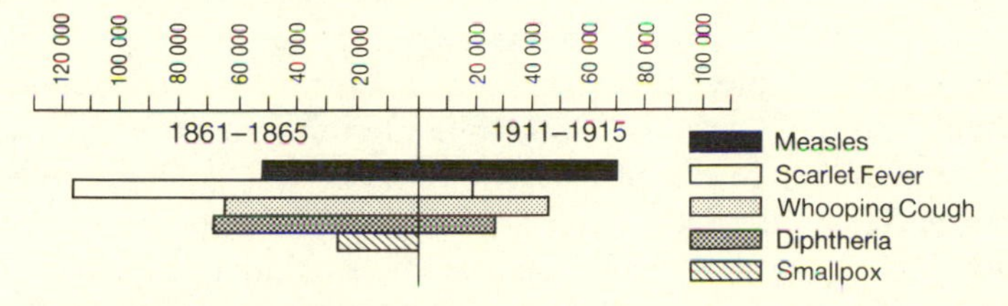

Mortality from measles, scarlet fever, whooping cough, diphtheria, and smallpox in Europe (except Russia and Balkan countries), 1900–1910.

	Measles	Scarlet Fever	Whooping Cough	Diphtheria	Smallpox
Total number of registered deaths	700 167	470 235	661 743	589 250	90 668
Death rate per million	254	171	240	214	33

Changes in annual death rates (per million) from measles, scarlet fever, whooping cough, diphtheria, and smallpox 1861/65–1906/10 in England & Wales, Belgium, and Sweden.

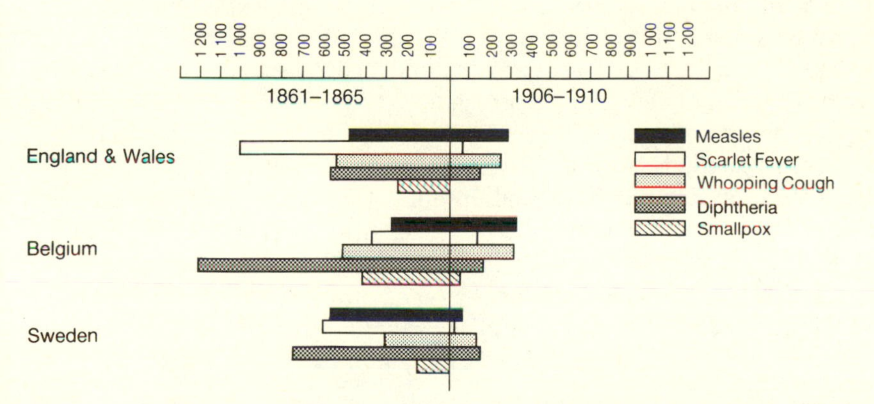

Fig. 11.2 Changes in death rates from the principal infectious diseases affecting children between the mid-nineteenth and early twentieth centuries in different European countries

Source: P. Huard and R. Laplane, *Histoire illustré de la pédiatrie* (Paris, 1983), vol. iii, p. 87.

had been virtually eliminated, and that from diphtheria and scarlet fever considerably reduced, though measles and whooping cough continued to claim victims, as they do at the present time in less developed countries. The pace of progress differed in different countries: it was considerable in Sweden and Denmark, average in England, and slow in Belgium. These differences can be explained in terms of the differences between the health standards of different populations, the number and distribution of medical personnel, and the state of medical science. In 1914 it was possible to treat smallpox and diphtheria, but not yet measles or whooping cough.

Recent researchers have made it possible to study the different pace of progress made by medicine in different social groups. At the beginning of the present century, town dwellers were at an advantage because of their proximity to medical personnel and institutions, at least among the élite groups who rapidly gained access to modern medical facilities; in the poorer quarters of the towns physicians were scarcer, and attitudes slower to change. Thus, in 1891, infant mortality in the poorer *arrondissements* in Paris was 71 per cent higher than in the wealthier; by 1911–13 the excess had become even larger and reached 135 per cent.[57] In Prussia, too, the difference between rates in different social groups continued to increase; there was an excess mortality amounting to 31 per cent among the children of manual workers compared to those of children of civil servants; in 1912–13 the excess was more than 91 per cent.[58]

4. Conclusion

There can be no doubt about the progress that has been achieved in methods of child-rearing and in paediatrics between 1750 and 1914. We have mentioned only some of these advances. One thing is certain: once physicians, midwives, and nurses had acquired the knowledge necessary to prevent the deaths of infants, they tried to persuade parents to bring up their children in accordance with certain rigorous rules and to convince them that the traditional methods were dangerous. They were not always listened to. Medicalization of childbirth and infant care was achieved in unequal measure in different countries, because of differences in the development of their social security and educational systems; it was, however, to make great strides after the First World War. However, in some regions old traditions remained dominant until the middle of the present century.

During the period 1750–1914, the first months of an infant's life came

[57] A. Perrenoud, 'Les Aspects médico-écologiques de la mortalité différentielle des enfants dans le passe', in IUSSP, *Proceedings of the International Population Conference*, ii (Manila (1981)), p. 33.

[58] R. Spree, 'Die Entwicklung der differentiellen Säuglingssterblichkeit in Deutschland seit der Mitte des 19. Jahrhunderts', in Imhof (ed.), op. cit. in n. 5.

increasingly to be supervised by medical or paramedical personnel. At the beginning, such supervision amounted to little more than good intentions, but later institutions were set up to make it a reality. Even if this degree of medicalization may not have been completely successful in changing attitudes, there can be no doubt that medical men were partly responsible for the fall in infant mortality, through their insistence on improved sanitary conditions, controls on the sale of milk, and the need for easily sterilized feeding-bottles, by popularizing hygienic measures and encouraging vaccination against smallpox, and introducing the serum treatment of diphtheria. It would not be right to refuse to recognize the part they played in the struggles to end this massacre of the innocents, and to improve the threatened lives of young children.

12 Pasteur, Pasteurization, and Medicine

JEAN-NOËL BIRABEN *Institut National d'Études Démographiques, Paris*

It is impossible to overestimate the revolutionary aspects of Pasteur's work in chemistry, biology, and medicine; his work has affected some of the most important aspects of people's lives, health, and longevity.

Before Pasteur's time very little was known about the causes of disease.[1] When Pasteur died, he had succeeded not only in providing an accurate explanation for a large part of human and animal pathology, but had also paved the way to immunology and the introduction of new treatments, and for advances which are still continuing in all branches of medicine, virology, and oncology.

It is less often realized how radically the struggle against micro-organisms, and the associated techniques of pasteurization, asepsis, and antisepsis have changed the conditions of human life, and that this remains true to the present day. Within the restrictions of this chapter we shall only deal with pasteurization and asepsis, and shall be content to describe only those aspects of antisepsis that are necessary for an understanding of our subject.

1. Pasteurization

When in 1854, Pasteur was appointed Dean of the Faculty of Science at Lille at the age of 32, his reputation was that of a chemist, who had done work on the deflection of light in tartaric acid and who had been Professor of Chemistry in Dijon and in Strasbourg. However, his interests were much more wideranging, but as he stated in his inaugural lecture: 'In the field of scientific observations, fortune only smiles on those who are prepared'.

Fortune did smile on him two years later, in the form of a Lille industrialist, M. Bigo, who was engaged in producing alcohol from beetroot, and who complained that a large part of his output was suffering from unexplained changes. Pasteur, visited Bigo's factory, had the method of producing alcohol explained to him, and sampled the beetroot juice at

[1] e.g. it had been recognized from 1627 onwards that mange was a disease caused by parasites, when the Hungarian physician Mate Czanaki established that the mite was responsible; Sir James Paget first observed in 1833 that trichinosis was caused by a nematode, and in 1839 Johan Lukas Schönlein described the microscopic fungus that caused ringworm.

various stages of manufacture. Looking at it under the microscope, he found that when fermentation proceeded normally, the juice contained round globules, which became elongated when fermentation was defective. Though some other chemists and biologists had anticipated Pasteur in this observation, they regarded these globules as being the result of spontaneous generation which could be observed in all organic media at current temperatures: any differences between them were assumed to have been caused by differences in the environment. The globules were not given a name and were ignored, because they were assumed to have no interest for scientists.

However, Pasteur considered them to be very important and asked himself questions about them. Were the globules always the same, or did they change in different nutritional media? Or were they of an entirely different kind? In order to study them, Pasteur provided different cultures for the first time: he cultivated the globules in glass vessels filled with a nutritive liquid the composition of which he was able to change at will. In this way he assisted their multiplication, but did not observe any changes in either their form or their nature: they remained different and identifiable. Pasteur went on to reverse the conventional way of thinking and concluded that it was these micro-organisms which were responsible for fermentation, rather than the other way round. They were the agents which induced fermentation, and different types of fermentation were produced by different organisms. It remained to prove the truth of this intuition, and in particular to show how these agents could enter the juice. Pasteur remembered Hippocrates and believed that these germs were carried in the atmosphere. He therefore conducted a number of experiments: he sterilized his vessels by heating them to a temperature of 110°C in a sterilizer, inserted a sterilized plug into the tube, and then pumped air through the tube so that the plug would trap the dust and the germs. He then put the plug into a sterile broth and kept his vessels closed at a temperature between 25 and 30°C. After two or three days, only the vessel with the cotton wool plug contained micro-organisms which were multiplying rapidly. When he put the sterile plug directly into the broth, without first pumping in the air, the broth always remained clear. Another experiment that was more relevant to the problem that he was dealing with, consisted of enclosing a bunch of grapes which had been washed in boiling water and then cooled in cotton wool until they ripened, so that no fermenting agents could settle on their surface. He found that although the juice of all other grapes fermented, that of the treated grapes did not.

Thus, Pasteur succeeded in demonstrating that not only beetroot juice, but also wine, vinegar, beer, and all other fermented beverages could be rendered unfit for consumption by the actions of specific micro-organisms which made wine taste bitter, gave a bad taste to beer, and destroyed vinegar. The protagonists of what was then the orthodox doctrine of spontaneous generation regarded all these experiments as an attack on their doctrine, and

Pasteur failed to be elected to membership of the Academy of Sciences when he was a candidate in 1857.

Pasteur, however, was certain of his results, continued his experiments, and devised a method for selecting benign germs by eliminating those which were harmful. He did this by heating a culture to a temperature of between 60 and 65°C for half an hour. He was thus able to convince the industrialists that their instruments, pipes, and dishes, indeed their whole plants, provided refuges for undesirable germs. They all needed to be washed and maintained in a state of meticulous cleanliness and were only to be used with pure fermenting agents which had been subjected to a process of controlled heating.

It took a long time to apply this process to the production of beer, wine, milk, and many other beverages. Pasteur was not looking for specific recipes; he was interested in obtaining a general understanding of the process and undertook a long and detailed study of its general aspects. The results of his researches were communicated in his lectures to the Chemical Society of Paris. In these lectures he reviewed and criticized the work of all his predecessors beginning with work done during the earliest periods of science on 'infinitely small animalcules' that caused disease. He considered the doctrine of spontaneous generation and its refutations, and considered possible applications for his work. He referred to Terentius Reatinus, the first man to have attributed disease to microscopic animals;[2] to the Italian physician Jerome Fracastor who took up this idea in 1546 and generalized it, so as to apply it to all cases of contagious disease; to the German Jesuit Athanasius Kircher who in 1658 attributed the plague which had ravaged Rome two years earlier to these creatures; to the Italian physician François Redi, who in 1688 was the first man to deny the doctrine of spontaneous generation through his convincing experiments; to the later observations by the French physicians Bertrand in 1720 and Deidier in 1725 who showed that it was possible to inoculate dogs with plague; to the English Catholic priest Needham, who in 1745 tried in London on Buffon's advice to sterilize by heat products placed in closed vessels; to the Italian naturalist Abbé Lazare Spallanzani who repeated Needham's and Buffon's experiments in Modena in 1765 and who actively denied the possibility of spontaneous generation; and more particularly to Nicolas Appert whom he regarded as his principal precursor.

Around 1780, Appert who had been steward to the Duc de Deux Points, and later to the Princesse de Forbach, came to live in Paris, and a few years later invented methods of preserving food in vessels which he had heated to boiling-point in a *bain-marie*. The first to benefit from his work were the

[2] 'In marshy places, minuscule animals multiply. They are so small that they cannot be seen with the naked eye, but enter the body with the breath, and cause grave illness.' Terentius Reatinus, *De re rustica*, trans. X. Rousselor (Paris, 1843), pp. 60–61.

housewives in his area. During the French Revolution the provisioning of the armies caused considerable problems, and the Directory offered a valuable prize for the best method that could be used to preserve food for the troops. Appert installed himself in Ivry in 1795, and devoted all the time that he could spare from his duties as a municipal councillor (he had been elected to this office on 7 Messidor of the year III) to putting his ideas into practice. His methods became widely known. Grimod de la Reyniere, at the time a *conseiller d'État*, in his *Almanac des gourmands* enthused about these products 'which remind one of May in wintertime, and which can even lead us to believe that we have mistaken the season, when the dishes are prepared by a skilful cook'. In 1804 Appert left Ivry for Massy in order to expand his activities, because the Navy had become interested in his products. However, it took a long time for the committee nominated by the Director of Supplies for the Navy to give a favourable opinion, The committee was set up in 1804, but did not report favourably until 15 March 1809. From 1804 onwards Appert employed some 25 to 30 female workers to shell the peas and beans, and to prepare fruits and vegetables in season, and his business prospered. The official committee consisting of Bardel, Gay-Lussac, Scipion-Perier, and Molard having reported favourably, the Minister for the Interior, Montalivet, informed Appert on 10 January 1810 that the Consultative Office of Arts and Manufactures had awarded him a prize of 12,000 francs, on condition that he published his method without delay.

Towards the end of 1810 Appert decided not to profit by his monopoly which was being attacked in the newspapers and published *The Art of Preserving All Animal and Vegetable Substances for Several Years*, and thus brought his method into the public domain. His principles were relatively simple: they consisted of:

1. enclosing the substances to be preserved in bottles or similar vessels;
2. sealing these vessels hermetically, and with great care; success depended on the sealing process being properly done.
3. exposing the enclosed substances to the action of boiling water in a *bain-marie* for shorter or longer periods, a specific method being used for each substance. It was this third condition which took longest to be adopted.

From Pasteur's point of view the importance of Appert's work consisted of the fact that – in contrast to the scientific orthodoxy of the time – he had correctly interpreted the evidence, whilst during the same year Gay-Lussac stated in a paper submitted to the Institute that

> animal and vegetable substances acquire a tendency to putrefaction by contact with the atmosphere; but if they are exposed to the effect of boiling water in properly sealed vessels, the oxygen absorbed by the process results in a new combination which

no longer leads to fermentation or putrefaction, and is fixed by heat, as in the case of albumin.[3]

Nicolas Appert, in his work, stated that:

the action of heat destroys, or at least neutralizes, all the fermenting agents which, in the natural order of things produce these changes, and by altering the constituent parts of animal or vegetable matter change their qualities.[4]

Thus, the scientists of the period believed that oxygen, fixed by heat, made the further generation of germs resulting from fermentation or putrefaction impossible, whereas Appert thought that these germs had existed before the process was begun and were destroyed or neutralized by heat, and that it was they who were responsible for fermentation.

It thus becomes clear why Pasteur cited Appert as having anticipated him no fewer than eleven times; preservation having already been invented, Pasteur proceeded to perfect what scientists abroad called 'pasteurization', (the term was used from 1872 onwards). The process consisted of varying the temperature used to control specific germs. Like Appert, Pasteur searched for the ideal temperature and length of the process of heating for different liquids, and he waited many months for the results to become apparent. As regards wine, for instance, he waited until 1865 before taking out a patent, which he immediately made available for public use. The required temperature was between 55 and 75°C depending on the wine's alcohol content and on the amounts of tannin and acid that were present. In principle, the pasteurizing of liquids at a high temperature for short periods was to be preferred to a longer process at lower temperatures. However, this would depend on the stability of the liquid's constituents and on its acidity: an acidic liquid did not require as high a temperature as a less acidic one. An organic liquid, e.g. milk, retained all its qualities and could be kept for use for a day or two, provided it had been raised to a temperature of 70°C for a period of 20 minutes and was then rapidly cooled to a temperature of 12°C.

As was the case with Appert's techniques, Pasteur's were improved, though the principle remained the same. From 1817 onwards, Appert had ceased using vessels made of glass, and used tin plate instead. To complete his researches on tin plate, he went to England, and later he tried autoclaving (for gelatinizing bones), a method which he preferred to the *bain-marie*. In the beginning, Pasteur, too, used a type of large cylinder heated by gas or steam passing through coiled tubes for the pasteurization of liquids in bulk.

Later, liquids were pasteurized after they had already been put into sealed

[3] Cited in Charles Nicolas Appert, 'Le Livre de tous les ménages, ou l'art de conserver pendant plusieurs années toutes les substances animales et végétales (2nd edn., Paris, 1811), p. 36.

[4] Appert, op. cit. in n. 3 above, pp. 45–48.

bottles (e.g. wine, beer, cider, fruit juices, etc.) in horizontal vessels in which the liquids were exposed to steadily increasing water temperatures, until they reached a temperature of between 65 and 75°C maintained for 20 to 30 minutes, which was then replaced by water that was gradually cooled down to a temperature of between 10 and 12°C. This method had the advantage that it could be operated continuously; its disadvantage was that the sterilizing vessels required were large and clumsy.

The introduction of these techniques led to a revolution in the method of production used in the industry which produced beverages for human consumption. Not only did they result in a considerable increase in productivity, but the quality of the finished product was also much improved. This is why Paul Bert, a physician and the pupil of Claude Bernard, presented Pasteur as an economic benefactor, when he made his report in 1874 to the Parliamentary committee that had been set up to assess Pasteur's work and fix his compensation.

> At that time the debt owed to Germany [the 5,000 million exacted as reparations in 1871] was largely covered by the value of Pasteur's discoveries. These millions came from a laboratory, which was linked to the teaching faculty at the Sorbonne. This laboratory must be maintained, and will be maintained, for him by vote of Parliament.

Although Pasteur's discoveries are more than a century old,[5] pasteurization has retained its original value and continues to be universally used in much the same way as in Pasteur's time, though with a few technical improvements. Since the 1960s, only milk destined for human consumption has been pasteurized in vessels or heat exchangers heated by plates or tubes (with hot water, steam, or electricity) made from inoxydable steel or by infra-red light, with a pre-heating from 42 to 60°C, pasteurization lasting for 30 minutes at 62°C, followed by a cooling-down period from 52 to 40 and later to 25°C. Milk that was destined for the food industry (for the production of condensed milk, powdered milk, chocolates, and confectionery, sent to creameries to be made into butter, and for other beverages) is now pasteurized in bulk in large vats that are raised to temperatures of between 72 and 75°C, but only for a period of 15 minutes. Finally, during the 1970s, the pasteurization of milk for human consumption has been replaced by new processes which make its long-term preservation possible (UHT procedures, filling under vacuum, sterilization by irradiation, etc.).

We must also mention the works of John Tyndall, a British physician, which followed on Pasteur and pasteurization. His aim was not to select

[5] It was only on 2 July 1935 that the pasteurization of milk, which originated from uncontrolled sources, was made compulsory in France, and on 21 May 1955 that the imprecise term 'pasteurization' was defined, and minimum conditions for the treatment of milk were laid down.

different germs, but to destroy them in order to sterilize the final product, without having to use temperatures which were so high that they damaged its components, which happened when Appert's methods were used. In 1882 he invented an original method which consisted of separate heat treatments. Depending on the nature of the product, he used three separate heatings at 24-hour intervals with a temperature of 70°C maintained for an hour, or alternatively five heatings to a temperature of 60°C. He showed that the bacterial spores were affected by the first treatment and destroyed by the later ones, but that the products, and particularly albumin, retained all their qualities. This method of sterilization which came to be called 'Tyndallization', was used particularly in pharmacological work, and for all products which tended to coagulate as boiling-point was approached.

2. Asepsis

The discovery that bacteria caused fermentation and putrefaction opened vast new vistas to Pasteur and provided scope for applying his methods to subjects other than pasteurization. In 1865 he was consulted by the silkworm breeders of southern France about a new disease which appeared to have infected their silkworms and which appeared to be contagious (*pébrine*) and he became convinced that this disease was caused by bacteria, as were all other contagious diseases that affected humans. Two years later Pasteur had succeeded not only in saving the silk industry by providing it with a method of overcoming this disease (and, indeed, a second silkworm disease *flâcherie*) but had provided a proof that microscopic organisms were responsible for an animal disease and confirmed that this also was true of human diseases. He also demonstrated the means available for the elimination of pathogenic germs: heat, filtration, or the use of antiseptics.[6] In the same year in Glasgow, Lister a Scottish surgeon who had read Pasteur's work decided to act, published a paper on the principles of antisepsis, and began to use phenic acid after several other attempts. From 1869 onwards, Lister did not perform any operations without having first disinfected his hands and all objects which came into contact with the wound. After the operation he covered the wound with a piece of gauze that had been dipped into a solution of phenic acid, which had been diluted so as not to cause irritation to the tissues. His results were remarkably good: not only was he able to avoid a long and damaging suppuration of the wound, but the mortality from operations which had been of the order of 6 per cent or higher, fell to 2 per

[6] In addition to simple substances, such as alcohol and ether, other antiseptic means such as a mixture of sodium chloride and chloride of lime had been used by the pharmacist Antoine Labarraque in 1825, and the disinfectant properties of phenic acid had been demonstrated by the chemist François Lemaitre in 1860.

cent or lower within a period of a few years,[7] and as mortality declined, Lister attempted operations and interventions that had not been attempted previously.[8] By 1871 Lister's method had triumphed and was widely used by other British surgeons.

However, in spite of all his precautions, Lister found that there persisted a relatively large number of infections among his patients. He began to spray phenic acid in the air above the wound, but, although he used antiseptics freely, infections supervened, and even in cases where they were overcome, the tissues which had been irritated by the antiseptics healed badly and left scars. In particular, Lister was as yet unable to sterilize catgut which was used in operations, and this caused him considerable difficulty.

Pasteur, who was not medically qualified himself, reflected on these problems and realized that it was possible to make progress by preventing the bacteria from settling on the wound, rather than attempt to destroy them once they had settled there.

Since the 1870s surgeons of the Lister school had used antiseptics that were efficient disinfectants, but their use resulted in complications, required a larger number of assistants for the surgeon, and prolonged the healing period. As Pasteur recognized, the objective was no longer to destroy bacteria which had caused the infection of the wound, but to exclude them from the site of the operation as far as was possible. Lister's methods were very rapidly adopted after 1875 by his professional colleagues in Germany, Austria, the Netherlands, Belgium, Scandinavia, and Russia.

Among French surgeons, Just Lucas-Championnière was a fervent protagonist of antisepsis[9] and invented a sprayer which was designed to disinfect the air in the operating theatre before the operation, but he was unsuccessful in attracting any followers. In 1878 Pasteur tried to convince the members of the Academy of Medicine of the importance of sterilizing their instruments before operating. In addressing the distinguished assembly of surgeons, he said:

> If I had the honour of being a surgeon, I would not only confine myself to using perfectly clean instruments, but I would, after having washed my hands very carefully, only use bandages which had previously been heated to a temperature of

[7] The mortality rate for amputation, which was the most dangerous operation, had been of the order of 60 per cent. Between 1867 and 1869, when Lister first began to use his new method, he performed 40 amputations, and only 4 of the patients died, i.e. a mortality rate of 10 per cent.

[8] Even before Pasteur and Lister, surgeons had noted that cleanliness reduced the numbers of infections and deaths. In particular, obstetricians, such as Oliver Wendell Holmes in Boston, and Ignaz Semmelweiss in Budapest in 1860, understood this, but theirs was a simple recognition of an empirical truth, and they were not aware of the true reason why cleanliness was efficacious.

[9] Another surgeon, Alfonse Guerin, was attracted by Pasteur's theories and during the siege of Paris in 1870–71 attempted to filter the air above the wounds of his patients by covering them with a thick sterile dressing, but his results did not live up to his hopes.

between 130 and 150°C, and I would only use water which had been heated to a temperature of 120°C.

The new methods of antisepsis were not all introduced simultaneously; they consisted of a number of small details that originated in all parts of the world, and only became a coherent whole around 1880. Octave Terillon brought them all together and began to apply them in 1883 under the name of asepsis. By using an operating theatre which had been kept scrupulously clean and disinfected, and by sterilizing all his instruments in boiling water he achieved excellent results, even though he did not use phenic acid, which had been employed until then. This new method began to be used in 1886 and from that date onwards sterilization of instruments in boiling water was replaced by dry sterilization at a temperature of between 120 and 130°C. The Berlin surgeon, Ernst von Bergman, introduced the sterilization of dressings by steam. By 1889 sterilization was done in autoclaves at a pressure of between two and three atmospheres, and in the same year, almost simultaneously in Baltimore and Paris, W. S. Holstead and Henri Chaput invented sterilized rubber gloves to be used by surgeons and their assistants. At the same time, Felix Terrier at the Bichat Hospital constructed the first operating theatre designed for use with an operating table and special lighting. In 1890 the white coat, the surgeon's cap, and face mask made their first appearance, the patient's skin was disinfected before operation and a method for sterilizing catgut came into use. It was only then that surgeons dared touch the peritoneum and to operate on the bowel, as until then such operations had almost invariably proved fatal. The major principles of aseptic surgery had been laid down, and later improvements were only those of detail.

Between 1885 and 1895 asepsis came to be accepted and was used by surgeons throughout the world, by the whole medical profession, and by the educated public. By 1895 knowledge of the procedure had spread to the general public, and although much was gained, there were also some excesses. Knowledge about microbes filtered down to the primary schools, and some families became obsessed with fear of bacteria: insects—flies, lice, midges, and mosquitoes—were hunted down, and the body was washed and disinfected with an ardour that sometimes resulted in dermatitis; laundry was sterilized as if it were to be used in surgical operations; and food was boiled to an extent that it lost some of its nutritional value. Babies were given milk that had been boiled so that its Vitamin C content was destroyed, and physicians were surprised to find cases of scurvy among children of economically well-off families.

Looking at the situation as a whole, these excesses were not dangerous, and the phobias lasted for a short time only: the disadvantages were small when compared to the gains achieved. In Western Europe mortality had begun to fall during the 1870s, but its decline reached unprecedented levels from 1885 onwards. As is clear from the tables in the Appendices, it was not vaccines or sera which were responsible for this fall that has continued into our own period, but the spread of cleanliness, disinfection, antisepsis, and asepsis.

Appendix 1

Changes in mortality recorded both in Paris and London show clearly that its fall accelerated at the time when asepsis and pasteurization were introduced, during the last decade of the nineteenth century; 1895 was the turning point. In London mortality fell by 19 per cent between 1861/70 and 1881/90, and by 25 per cent between 1881/90 and 1901/05. In Paris, the falls during the same period were 7.2 and 32.1 per cent respectively; antisepsis was introduced earlier than in London.

Table 12.1 Death rates per 1,000 population

Year	London	Paris
1861–65	24.4	25.7
1866–70		27.0
1871–75	22.5	22.4
1876–80		23.7
1881–85	20.5	24.4
1886–90		22.9
1891–95	19.6	21.1
1896–1900	16.4	19.1
1901–05		17.9

Appendix 2

Changes in cause-specific death rates in Paris show more clearly than changes in the overall death rate, the very considerable decline that occurred in the death rate from most diseases and which was caused by the reduction in complications due to infection. Hygiene, supported by the concepts of asepsis and antisepsis became more and more effective.

Table 12.2 Mortality in Paris per 100,000 population from principal causes of death between 1876/1880 and 1901/1905

Cause of death	Mortality rate per 100,000						Difference	
	1876–80	1881–85	1886–90	1891–95	1896–1900	1901–05	1876/80–1886/90	1886/90–1901/05
Typhoid fever	69	88	41	22	19	12	−28	−29
Smallpox	35	21	9	4	5	−26	−24	−4
Measles	39	54	56	34	32	20	+17	−36
Scarlet fever	7	9	10	7	6	4	+3	−6
Whooping cough	17	19	19	15	12	12	+2	−7
Diphtheria	94	88	70	44	13	17	−24	−53
Sub-total	264	279	205	126	84	70	−56	−135
Tuberculosis[a]	443	476	499	489	472	456	+56	−43
Cancer	94	95	99	99	105	109	+5	+10
Diabetes	5	8	12	13	15	15	+7	+3
Meningitis	115	110	77	58	45	36	−38	−41
Congestion, paralysis	156	162	139	128	126	117	−17	−22
Heart disease	124	126	126	126	122	118	+2	−2
Respiratory disease	435	410	435	410	330	294	—	−141
Diarrhoea enteritis	} 290	237	176	146	119	89	} −63	−87
Congenital debility		58	51	54	48	46		−5
Diseases of liver	39	41	38	37	34	37	−1	−1
Nephritis	21	25	34	42	47	49	+13	+15
Senility	62	62	67	68	71	69	+5	+2
Violence	65	70	65	70	67	61	—	−4
Sub-total	2,110	2,159	2,023	1,864	1,685	1,556	−87	−457
Other causes	262	281	264	248	224	229	+2	−35
All causes	2,372	2,440	2,287	2,112	1,909	1,795	−85	−492

[a] all sites

13 Public Health and Public Hygiene: The Urban Environment in the Late Nineteenth and Early Twentieth Centuries

ROBERT WOODS *University of Liverpool*

Both Gustave von Aschenbach and Dr Bernard Rieux would have known exactly what was meant by public hygiene, and how its breakdown might have disastrous consequences for public health, consequences that were initially disguised by administrative inaction, even duplicity. But in the late twentieth century it is all too easy to take for granted that those conditions which cost Aschenbach his life and the lives of many of Rieux's friends have been banished once and for all. We now assume that our piped water supply is not contaminated; that sewage is effectively removed from our homes and treated; that food and drink are not adulterated; that streets are paved, lighted, and cleaned. While some people in some places at some times are not able to make these assumptions, for most of us in the industrialized countries at least these elements of environmental quality are guaranteed. The same could not be said of any period before the First World War. Indeed, it would seem that, for many, the rise of great cities during the eighteenth and nineteenth centuries meant deteriorating public hygiene. The securing of public health through public hygiene represents a long and complicated story in which many individuals, organizations, and institutions played prominent roles. Not only is it difficult to see who is responsible for what, but the entire contribution of public hygiene, in relation to other advances, is still open to question.

In this chapter we deal with four issues in the long debate on the form and causes of the decline in mortality between 1700 and 1914, issues which are especially associated with the contribution of public hygiene. The first concerns the nature of public hygiene as an element of public health, including the various forms of environment and environmental change which have come to be linked with notions of public health. The second is concerned with the urban environment, urbanization, and the high level of mortality experienced by the inhabitants of most large towns. The third deals with the issue of public responsibility. Finally, the role of medical intervention is considered as it influenced, or otherwise, public health.

1. Public Hygiene and Public Health

The daily lives of ordinary citizens during the eighteenth and nineteenth centuries brought them into contact with a number of different environments, each of which held its own particular dangers for health. The sleeping, food-preparation, eating, and living spaces of the home (often a single space) were each potential areas for germ transmission. Under what circumstances was food prepared? Was a supply of clean water readily available? Were there facilities for washing? How were human excreta removed from the dwelling? Of what material were beds constructed, and could bedding be changed or cleaned? Were floors made of earth, stone, or board; were they covered and could they be cleaned? How many people of what ages lived and slept together? While we cannot be exact in our answers to many of these questions—especially for particular groups, periods, and places—it seems likely that for the majority the home environment in the twentieth century differed substantially, and for the better, from that of the eighteenth.[1] By 1900 the home environment for most was at least different from what it had been for earlier generations, and for many it was less dangerous and far more comfortable. More rooms, piped water, effective sewage and refuse disposal, easier-to-clean surfaces, these were all important features. But the homes themselves were likely to be closer together, if not actually on top of one another. What was gained in the private family environment could be lost once across the threshold in the wider community environment.

The daily activities of Edwardian adults took them to work, to shops, and to places of entertainment which required them to make journeys on foot, by horse or carriage, or more probably by some form of public transport. For the remaining rural population little had changed in these respects: cottage, farm, village, and market town were the daily round, as they had always been with labourers or peasants moving individually through deserted fields. Edwardian children faced new perils in the schoolroom where crowding and poor hygiene could easily prove hazards to health.[2]

Thinking in terms of daily-activity spaces helps to suggest the form of

I would like to thank Osamu Saito, Patti Watterson, and members of the Institute for European Population Studies, University of Liverpool, for their helpful comments on an earlier draft of this chapter, and the Wellcome Trust for its financial support.

[1] Interesting contrasts are found in Pierre Goubert, *The French Peasantry in the Seventeenth Century* (Cambridge, 1986) and Martine Segalen, *Love and Power in the Peasant Family: Rural France in the Nineteenth Century* (Oxford, 1983) for rural France.

[2] On infant and child mortality in England and Wales see R. I. Woods, P. A. Watterson, and J. H. Woodward, 'The Causes of Rapid Infant Mortality Decline in England and Wales 1861–1921: Parts I and II', *Population Studies*, 42(3) (1988), pp. 343–64 and 43(1) (1989), pp. 113–32, and on schooling and infectious diseases, Randall Reves, 'Declining Fertility in England and Wales as a Major Cause of the Twentieth Century Decline in Mortality: The Role of Changing Family Size and Age Structure in Infectious Disease Mortality in Infancy', *American Journal of Epidemiology*, 122 (1985), pp. 112–126.

environment which individuals with period, residence, or age in common would have experienced. It highlights both the particular and the general in the relationships between public hygiene, public health, and the decline of mortality.

First, the state of public hygiene would affect individuals at three distinct nodes of their daily activity—at home, at work, in places of public assembly (theatres, churches, sporting events, even schools, for example)—and as they moved between these nodes along public highways (or, if children, as they played in local courts and streets). The normal daily-activity space contains a number of distinct environments which are entered and exited in far from simple patterns and with durations of stay determined by personal characteristics.[3] The effects of improvement in one environment could be offset or nullified by deterioration in another. General health may have been affected more by conditions in the worst environment, rather than by those in the others, however good. Consider the examples of restrictions on spitting in public places, and the gradual substitution of motor vehicles for horses in urban streets.

Secondly, while the words 'hygiene' and 'health' have similar origins and meanings, notions of public hygiene have come to be associated with drainage and sewage disposal, that is with sanitation. Public health now represents a far broader concept but, for Victorians, sanitary reform alone became the means to advance public health almost to the exclusion of other problems, such as air pollution and dangers to the public from accidents, although vaccination and the problems associated with it were prominent. Even the best form of sanitary system would have only a limited impact while other dangers to public health persisted.

Thirdly, whatever the period, Western urbanism has been characterized by higher mortality in the largest urban centres.[4] Level of mortality and position in the urban hierarchy show a persistently strong and positive relationship. On the one hand, urbanization is likely to have a deleterious effect on public hygiene, but, on the other, once investments have been made in sanitary provision, the effects should be immediate, substantial, influence large numbers of citizens, and thus prove more cost-effective than similar units of investment in sanitary facilities for a scattered rural population.[5]

Fourthly, private and public environments are socially divided in forms

[3] For an introduction to the literature on activity-spaces and time geographies see K. Lynch, *The Image of the City* (Cambridge, Mass., 1960) and D. J. Walmsley, *Urban Living: The Individuals in the City* (London, 1988).

[4] Compare Susan B. Hanley, 'Urban Sanitation in Preindustrial Japan', *Journal of Interdisciplinary History*, 18 (1987), pp. 1–26 with R. I. Woods and P. R. A. Hinde, 'Mortality in Victorian England: Models and Patterns', *Journal of Interdisciplinary History*, 18 (1987), pp. 27–54.

[5] See Jan de Vries, *European Urbanization 1500–1800* (London, 1984) and R. I. Woods and J. H. Woodward (eds.), *Urban Disease and Mortality in Nineteenth-Century England* (London, 1984).

that have always required the reconciliation of private and public interests, particularly in respect of property rights.[6] Substantial advances in public hygiene therefore require the political élite to take overall responsibility for the general good. This intervention would be encouraged if a particular form of altruistic moral code were adopted; if a universal franchise made social responsibility politically advantageous; of if the environment used by the élite was itself affected in a way detrimental to the health of that group. In short, advances in public hygiene require changes in the politics of public responsibility.

These four points do, of course, require elaboration, but in order to identify the role of medical intervention in the decline of mortality through its influence on public hygiene, illustrations must be drawn where the characteristics of environment, mortality patterns, and medical intervention are most clear. In the next section we attempt a sketch with the urban environment as its canvas.

2. The Urban Environment and Sanitation

Dr Thomas Legge's survey of sanitary conditions in six European capitals, which was conducted during the early 1890s, gives an interesting description not only of comparative provision, but also of a contemporary's reaction to the eccentricities of sanitary practice.[7] Legge was clearly impressed by the architectural grandeur of Paris's main sewers, yet dismayed by the extent to which the Seine below Paris was polluted by untreated sewage. Legge also remarked on the practice, common in the late 1880s, of supplementing depleted water supplies during the summer months with water taken directly from the Seine. To demonstrate his point, Legge also quoted the saying 'Pas d'eau de Seine, pas de choléra' in his reference to the cholera outbreak of 1892.[8] Many of these difficulties had been removed by the early 1900s with the completion of the sewer system and the creation of extensive sewage farms, but even in 1911 Paris was particularly badly afflicted by an epidemic of summer diarrhoea.[9]

[6] Gerry Kearns, 'Private Property and Public Health Reform in England 1830–70, *Social Science Medicine*, 26 (1988), pp. 187–99.

[7] Thomas M. Legge, *Public Health in European Capitals* (London, 1896). Sir Thomas Legge (1863–1932) was later knighted for his work as Medical Inspector of Factories, but some of his early career was spent in Brighton with Sir Arthur Newsholme, to whom his 1896 publication was dedicated.

[8] Ibid. 52.

[9] On the French situation in general see J.-P. Goubert, 'Public Hygiene and Mortality Decline in France in the Nineteenth Century', in T. Bengtsson *et al.* (eds.), *Pre-Industrial Population Change* (Stockholm, 1984), pp. 151–59; on the 'Eiffel Tower effect' of late summer diarrhoea, see Pierre Budin, *The Nursling* (London, 1907), originally published as *Le Nourrisson* (Paris, 1900), and, more recently, Deborah Dwork, *War is Good for Babies and Other Young Children: A History of the Infant and Child Welfare Movement in England 1898–1918* (London, 1987), pp. 96–97.

Legge was highly complimentary about sanitary conditions in Brussels, a state of affairs he attributed almost entirely to the wide ranging powers of the Burgomaster; the creation of a Bureau d'Hygiène in 1874 and the ability of its chief inspector Dr Eugène Janssens. The significance of Dr Janssens's office lay in its combination of ten vital functions, among which the medical inspection of prostitutes and of children in state schools; the analyses of water and food; the preparation of demographic analysis from the certification of births and deaths; and the supervision of dangerous occupations were some of the most important. For English readers, Legge stressed the inspection and supervision of prostitutes. Apart from the need for a separate isolation hospital, Brussels in 1894 had a particularly high reputation for public health.[10] In Legge's view 'This sanitary organization developed by Dr Janssens deserves the more attention, because it is probable that future improvements in the public health service abroad will be made by adopting its methods, rather than those of Great Britain'.[11]

The Scandinavian capitals visited by Legge also had a good deal to recommend them, particularly the care taken with the milk supply in Denmark and Sweden. But in Copenhagen sewage was being discharged directly into the harbour, and in Christiania, despite the existence of a health office or *Sundhedskommission* since 1860, sections of the town were unpaved and undrained, and the sewage disposal system was inadequate.

The sixth European capital, Berlin, was particularly commended for the advances made between 1872 and 1892. Robert Koch's advocacy of sand filtration for the purification of water was being put to good effect, while the problems caused by low altitude and a high water table forced the construction of sewage farms served by a radial system of sewers and collection-points. Berlin was not without its sanitary problems in the 1890s, but in spite of its natural environment it passed the test posed by cholera in 1892, unlike Hamburg and Paris.[12]

Although Legge himself refused to draw any general conclusions from his survey, several are clear. First, even during the late nineteenth century the natural environment of Europe's cities imposed certain restrictions on the provision of adequate sanitation. Winter frost, summer drought, the proximity of mountain streams, a high water table, impermeable soil, and low elevation were each likely to impose costs or confer benefits which during the early history of public hygiene would create differences in morbidity and mortality regardless of official policy. Secondly, the availability of a substantial river, or a conveniently placed stretch of tidal water, might encourage their use as open sewers, whereas those inland cities on insubstantial waterways would be forced to seek alternative means of sewage

[10] L. Verniers, *Bruxelles et son agglomération de 1830 à nos jours* (Brussels, 1958).

[11] Legge op. cit. in n. 7, p. 128.

[12] On mortality in Berlin, see A.E. Imhof, 'Mortalität in Berlin vom 18. bis 20. Jahrhundert', *Berliner Statistik*, 31 (1971), pp. 138–45.

disposal, despite the higher cost. Thirdly, even when the political will to improve sanitation was present the bureaucratic machinery might be inadequate, but where both existed and worked together, as appeared to be the case in Brussels, much could be achieved. The absence of both could prove disastrous.

These points, though expressed too simply, help us to focus on those factors that were important for the advance of public health. In the remainder of this section we deal with two additional issues. First, progress made in Berlin, Brussels, or Paris can be placed in context once one considers what could, and in the case of Hamburg did, happen when local politicians and medical men were indifferent to the fundamental principles of public hygiene. Secondly, although one would be entirely justified in assuming that improvements in the sanitary environment should have a direct bearing on the pattern and level of mortality, the relationship still requires to be demonstrated, since mortality decline may have been more the consequence of several other coincidental developments. Here we have the central point for debate, one to which we shall return repeatedly. Recent discussion harks back to the analysis presented by Thomas McKeown in *The Modern Rise of Population*[13] in which he argued that about a quarter of the decline in mortality in England and Wales between the middle of the nineteenth century and 1901 was due to the specific measures of the sanitary reformers as they affected public, but also to some extent personal, hygiene through their effects on the water- and food-borne diseases. But the argument has wider implications, not only for the rest of Europe and America, but also for general issues of method. How is impact to be assessed if it cannot be measured directly? Hamburg and Birmingham provide the setting for a brief examination of these points.

The population of Hamburg in 1892 was about 625,000. The cholera epidemic of that year affected at least 16,926 (the number of officially reported cases) and killed at least 8,605 persons. How could such a disaster have struck a large west European city eight years after the discovery of the cholera bacillus? The answer appears to lie in the 'indissoluble connection between medical science, economic interest, and political ideology'.[14] Cholera was brought to Hamburg by Russian emigrants who intended to proceed to America. It entered the unfiltered water-carriage system from the Elbe, the first case was reported on 16 August, and twelve days later, on

[13] Thomas McKeown, *The Modern Rise of Population* (London, 1976) and originally Thomas McKeown and R.G. Record, 'Reasons for the Decline in Mortality in England and Wales during the Nineteenth Century', *Population Studies*, 16(2) (1962), pp. 94–122. Thomas McKeown (1912–88) has had an important influence on the debate about advances in public health: see Simon Szreter, 'The Importance of Social Intervention in Britain's Mortality Decline *c*.1850–1914: A Re-Interpretation of the Role of Public Health', *Social History of Medicine*, 1 (1988), pp. 1–37.

[14] Richard J. Evans, *Death in Hamburg: Society and Politics in the Cholera Years 1830–1919* (Oxford, 1987), p. 275.

27 August, more than 1,000 cases a day were being reported (the bacillus was probably in the harbour on 13 August and in the water system on 19 August). The local administration and the medical profession of Hamburg failed its inhabitants through indifference, self-interest, and ignorance. Hamburg, always individualistic and antagonistic to Berlin, rejected the work of Koch and the bacteriologists. The merchant élite which dominated local politics was largely geographically isolated from, and indifferent to, the needs of the labouring classes who occupied their own wretched environment in the old town close by the harbour. Worse still, there was no particular policy to deal with epidemics. Little had been learned from previous cholera outbreaks, or for that matter from the devastating smallpox epidemic of 1871. Indeed, the first reaction in August 1892 was to conceal the existence of Asiatic cholera so that the Imperial Health Office in Berlin would not impose quarantine, thus disrupting trade. Certainly, everything that could go amiss did so in Hamburg in 1892, although those responsible were not, of course, the ones to suffer most. Richard Evans's analysis clearly shows that cholera morbidity and mortality rates were both significantly and inversely related to income. Yet the question remains, why were the Russian emigrants forced to travel in sealed trains across Prussia, but allowed to disembark in Hamburg?

In 1891 the population of Birmingham was 430,000. In the annual league table of urban death rates it occupied a central position, better than Liverpool, Manchester, and Sheffield, but not as healthy as several smaller towns, Bristol among them. Hennock has argued that this middling position meant

> Advocates of a more vigorous sanitary policy were met with evidence furnished by the comparative statistics. The lack of uniformity, which characterised local administration in England, meant that the best work was frequently done in the worst places, while in less unsatisfactory districts the stimulus to action was lacking. This gave the administrative measures that were taken the character of first-aid work, and did little to raise the general standard of health expected from a town. Places like Birmingham were able to treat their favourable topographical conditions as a substitute for administrative action, instead of making them a springboard to a higher standard.[15]

The point is well made, yet even with an effective local administration it is difficult to see how the year-on-year comparative statistics can be used to assess the impact of a vigorous sanitary policy.[16]

[15] E.P. Hennock, *Fit and Proper Persons: Ideal and Reality in Nineteenth-century Urban Government* (London, 1973), pp. 112–13.

[16] Compare e.g. Sir Arthur Newsholme, 'The Measurement of Progress in Public Health, with Special Reference to the Life and Work of William Farr', *Economica*, 9 (1923), pp. 186–202, with George Rosen, 'Problems in the Application of Statistical Analysis to Questions of Health 1700–1880', *Bulletin of the History of Medicine*, 29 (1955), pp. 27–45, on the use of statistical analysis. The former, following William Farr, was optimistic, while the latter was much more cautious.

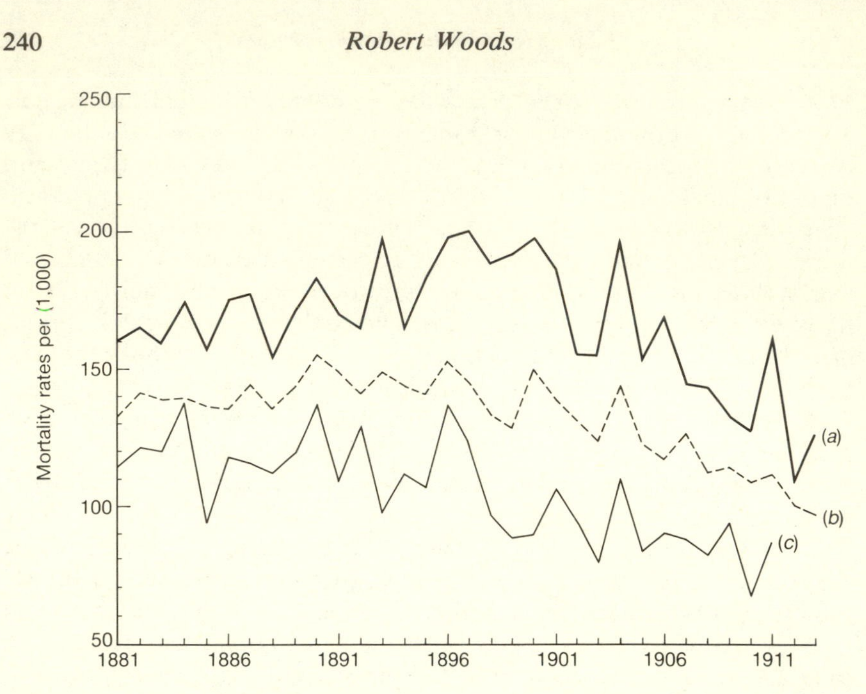

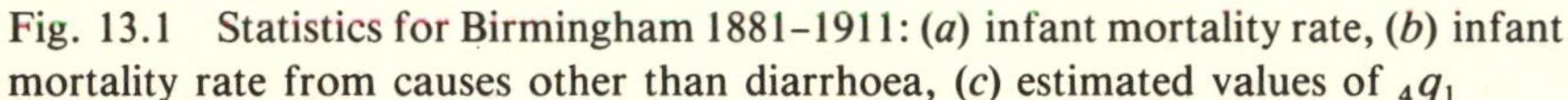
Fig. 13.1 Statistics for Birmingham 1881–1911: (*a*) infant mortality rate, (*b*) infant mortality rate from causes other than diarrhoea, (*c*) estimated values of ${}_4q_1$

Consider the pattern of mortality in Birmingham during the 1880s, 1890s, and 1900s, especially that for infants and young children, arguably the age groups most vulnerable to defective sanitation. In Fig. 13.1 we show the infant mortality rate (q_0), the infant mortality rate from diseases other than diarrhoea, and estimates of ${}_4q_1$ between 1881 and 1911. What does it tell us about sanitary conditions in Birmingham? There is no clear picture. Infant mortality remained at a high level throughout the 1880s and 1890s.

It even increased during the latter period, but had it not been for higher levels of mortality from diarrhoea and enteric fever it would have declined during the 1890s, as did childhood mortality. If one looks more closely at particular years, 1892 and 1911 for example (the former a cholera year, the latter the year of *Der Tod in Venedig*), more of the picture may be revealed. Figs. 13.2 and 13.3 show the total number of deaths and the number of infant deaths per week in Birmingham in 1892 and 1911, as well as the deaths of those aged 1 to 4, and deaths from diarrhoea. Neither 1892 nor 1911 was a cholera year in Birmingham, indeed, mortality in the former was highest in the first, second, and fourth quarters, although in 1911 there was a severe outbreak of epidemic diarrhoea which particularly afflicted infants, but was also reflected in a peak for total deaths during the third quarter of the year.

Several contemporary and modern demographers have noted this 'Eiffel Tower effect', but Cheney, working with data for Philadelphia, has argued that while infant mortality may have stayed high at the end of the nineteenth

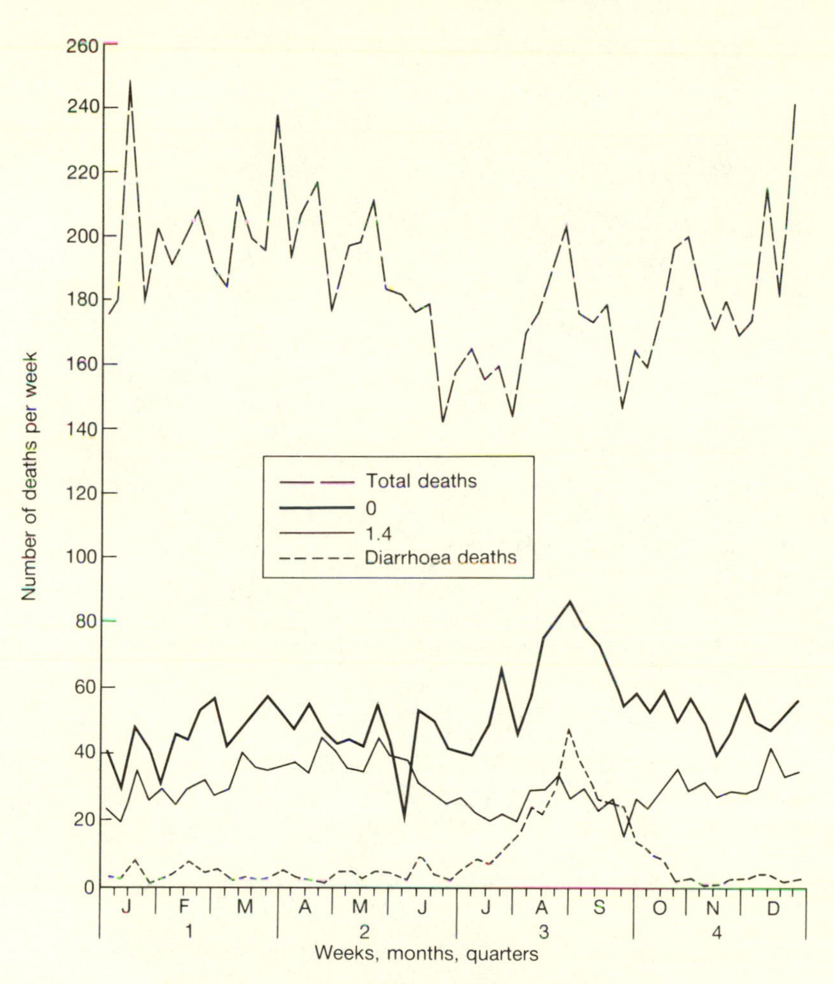

Fig. 13.2 Weekly deaths in Birmingham 1892

century, mortality during the second year of life fell in response to improvements in nutritional status.[17] If appropriate, such an argument could be applied equally well to Birmingham (${}_4q_1$ contains q_1 in Fig. 13.1). However, contemporary British observers, like Arthur Newsholme, were preoccupied with the way in which epidemic diarrhoea sought out those towns

[17] On Paris, see Budin, op. cit. in n. 9, but also Etienne van de Walle and Samuel H. Preston, 'Mortalité de l'enfance au XIXe siècle à Paris et dans le département de la Seine', *Population*, 29(1) (1974), pp. 89–107, on the quality of French data; on Belgium, E. Vilquin, 'La Mortalité infantile selon le mois de naissance: Cas de la Belgique du XIXe siècle', *Population*, 11 (1978), pp. 1137–50; R. A. Cheney, 'Seasonal Aspects of Infant and Childhood Mortality: Philadelphia 1865–1920', *Journal of Interdisciplinary History*, 14 (1984), pp. 561–85.

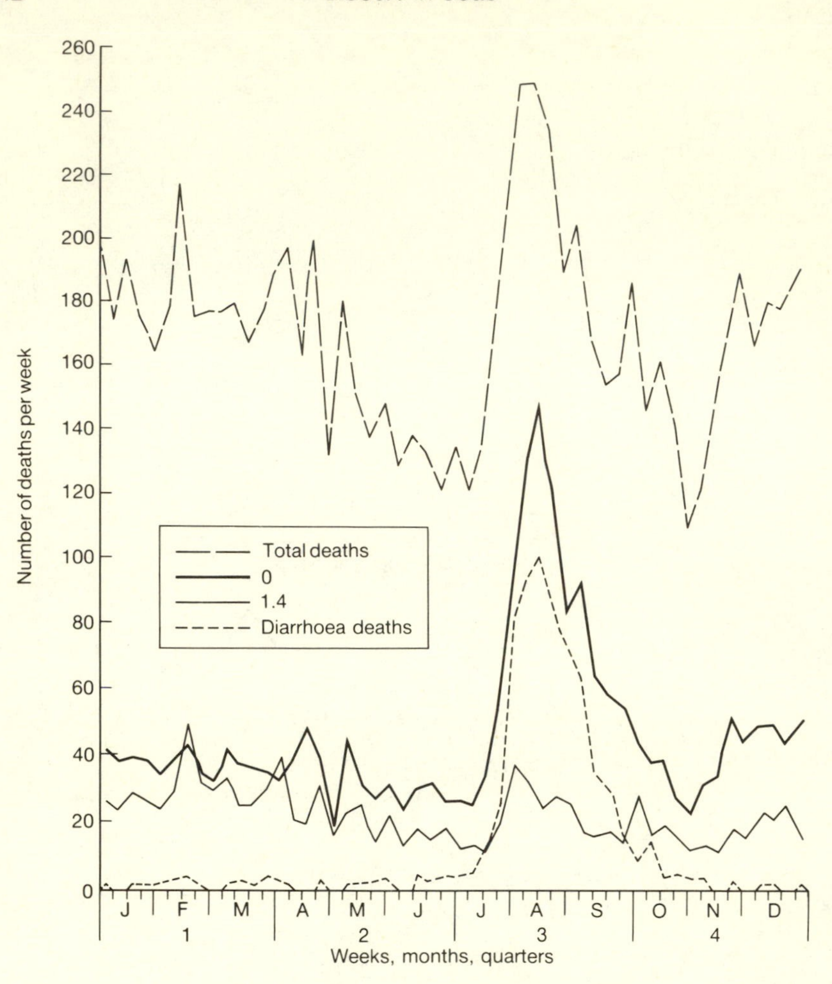

Fig. 13.3 Weekly deaths in Birmingham 1911

with the least satisfactory systems of sewage and house-refuse disposal in years with high temperature and low rainfall in the third quarters (not 1892, but 1911). Newsholme clearly saw this as a means of evaluating the effectiveness of sanitary provision in towns.[18] Huddersfield and Halifax (lowest mortality) could easily be distinguished from Preston and Leicester (highest mortality). But any attempt to judge progress from trends is bound to encounter certain obvious problems. First, the three curves in Fig. 13.1 tell different stories. Infant mortality only began to decline after 1900, but

[18] Arthur Newsholme, 'A Contribution to the Study of Epidemic Diarrhoea', *Public Health*, 12(3) (1899), pp. 139–213.

the downward trend was broken in 1904, 1906, and 1911. Between the early 1880s and the late 1890s q_0 increased from 0.16 to 0.20. Did sanitary conditions improve, then deteriorate, then improve dramatically? Secondly, if one looks at Figs. 13.2 and 13.3 in isolation, what conclusions would one draw about the state of public hygiene in Birmingham? Clearly Birmingham failed the test in 1911, but then so did most British and many other European cities.

On a cross-sectional basis there is some justification for taking Newsholme's comparative view. Birmingham fared better in the summer of 1892 than Paris or Hamburg for example, but the use of such mortality series to evaluate changes over time represents a very crude device, fraught with difficulties of interpretation and confounding variables.[19]

3. Public Responsibility

The third issue raised in the introduction was concerned with the question of what could be done to change the environment. Although some aspects of the answer have already been touched on in passing, the question still remains to be considered directly.

In terms of technology, there certainly were advances during the nineteenth century. The ability to tunnel for long distances, to pump water, to construct reservoirs, sewage farms, destructors for refuse disposal water-filtration works, and to manufacture connecting pipes and sanitary ware, all increased the possibility of altering the urban sanitary environment and, of redressing the balance against urbanization.[20] But each of these innovations had its own diffusion curve in which the lag time to adoption was affected by circumstances beyond the control of engineers, thus ensuring uneven progress. There are many examples of sanitary engineers' plans being rejected or under-financed as a consequence of local political decisions even where the technology was available.[21] On other occasions, such as Koch's insistence on the filtration of drinking water, the scientific arguments themselves were still under debate. Where river- or sea-pollution was concerned, local administrations were tempted to take the easy way out and export their problems to neighbouring authorities.

The history of urban health during the nineteenth century is surely one of the union between technical possibility and public responsibility. But

[19] See also Woods *et al.*, op. cit. n. 2, for additional examples.

[20] There are valuable surveys in Sir John Simon, *English Sanitary Institutions Reviewed in their Course of Development and in some of their Political and Social Relations* (London, 1890); A. Palmberg, *A Treatise on Public Health and its Application in Different Countries of Europe* (London, 1893); and more recently A. S. Wohl, *Endangered Lives: Public Health in Victorian Britain* (London, 1983).

[21] Evans op. cit. in n. 14, p. 152, relates the case of the English sanitary engineer William Lindley whose work in Hamburg was thwarted by local parsimony.

what could account for the rise of public responsibility? Some of the most likely reasons have already been touched on—morality, electoral appeal, élite self-interest—yet none may be isolated with impunity as the critical element in the development of a collective ideology, which, by the 1900s, had come to be taken for granted by Europeans at home and overseas. Governments, whether local or national, accepted their responsibility to provide and monitor basic public-health facilities. Although methods of finance—taxation or direct charges to customers—varied, the goal remained the same: a safe and sufficient water supply, effective sewage and refuse disposal without pollution, clean and paved streets.

Hennock's account of local government in Victorian Birmingham provides an insight into the individuals involved, their interests, and objectives.[22] National legislation forced Birmingham to appoint its first Medical Officer of Health in 1872 and during the following year not only was a new sanitary committee elected on a broader franchise (18 per cent of the population were electors in 1871, rather than only 3 per cent in 1861), but Joseph Chamberlain became mayor for the first of his three terms. In 1874 Sir William Cook began his chairmanship of the Sanitary Committee which he retained for 34 years. The coming together of these elements began a period of long-overdue reform which had implications for public hygiene as well as housing. Yet, as we have already seen, the consequences for mortality were neither immediate nor obvious.

4. Medical Intervention and Public Hygiene

There would appear to be four ways in which members of the medical profession could have intervened to promote the cause of public health during the nineteenth century. First, the medical profession as a whole, through its various professional bodies, could lobby for reform. The effectiveness of such action would depend upon group cohesion—speaking with one voice—and the status of the medical profession. The former was beyond organization for much of the nineteenth century in such an individualistic, hierarchical, internally fragmented, and social-status-conscious profession.[23] The latter was not high, until medical science made its great advances in this century.

Secondly, individual practitioners could make great personal contributions either by direct intervention, as for instance with the famous case of Dr John Snow and the Broad Street pump, or by becoming local or national health officials. There are numerous examples of full-time salaried health

[22] Hennock, op. cit. in n. 15.

[23] See e.g. M. Jeanne Peterson, *The Medical Profession in Mid-Victorian London* (Berkeley, Calif., 1978).

officials who as medical officers of health or directors of health offices were able to use their medical or administrative skills to change the sanitary environment for the better, but who were often hampered by conservative town councils whose commitment to the minimum of intervention and sectional self-interest was notorious.[24]

Thirdly, several medically qualified individuals acted as early medical statisticians and demographers. One of the most important of these was Dr William Farr, but he was succeeded as Compiler of Statistics in the General Register Office, London, by Drs Ogle, Tatham, and Stevenson. Each of these medical men made his greatest contribution to public health as a medical statistician. Farr, in particular, seems to have been influenced by the work and teaching of Gabriel Andral, Pierre Louis, and Louis René Villermé during his stay in Paris in 1829–30. Villermé even gave a course of lectures on population and hygiene in 1829. These medical statisticians cum demographers formed a very important group. One can trace the links between Louis and his 'numerical method', the founding of *Annales d'hygiène publique* in Paris also in 1829 (early issues of which contained papers on occupational health and urban mortality by Villermé, the Belgian statistician Adolphe Quetelet, and the Brussels medical officer Eugène Janssens).[25] In England the line continues by way of Farr to Sir Arthur Newsholme and Sir Thomas Legge. Koch's founding of the *Zeitschrift für Hygiene und Infektionskrankheiten* in Berlin in 1880 may be part of a separate line.

Fourthly, physicians also came to be involved as medical researchers, as laboratory-based experimental scientists in the way we now understand the specialism. Perhaps Robert Koch's work in Berlin, where from 1880 he had his own laboratory in the Imperial Health Office and from 1885 was Professor of Hygiene, provides the best example. The early work of Max von Pettenkofer in Munich may also be included. But physicians and their assistants also undertook the more humble tasks of public analysts, monitoring the quality of water, milk, and food supplies.

Set against these four points we have also to recognize that medical men and organizations were not only not alone in their advocacy of

[24] P.E. Brown, 'John Snow—The Autumn Loiterer', *Bulletin of the History of Medicine*, 25 (1961), pp. 512–28, and Sir Arthur Newsholme, *Fifty Years in Public Health* (London, 1935) give good examples.

[25] There is only circumstantial evidence for this connection, yet its importance for the statistical analysis of health and mortality would seem to have been profound. See J.M. Eyler, *Victorian Social Medicine: The Ideas and Methods of William Farr*, (Baltimore, 1979); E.H. Ackerknecht, 'Hygiene in France 1815–1848', *Bulletin of the History of Medicine*, 22 (1948), pp. 117–55; id., 'Villermé and Quetelet', *Bulletin of the History of Medicine*, 26 (1952), pp. 317–29. The flavour of Villermé's work is represented in 'De la mortalité dans les divers quartiers de la ville de Paris, et des causes qui la rendent très différente dans plusieurs d'entre eux, ainsi que dans les divers quartiers de beaucoup de grandes villes', *Annales d'hygiène publique*, 3 (1830), pp. 294–339. The first English text on the subject also appeared in 1829: F. Bisset Hawkins, *Elements of Medical Statistics* (London, 1829).

public hygiene, but that many were often at best apathetic and at worst antagonistic. Consider the career of Sir Edwin Chadwick, a lawyer by training, who used his position as secretary of the Poor Law Board to influence the preparation of documents like the *Report on the Sanitary Condition of the Labouring Population of Great Britain* (1842) to lobby for public-health legislation.[26] However, Chadwick's almost Messianic drive to improve sanitation stemmed from his conviction that disease must be reduced because it caused destitution, rather than from a desire to see the health of the population improved for its own sake. We also have the case of Dr Johann Kraus who became Hamburg's chief medical officer in 1871 and was still in office in 1892. His adherence to Pettenkofer and his fatalistic view of cholera could not have improved public hygiene in a city so dominated by mercantile self-interest.[27]

It is also worth observing that during the nineteenth century medical intervention by practising physicians was far more likely to be concerned with caring and curing, than with prevention, while social administrators, like Chadwick and others of a Benthamite persuasion, who ran the system of poor-law relief would have been preoccupied with the financial burden of morbidity on the family, local ratepayers, and ultimately the State. In these circumstances, it is perhaps surprising that so many medical men also became involved in advocating the preventive measures associated with public health, whether as statisticians, scientists, or full-time health officials.

There can be little doubt that medical intervention, broadly defined, did assist the cause of public hygiene, particularly during the late nineteenth century, that public hygiene represented an important part of public health at that time and, further, that advances in public health assisted the decline of mortality. What we do not know, and can never know, is the extent to which each contributed to the other. We are coming closer to understanding, the variety of forms these relationships can take, but our ability to measure contributions exactly is woefully inadequate.

5. Return to McKeown's Problem

It would be misleading to conclude this chapter on a completely negative note since there are probably certain ways in which we would come closer to solving McKeown's central problem: how to ascribe relative numerical weights to the individual component causes of mortality decline. McKeown's own solution was epidemiological, to use cause-of-death statistics to trace likely ultimate causes. By this means, about one-quarter of the mortality

[26] M.W. Flinn (eds.), *Report on the Sanitary Condition of the Labouring Population of Great Britain by Edwin Chadwick 1842* (Edinburgh, 1965).

[27] Evans op. cit. in n. 14, pp. 252–53.

decline in England and Wales between the mid-nineteenth century and 1901 could be directly related to the sanitary revolution. Although there is spurious precision here, and the logic with which it is derived is probably flawed, the prospects of substituting a superior figure based on sound logic are limited. The quality of nineteenth-century vital statistics and population censuses handicaps those who attempt to use numerical methods with changes of accuracy and reporting conventions. One strategy would be to trace the progress of a particular disease chosen to provide a sensitive indicator of public health advances. Typhoid and epidemic diarrhoea would seem sensible choices. A second possibility would be to trace the morbidity and mortality of a particular age group known to be prone to inadequate hygiene. A third possibility would direct attention to detailing the history of a distinctive environment in which the administrative history of sanitary reform can be particularly well documented.

Each of these approaches has been attempted with varying degrees of success. Let us briefly consider the second. The secular decline of infant mortality in England and Wales during the late nineteenth and early twentieth centuries has been studied in some detail recently.[28] The principal conclusions appear as follows. First, infant mortality certainly was highest in those urban areas with the worst public-health conditions. Secondly, the precipitous decline of infant mortality post-1899 appears more striking because infant deaths increased during the 1890s compared with the 1880s. Epidemic diarrhoea appears to have been an important contributor to retarding the secular decline of infant mortality during the 1890s. Despite obvious and substantial improvements in urban hygiene from the mid-nineteenth century these were not sufficient to counter entirely the effects of a short run of hot, dry summers, but without such advances, mortality might have been far worse. Thirdly, although the true origins of the secular decline of infant mortality do lie in the nineteenth century it seems most likely that the contribution of public hygiene was felt by infants during the twentieth century; the matter is still obscure.

There is reason to believe that we will in future move closer to solving McKeown's problem in societies in which statistics are well developed and that one, or a combination, of the three approaches mentioned above will at least assist our endeavours in circumstances where, although there are many numbers and much political arithmetic, the value of our knowledge is only just being brought into question.

[28] Woods and Woodward, op. cit. in n. 5, and Woods *et al.*, op. cit. in n. 2, contain examples of recent attempts, often thwarted, to follow the line established in 1829.

14 The Personal Physician and the Decline of Mortality

STEPHEN J. KUNITZ *University of Rochester Medical Center*

1. Introduction

My topic is the contribution of the personal physician system to the historical decline of Western mortality. In a sense the subject may be disposed of quickly. With the exception of vaccination against smallpox at the beginning of the nineteenth century, and diphtheria antitoxin at the end of the century, there was until the 1940s no preventive or therapeutic treatment a practitioner could provide for a substantial number of patients which could have had a measurable impact on mortality rates in an entire population. Moreover, until the 1940s virtually no one, physician or non-physician, would have accorded the lion's share of credit for declining mortality to the personal-physician system. And yet during the past ten or twenty years, sorting out the 'medical contribution' to the historical decline in Western mortality has become a thriving cottage industry. Why has this happened? Why, that is, has it seemed important to answer a question which most knowledgeable contemporaries with first-hand experience do not seem to have considered to be of major importance?

That is a question which cannot be disposed of so easily. The answer has to do with the changing place of science and medicine in Western societies. Indeed, I shall argue in this paper that in asking such a question, which did not exercise the minds of our predecessors, we are projecting on to the past, debates that are of contemporary relevance to us, and are using the past to justify present policies. That is not unprecedented. Politicians do it all the time. That in itself should be enough to raise suspicions about its appropriateness.

What I should like to do, then, is discuss first the various things physicians do in practice. I shall emphasize the seemingly obvious point that stamping out death is generally not high on the list. Secondly, I shall describe briefly the changes and conflicts within medicine from the end of the nineteenth century to the end of World War II, during which time a major epistemo-

I am grateful to Theodore M. Brown and Russell C. Maulitz for helpful comments on an early version of this chapter.

logical revolution occurred, unaccompanied by a therapeutic revolution of equal magnitude. Thirdly, I shall discuss some of the consequences of and reactions to the therapeutic revolution of the 1940s and 1950s. It is in the reactions to this revolution that questions relating to the historical effectiveness of medicine are rooted.

2. What Physicians Do

Thomas McKeown has rightly observed that 'Historical interpretation of changes in health must rely largely on knowledge of the behaviour of the death rate and the contribution made to it by different causes of death.'[1] This is so, because mortality is more easily measured than morbidity, particularly in the past, but also in the present. The difficulty is that as a result mortality has become the sole measure of whether or not any particular phenomenon contributed to improved health. When considering the care provided by individual physicians to particular patients, however, the concern goes much beyond prevention of premature death, and always has.

Therapy has always been central to what healers have to offer, and it is conventional wisdom that most of the therapy that was provided was effective—if at all—as a consequence of its placebo effect, not simply on the patient but on the physician as well. We shall never know whether the placebos given to our ancestors measurably lengthened or shortened their lives, but surely all the dosing, purging, cupping, and bleeding they endured encouraged them to believe that something was being done for them. At least as important, these therapeutic activities allowed physicians to believe that they were being effective. In 1924, Charles Minor, a physician in Ashville, North Carolina, observed that the scepticism and therapeutic nihilism so prevalent in his day had served a useful purpose 'in that it tended to prevent us from too blindly trusting to drugs'. But, he continued, 'I found I could not leave it all up to nature. I found that the best diagnosis was of little use unless it led up to an active, resourceful treatment, unless I understood the use of drugs, and that, moreover, my familiarity with them had a distinct value in giving me that confidence in myself without which a therapeutic result cannot be had.'[2] Which is to say, if the physician did not believe in his therapeutic intervention, he could not believe in himself; and if he did not believe in himself, he would be unable to use himself as a therapeutic

[1] T. McKeown, 'A Historical Appraisal of the Medical Task', in G. McLachlan and T. McKeown (eds.), *Medical History and Medical Care: A Symposium of Perspectives* (Oxford, 1971), p. 30.

[2] C.L. Minor, 'The Confessions of a Therapeutist, or Some Meditations on Modern Therapy', *Transactions of the American Climatological and Clinical Association*, 40 (1924), pp. 7–15.

instrument with which to inspire hope. 'Patients come to us hoping that we can do something for them, and not merely to give us an opportunity for scientific study of their interesting cases, and we have not done our duty by them until by drugs, by other measures, by suggestions, by building up hope, we have helped to cure them or at least aided them to meet the end bravely.'[3]

Though perhaps more sophisticated and perceptive than most of his contemporaries and predecessors, Minor was in fact speaking for an old and central tradition in medicine. Therapy has always been a crucial part of the physician's task: not simply for the sake of the patient but for the sake of the physician, whose sense of efficacy was validated by the physiological response of his patients to his ministrations. The shared belief of physician and patient in the therapeutic efficacy of the physician's intervention helped give meaning and a sense of control to the experience of sickness.[4]

Just as diagnosis without therapy was sterile, so was diagnosis without prognosis. The purpose of diagnosis, in fact, is to classify the patient's experience in such a way as to make sense of it; to explain both its origin and its likely outcome.[5] Again this is central to the physician's task; it may well have an impact on the illness experience; but it is an activity the results of which are not reflected in deflections of the curve of mortality rates.

And finally, physicians have often served as agents of cultural and behavioural change, for often they have been the intermediaries between bourgeois society and the working classes. Before the germ theory of disease was enunciated, much that they taught about hygiene and breast-feeding may have been based partly on clinical observation and largely on the diffusion of manners and 'civilized behaviour' from the upper classes, all legitimated by their status as physicians. Such acculturation to different modes of behaviour may well have had a significant but unmeasurable effect.[6] Indeed, it has been argued that one of the important consequences of the creation of national health insurance in Germany in the 1880s was precisely to make middle-class physicians more accessible to working-class patients and thus to 'medicalize' childbirth and child-rearing, sexual behaviour, education, diet, and manners.[7] It seems likely that something

[3] C.L. Minor, 13.

[4] C.E. Rosenberg, 'The Therapeutic Revolution: Medicine, Meaning, and Social Change in Nineteenth-Century America', in M.J. Vogel and C.E. Rosenberg (eds.), *The Therapeutic Revolution: Essays in the Social History of American Medicine* (Philadelphia, 1979).

[5] S.J. Kunitz, 'Classifications in Medicine', in R.C. Maulitz and D.E. Long (eds.), *Grand Rounds: One Hundred Years of Internal Medicine* (Philadelphia, 1988).

[6] N. Elias, *The Civilizing Process: The Development of Manners* (New York, 1978), id., *The Civilizing Process: State Formation and Civilization* (Oxford, 1982). See also J. Frykman and O. Lofgren, *Culture Builders: A Historical Anthropology of Middle-Class Life* (New Brunswick, 1982).

[7] A. Labisch, 'Doctors, Workers and the Scientific Cosmology of the Industrial World: The Social Construction of "Health" and the "Homo Hygienicus" ', *Journal of Contemporary History*, 20 (1985), pp. 599–615, U. Frevert, 'Professional Medicine and the Working Classes

similar occurred elsewhere in Europe as national health insurance schemes became widely diffused. Again, however, it is impossible to measure the impact of such changes on either mortality or morbidity.

All these activities—therapy, diagnosis, prognosis, acculturation—are central to the healer's task. It is likely that sometimes they will have resulted in increased, and at others, decreased risk of death. It is even more likely that they would have had an impact on the incidence and experience of sickness. In either case, however, the effects on rates of mortality would have been undetectable. This does not mean that the historical contribution of medical practice to health was insignificant. It means that it is unmeasurable, because the only way we have to measure health in the past is by death rates from different causes, and these are, at best, an inadequate reflection of the experience of disease. The fact that the impact of personal physicians on the health of populations in past times is unmeasurable does not mean that the effect will always be unmeasurable, or that it is entirely unmeasurable even now.

3. The Epistemological Revolution

During the nineteenth century a major transformation occurred in the way disease causation was understood in Western medicine.

> Assumptions about disease shared by doctor and patient and oriented toward visibly altering the symptoms of sick individuals, began to be supplanted by strategies grounded in experimental science that objectified disease while minimizing the differences among patients. Concurrently the bases of physicians' professional identity were also transformed. Through the mid-nineteenth century professional identity was based on proper behaviour and on a medical theory that stressed the principle of specificity the notion that treatment had to be matched to the idiosyncratic characteristics of individual patients and their environments. During the last third of the century a new conception of professional identity defined by allegiance to knowledge generated and validated by experimental science and characterized by universalized diagnostic and therapeutic categories was clearly in ascendance.[8]

There are many reasons for the transformation described in the passage quoted above. I shall do no more than list two which are particularly important for my purposes. One is the growth of physiological research based on assumptions nicely captured in the following remark by Claude Bernard, the great French physiologist, in his classic treatise *An Introduction to the Study of Experimental Medicine* (1865):

---

in Imperial Germany', *Journal of Contemporary History*, 20 (1985), pp. 637–58; R. Spree, *Health and Social Class in Imperial Germany* (Oxford, 1988).

[8] J. H. Warner, *The Therapeutic Perspective: Medical Practice, Knowledge, and Identity in America, 1820–1885* (Cambridge, Mass., 1986), p. 1.

If based on statistics, medicine can never be anything but a conjectural science; only by basing itself on experimental determinism can it become a true science: i.e. a sure science. I think of this idea as the pivot of experimental medicine, and in this respect experimental physicians take a wholly different view from so-called observing physicians . . . Most physicians seem to believe that, in medicine, laws are elastic and indefinite. These are false ideas which must disappear if we mean to found a scientific medicine.[9]

Such determinism clearly struck at the very roots of the physician's skills, which were grounded precisely in his knowledge of the unique characteristics of each patient.

'Observing physicians' did attempt to classify diseases, of course, because it was clear that people often fell ill with afflictions that physicians had seen before. Indeed, diagnosis is a matter of matching the patient's disease to an existing category. But Bernard objected that classification should not be mistaken for explanation:

It would be a grave illusion for physicians to believe they know diseases by giving them names, because they classify and describe them, just as it would be an illusion for zoologists or botanists to believe they know animals and vegetables because they have named them, catalogued, dissected, and shut them up in museums after stuffing, preparing, or drying them. Physicians will not know diseases until they can act on them rationally and experimentally, just as zoologists will not know animals until they explain and regulate the phenomena of life.[10]

Thus, another essential of the physician's task, diagnosis and classification, was diminished. Clearly they could not be regarded as sufficient if the physician was truly to understand diseases.

Another reason for the change from particularism to universalism was the change in ideas of causal attribution that followed upon the elaboration of the germ theory in the 1880s. K. Codell Carter has shown that until that time, when Robert Koch enunciated the postulates that now bear his name, physicians explained diseases in terms of multiple weakly sufficient causes.[11] A sufficient cause is one which is followed by a particular effect. A weakly sufficient cause is one which is sometimes followed by the effect. Nineteenth-century physicians believed that diseases might be caused by a variety of factors, that a common cause could not be inferred from a common effect, and that diseases might blend into one another.

With the work of Koch and other bacteriologists, the idea of necessary cause of disease was introduced for the first time. A necessary cause is one without which an effect cannot occur. Without the tubercle bacillus there

[9] C. Bernard, *An Introduction to the Study of Experimental Medicine*, trans. H.C. Greene (New York, 1949), p. 139.

[10] Ibid. 144.

[11] K.C. Carter, 'Koch's Postulates in Relation to the Work of Jacob Henle and Edwin Klebs', *Medical History*, 29 (1985), pp. 353–74.

can be no tuberculosis. As I have argued elsewhere, 'the result was a subtle but far-reaching change. Many diseases could now be classified etiologically as well as anatomically or symptomatically. Disease specificity became increasingly possible, and with it the possibility of disease-specific interventions that would be applicable in all places and among all people, regardless of topography, climate, or culture.[12]

This change in ideas of causal attribution made possible by exposure to German research methods, by major changes in medical education, and by the growing possibility of academic careers in medical research in the United States, all combined at the end of the nineteenth century to cause a major epistemological revolution. Diseases were now to be explained at a deep level, not simply described and classified. Increasingly, disease processes, not unique patients, became the focus of attention for the rising élite in medicine.[13] This élite was not numerous, but held prestigious posts in the newly established, as well as in the old transformed, medical schools that were emerging during the early decades of this century. The possibility of stable careers in academic medicine was new in this century in the United States, and for the men who entered these careers in increasing numbers as the century wore on, the interpersonal and clinical skills of the physician were devalued as a new kind of knowledge—of disease mechanisms common to all patients—became increasingly important.

There were a number of responses to this revolution. I have already described one, the 'therapeutist's' reaction. Dr Minor in 1924 described the behaviour of one of the new élite of German-trained American academics.

> Years ago, in the clinic of a great medical school, I saw a good example of the different attitude toward disease of the ultramodern physician and that of his great predecessors. A keen diagnostician demonstrated the interesting case of an old darky [*sic*] with faultless thoroughness and, doubtless considering treatment useless or hopeless, and forgetting the value of suggestive therapeutics and his duty as a doctor to consider his patients, dismissed the class without laying out any plan of treatment, leaving the impression on their minds that diagnosis alone was valuable. When the patient saw the doctors going away and nothing done for his malady he called out plaintively: 'But, doctor, what is yo' going to *do* fo' me?' This physician deduced the inutility or unimportance of treatment for this case, thought of it merely as a 'case' for diagnosis, which is the almost universal habit in Germany, and not as a suffering human being needing help, and forgot that even if this deduction of his was right, he had still failed to be humane, or to consider the psychology of the case, or to remember that to encourage the discouraged, to hearten the hopeless, even if but with a placebo, is no mean or negligible part of the doctor's work.[14]

[12] S. J. Kunitz, 'Explanations and Ideologies of Mortality Patterns', *Population and Development Review*, 13 (1987), p. 380.

[13] Id., 'The Historical Roots and Ideological Functions of Disease Concepts in Three Primary Care Specialties', *Bulletin of the History of Medicine*, 57 (1983), p. 414.

[14] Minor, op. cit. in n. 2, p. 13.

Another response was made by Knud Faber, a Danish physician, in his history of medical classifications. Arguing against Bernard's dismissal of the taxonomizing engaged in by 'observing physicians', he wrote: 'To the physiologist and the worker in the laboratory morbid categories are subordinate concepts, but to the physician, to the clinician, the reverse is the case: he cannot live, cannot speak, cannot act without them.'[15] This was so because naming and classifying were necessary both for prognostic purposes and for guiding therapy.

Yet a third response was a growing concern with psychosomatic medicine on the part of a number of established academic physicians, called by Theodore Brown 'the holistic elite'.[16] These were men like Lewellys Barker, Francis Weld Peabody, and G. Canby Robinson who believed that concern with disease mechanisms was drawing attention away from concern for the patient as a person—the title of an influential book by Robinson.[17] In a seminal address to medical students in 1927 Peabody said: 'The most common criticism made at present by older practitioners is that young graduates have been taught a great deal about mechanisms of disease, but very little about the practice of medicine—or, to put it more bluntly, they are too "scientific" and do not know how to take care of patients'. He estimated that, excluding patients with acute infections, half the remaining patients seen by physicians 'complained of symptoms for which an adequate organic cause could not be discovered . . . Here . . . is a great group of patients in which it is not the disease but the man or the woman who needs to be treated.'[18]

There are two related points to be made here. First, the epistemological revolution beginning in the 1880s was, with a few promising exceptions (e.g. diphtheria antitoxin, insulin for diabetes, liver extract for pernicious anaemia, nicotinic acid for pellagra), unaccompanied by a therapeutic revolution. The therapeutic nihilism of the German-trained American academic described by Dr Minor was the nihilism of a man who did not yet have anything but a causal explanation to offer, and whose career depended on salary rather than fees for clinical service. Secondly, the response of many physicians, who needed to earn their living in practice, to such nihilism was not to assert that they were in fact saving lives by the thousands but that they were caring for patients as individuals, hopefully curing some, but at least comforting all.

[15] K. Faber, *Nosography: The Evolution of Clinical Medicine in Modern Times* (New York, 1930), p. 211.

[16] T.M. Brown, 'The Holistic Elite: A Network of American Medical Humanists in the Early Twentieth Century', Lecture presented at the Institute of the History of Medicine, The Johns Hopkins University, Baltimore, Md., 2 Mar. 1989.

[17] G.C. Robinson, *The Patient as a Person* (New York, 1939).

[18] F.W. Peabody, 'The Care of the Patient', *Journal of the American Medical Association* 88 (1927), pp. 877–80.

4. The Therapeutic Revolution

In his autobiography Lewis Thomas describes the several months during the 1930s that he spent as a fourth-year medical student with Dr Hurman Blumgart, a famous physician at the Boston City Hospital.

So far as I know, from that three months of close contact with Blumgart for three hours every morning, he was never wrong, not once. But I can recall only three or four patients for whom the diagnosis resulted in the possibility of doing something to change the course of the illness, and each of these involved calling in the surgeon to do something—removal of a thyroid nodule, a gall bladder, an adrenal tumor. For the majority, the disease had to be left to run its own course, for better or worse.[19]

But, Thomas continues, 'As early as 1937 medicine was changing into a technology based on genuine science.'[20] Even then, however, 'For most of the infectious diseases on the wards . . . there was nothing to be done beyond bed rest and good nursing care. Then came the explosive news of sulfanilamide, and the start of the real revolution in medicine.'[21]

Walsh McDermott has argued that there was a discernible downward deflection in mortality rates beginning in 1937, and that it was attributable to the rapid diffusion of sulpha drugs and antibiotics, but that the real revolution was in the kinds of diseases treated in hospitals.[22] During the 1930s, patients moribund with pneumococcal pneumonia, in congestive heart failure from syphilitic or rheumatic heart disease, dying from streptococcal bacteraemia, at bed rest with pulmonary tuberculosis, or suffering from peritonsillar abscesses, mastoiditis, or subacute bacterial endocarditis, made up the bulk of the patients in the medical wards. Within two decades the spectrum of disease common in hospitals during the early 1930s had largely changed.[23]

Lewis Thomas has suggested that

The professionals most deeply affected by these extraordinary events were, I think, the interns. The older physicians were equally surprised, but took the news in stride. For an intern, it was the opening of a whole new world. We had been raised to be ready for one kind of profession, and we sensed that the profession itself had changed at the moment of our entry. We knew that other molecular variations of

[19] L. Thomas, *The Youngest Science: Notes of a Medicine-Watcher* (New York, 1984), p. 31.

[20] Ibid., p. 32.

[21] Ibid., p. 35.

[22] W. McDermott, 'Absence of Indicators of the Influence of its Physicians on a Society's Health', *American Journal of Medicine*, 70 (1981), pp. 833–43; id., 'Social Ramifications of Control of Microbial Disease', *Johns Hopkins Medical Journal*, 151 (1982), pp. 302–12.

[23] A similarly profound impact has been described for paediatric practice. J. R. Boulware, 'The Composition of Private Pediatric Practice in a Small Community in the South of the United States', *Pediatrics*, 22 (1958), p. 55.

sulfanilamide were on their way from industry, and we heard about the possibility of penicillin and other antibiotics; we became convinced, overnight, that nothing lay beyond reach for the future. Medicine was off and running.[24]

This generational phenomenon is significant, for the young men who were interns in the 1930s returned from World War II to assume careers in practice and in academic medicine. During the post-war years when support for hospital construction and biomedical research flowed freely, and when third-party reimbursement became increasingly available, their careers flourished. In Great Britain the situation was, of course, different, but there, too, hospitals and specialty services received the bulk of support.[25]

The result of the therapeutic revolution in both the United States and Great Britain was increasing specialization, increasing dependence upon hospitals, and increasing costs. Therapeutic nihilism was no longer the problem. If anything, therapeutic adventurism—the emphasis on cure, or attempted cure, rather than care—replaced it. The epistemological revolution had now been justified by a therapeutic revolution which weakened those who had been critical. It was one thing to be critical of the new medicine when it had nothing but arid explanations, sometimes less than humanely offered. It was quite another to be critical when dramatic cures and treatments had begun to emerge.

5. The Counter-Revolution

And yet there were, and continue to be, critics both lay and professional. In the United States they were found most prominently in the ranks of those who, with the support of private philanthropies, espoused the development of what was called 'comprehensive care' during the 1950s and early 1960s, and 'family medicine' and 'primary care' since the mid-1960s.[26]

In Great Britain, the early critics were found mostly among the ranks of epidemiologists.[27] During the war, methods of randomized controlled trials had been developed which were applied to therapeutic agents. Increasingly, epidemiologists argued that clinicians could not justify much of what they did on the basis of numbers, but that, given the limited resources of the National Health Service, they should be required to do so. The randomized controlled trial, the principal method of what has come to be called experimental epidemiology, was the recommended study design.

[24] Thomas, op. cit. in n. 19, p. 35. For a more detailed account of this era see P. B. Beeson and R. C. Maulitz, 'The Inner History of Internal Medicine', in Maulitz and Long (eds.), op. cit. in n. 5.

[25] D. M. Fox, *Health Policies, Health Politics: The British and American Experience 1911-1965* (Princeton, NJ, 1986), pp. 169–70.

[26] T. M. Brown, 'American Medicine and Primary Care: The Last Half-Century', in S. J. Kunitz (ed.), *The Training of Primary Physicians* (Lanham, Md., 1986).

[27] Fox, op. cit. in n. 25, pp. 179–80.

In some respects the agenda of the American and British critics differed, and the precise timing of their critiques differed as well. None the less, what they shared was an adverse reaction to the emergence of high-cost, high-technology medicine, particularly since it devalued interpersonal skills and modes of causal attribution that they believed were at the core of good medical care.

The British epidemiologist who argued the case for randomized controlled trials most eloquently was Archibald Cochrane. He wrote that the importance of the randomized controlled trial (RCT) 'cannot be exaggerated. It opened up a new world of evaluation and control which will, I think, be the key to a rational health service. Freud in his *Zukunft einer Illusion* put his hopes on the gentle voice of intelligence producing order out of another more general chaos. I believe the RCT, suitably applied, may have a similar effect in producing an effective, efficient health service.'[28]

Cochrane listed the benefits to therapy of RCTs: Mather's study of home care compared with hospital care for acute myocardial infarctions; the multi-centre trial of oral antidiabetic therapy; and several others. Moreover, he suggested a number of investigations that might usefully be undertaken to determine whether services were being used efficiently. These included studies of the place of treatment and lengths of stay for a variety of conditions, the most appropriate use of screening tests, and the effectiveness of psychotherapy.[29]

It was Cochrane's belief that there was a marked imbalance between the 'care' and 'cure' sectors of the National Health Service, with the latter getting by far the lion's share of resources, without, however, having been forced to justify the expenditures based upon the rigorous evaluation required by a randomized controlled trial. Without the use of RCTs, he argued, there would inevitably be inflation of costs in the 'cure' sector of the Health Service, a widening of the gap with the 'care' sector, and, he wrote presciently, 'inevitably the return of much of the "cure" sector to the forces of the market place'.[30]

It was in this same reaction of epidemiologists to the inflation of the 'cure' sector of the National Health Service that Thomas McKeown's work was grounded. His early research during the 1930s had been with the famous Canadian investigator of stress, Hans Selye.[31] Selye's work was primarily concerned with the typical response to different kinds of stressful stimuli which he called the General Adaptation Syndrome.[32] For my purposes here

[28] A. Cochrane, *Effectiveness and Efficiency: Random Reflections on Health Services* (London, 1971), p. 11.

[29] Ibid., pp. 29–32.

[30] Ibid., p. 85.

[31] H. Selye and T. McKeown, 'Production of Pseudo-Pregnancy by Mechanical Stimulation of the Nipples', *Proceedings of the Society of Experimental Biology*, 31 (1934), p. 683.

[32] H. Selye, *The Stress of Life* (New York, 1956).

two points are relevant. First, this research partook of the general reaction to the epistemological revolution I described previously, for it was concerned with the total response of the organism to a wide variety of stresses, and as such had a profound impact on psychosomatic medicine. And secondly, it implicitly relied upon an earlier paradigm: that a common effect (the General Adaptation Syndrome) could have many different causes. It was not a uni-causal explanation.

This is relevant, because it suggests that McKeown, unlike people of his generation who had been profoundly influenced by the epistemological and therapeutic revolutions, adhered to an alternative tradition: one in which uni-causal explanations were less acceptable than multi-causal explanations: and in which disease was conceived of as the result of complex problems of adaptation of an organism to its environment. These are themes that permeate his work, that underlie his suspicion of the claims of curative medicine, and that inform his analysis of the historical contribution of medical care to the decline of Western mortality.

McKeown's analyses of the ineffectiveness of medical intervention are too widely known to require repetition.[33] My purpose here is twofold: to indicate that virtually no one had claimed that medical treatment had made a substantial impact on the European mortality decline; and to suggest that in his historical work McKeown was arguing not merely about the past, but about the present as well.

In respect of the first point, the only author McKeown cites as asserting the historical significance of the medical contribution is G. Talbot Griffith.[34] This is not entirely fair to Griffith, who claimed that drainage of marshes for agricultural purposes, increased food production, decreased consumption of alcohol, and gradual improvements in urban public health were important factors, together with the growth of hospitals and dispensaries, improvements in midwifery, and the spread of smallpox vaccination. Griffith's was a multi-factorial explanation, without weight of relative significance attached to any of the factors. He was not unique. Others during the inter-war years, for example M.C. Buer and A.M. Carr-Saunders, took an equally broad view of the factors contributing to declining mortality in the eighteenth and nineteenth centuries.[35]

It was only after the war that the multiplicity of causes invoked by earlier writers began to be disaggregated. In the same volume of *Population Studies* in which KcKeown and Brown's article on the medical contribution appeared

[33] T. McKeown and R.G. Brown, 'Medical Evidence Related to English Population Changes in the Eighteenth Century', *Population Studies*, 9 (1955), pp. 119–41; T. McKeown, *The Modern Rise of Population* (New York, 1976).

[34] G.T. Griffith, *Population Problems in the Age of Malthus* (Cambridge, 1926).

[35] M.C. Buer, *Health, Wealth, and Population in the Early Days of the Industrial Revolution* (London, 1926), A.M. Carr-Saunders, *World Population: Past Growth and Present Trends* (London, 1936).

in 1955,[36] George Stolnitz wrote that it had been common to explain 'increasing life chances' in Western nations 'by reference to two broad categories of causes: rising levels of living on the one hand (income, nutrition, housing, literacy) and, on the other, technological advances (medical science, public health, sanitation)'. The usual approach was to assume that they were interdependent. The same approach had characterized explanations of mortality decline in other parts of the world. But, he said, 'The introduction of new disease-control methods in the region [Latin America–Africa–Asia], usually unaccompanied by any important shifts in socioeconomic conditions, has led to drastic mortality declines in the last few years. It is worth noting, therefore, that a similar causal process may have been operative in acceleration of Western survivorship a good deal earlier.[37] In other words, not only was the therapeutic revolution having an important impact in the West, but the impact of public-health technologies in former colonies had begun to make demographers wonder whether the same sort of impact of public health might not also have occurred in the past experience of Western nations. In each case, technology isolated from social and environmental factors was being viewed as the cause of declining mortality.

As regards the second point (that McKeown was really arguing not so much about the past as about the present), we may turn to his publications from the early and mid-1960s.[38] In them, he argued that the decline of mortality during the nineteenth century had been the result of (1) a rising standard of living that led to improved diets and enhanced resistance to several diseases, of which tuberculosis was the most important; (2) public hygiene resulting in control of the environment; and (3) 'a favourable trend in the relationship between infectious agent and host' (i.e., scarlet fever and perhaps tuberculosis, typhus, and cholera). During the twentieth century, he continued, 'the outstanding feature has been the reduction of infant mortality. Because of the introduction of more effective forms of therapy, and of the personal health and social services, the task of interpretation is more complex.' None the less, improvements in the standard of living and protection from environmental hazards continued to be most important. 'We conclude that the advance in health since the eighteenth century has been due to a rising standard of living from about 1770; sanitary measures, from 1870; and therapy during the twentieth century.'[39]

The consequences of changes in health were twofold, and they were

[36] McKeown and Brown, op. cit. in n. 33.

[37] G. Stolnitz, 'A Century in International Mortality Trends: I', *Population Studies*, 9 (1955), pp. 28–9.

[38] T. McKeown, 'The Hospital and Related Services', in J. Pemberton, (ed.), *Epidemiology: Reports on Research and Teaching 1962* (Oxford, 1963); T. McKeown, *Medicine in Modern Society* (London, 1965).

[39] Id., (1965), op. cit., in n. 38, p. 58.

related: changes in causes of sickness, and changes in the age structure. The non-infectious diseases, including mental illness, in an ageing population posed the most important problems. At the same time, the system of care that had been developed to deal with the diseases of an earlier era was not appropriate to deal with the problems of the contemporary world. The legacy of the past, by then built into the National Health Service, was to separate acute from chronic patients, domiciliary from hospital practice, and preventive from curative services. All of these resulted in failure to deal adequately with problems of emerging significance. Indeed, McKeown's argument was very much like Cochrane's; that specialist, hospital-based services were inappropriately dominating the provision of health services and failing to deal with the most pressing problems, which were fast becoming those of caring for the chronically mentally ill and the infirm aged.

He expanded and subtly changed his argument in his Rock-Carling monograph *The Role of Medicine*[40] in which he argued from historical evidence that the reduction of mortality in past times had not depended upon knowledge of mechanisms of disease but upon the control of the origins of disease. 'In order of importance the determinants of health were nutritional, environmental, and behavioural in the past, and will probably be behavioural, environmental and nutritional in the future, at least in developed countries.'[41] It had not been necessary to understand the mechanisms of disease in order to control them in the past, nor would it be crucial in future. Understanding their origins, or risk factors, was sufficient.[42] Medical therapy had received favourable mention in his 1965 volume. It was dropped ten years later.

McKeown's interpretation of mortality decline in the past had important implications for the organization and provision of health care, for the education of physicians, and for the kind of research that should be supported. He wrote: 'In light of the interpretation of disease discussed [previously] I suggest that the role of medicine should be conceived as follows: To assist us to come safely into the world and comfortably out of it, and during life, to protect the well and care for the sick and disabled.'[43] He carefully avoided mention of cure. Like Cochrane, McKeown emphasized the caring function of medicine as a counterweight to the more usual emphasis on what he conceived of as mechanistic, high-technology, highly specialized, hospital-based medicine which was inappropriately attracting funds that could more usefully be spent on other kinds of services.

Cochrane and McKeown were not nearly as hostile to physicians as many have assumed. They were, instead, using techniques of experimental and historical epidemiology in the service of an old ideal based upon an earlier

[40] Id., *The Role of Medicine: Dream, Mirage, or Nemesis?* (London, 1976).
[41] Ibid., p. 147.
[42] Kunitz, op. cit., in n. 12.
[43] McKeown, op. cit. in n. 40, p. 173.

epistemology and a traditional view of what physicians do best and how they may make their most significant contributions. The older epistemology was based upon the notion of multi-causality—what are now called risk factors. The traditional idea of what physicians do best is the exercise of what Cochrane often called the 'caring' function; the effectiveness of the 'curing' function having been much overemphasized, according to him and McKeown.[44] It is for this reason that I have called this section 'counter-revolution'.

6. Conclusion

I have argued that the question about medicine's historical contribution to the decline of mortality in the West is not a particularly important one. Very few people ever thought it was. For those who did think medicine's contribution was significant, however, McKeown's work should have provided convincing evidence that it was not.

The more interesting question is why McKeown and others believed it was important to prove that medicine's past contribution had been trivial. The answer, I have said, is to be found in the epistemological revolution which occurred during the last decades of the nineteenth century and the first decades of the twentieth, and the therapeutic revolution which began during the late 1930s. The result was a new way of thinking about diseases, their causes, treatments, and victims. Many thought the focus upon universal mechanisms had distorted the way resources were allocated and medical practitioners trained. The care of the individual had been lost from view.

Medicine's past ineffectiveness thus was a way of addressing contemporary concerns. The concerns were valid. And the interpretation of the past was largely valid as well. What was questionable was the extrapolation from past ineffectiveness to present and future ineffectiveness. There is some evidence that mortality during the last twenty years has been favourably influenced by preventive and curative medical interventions.[45] It would thus be unwise to project the past of our grandparents onto the future of our grandchildren.

[44] This has been a particularly contentious issue. No one has disagreed about the importance of the 'caring' function, but there has been much debate about the contemporary effectiveness or lack of effectiveness of the 'curing' function. See the articles in the summer 1977 issue of the *Milbank Memorial Fund Quarterly* as well as the following: A. F. Lever, 'The Role of Medicine', *The Lancet* (1977), (i), pp. 352–55; L. Black, 'What should Doctors be doing?', *The Lancet* (1980) (ii), pp. 304–06.

[45] J. R. H. Charlton and R. Velez, 'Some International Comparisons of Mortality Amenable to Medical Intervention', *British Medical Journal*, 292 (1986) pp. 295–301, K. Poikolainen and J. Eskola, 'The Effect of Health Services on Mortality: Decline in Death Rates from Amenable and Non-Amenable Causes in Finland 1969–1981', *The Lancet* pp. 199–202, J. P. Mackenbach, 'Mortality and Medical Care' Ph.D. thesis (Erasmus Univ., Rotterdam, 1988); J. Hadley, *More Medical Care, Better Health?* (Washington, DC, 1982).

Finally, it is worth observing that the epidemiological critique of medicine's role was made with an eye to re-allocating and humanizing health care. It is thus a sad irony that McKeown's historical work and Cochrane's advocacy of randomized controlled trials gained popularity during a period of growing concern over the costs of health services in the United States, Great Britain, and other Western societies, for both these bodies of work have been used as a way of containing costs and providing a rationale for doing so, without at the same time sharing the concern of the authors for humane and equitable care.

Index